2011
YEAR BOOK OF
PATHOLOGY
AND LABORATORY
MEDICINE®

The 2011 Year Book Series

Year Book of Anesthesiology and Pain Management™: Drs Chestnut, Abram, Black, Gravlee, Lien, Mathru, and Roizen

Year Book of Cardiology®: Drs Gersh, Cheitlin, Elliott, Gold, Graham, and Thourani

Year Book of Critical Care Medicine®: Drs Dellinger, Parrillo, Balk, Dorman, Dries, and Zanotti-Cavazzoni

Year Book of Dermatology and Dermatologic Surgery™: Dr Del Rosso

Year Book of Diagnostic Radiology®: Drs Osborn, Abbara, Elster, Manaster, Oestreich, Offiah, Rosado de Christenson, Stephens, and Walker

Year Book of Emergency Medicine®: Drs Hamilton, Bruno, Handly, Mullin, Quintana, and Ramoska

Year Book of Endocrinology®: Drs Schott, Apovian, Clarke, Eugster, Ludlam, Meikle, Ovalle, Schinner, Schteingart, and Toth

Year Book of Gastroenterology™: Drs Talley, DeVault, Harnois, Pearson, Picco, Scolapio, Smith, and Vege

Year Book of Hand and Upper Limb Surgery®: Drs Yao and Steinmann

Year Book of Medicine®: Drs Barker, Garrick, Gersh, Khardori, LeRoith, Seo, Talley, and Thigpen

Year Book of Neonatal and Perinatal Medicine®: Drs Fanaroff, Benitz, Donn, Neu, Papile, Polin, and van Marter

Year Book of Neurology and Neurosurgery®: Drs Klimo and Rabinstein

Year Book of Obstetrics, Gynecology, and Women's Health®: Drs Dungan and Shulman

Year Book of Oncology®: Drs Arceci, Bauer, Gordon, Lawton, and Thigpen

Year Book of Ophthalmology®: Drs Rapuano, Cohen, Flanders, Hammersmith, Milman, Myers, Nelson, Penne, Pyfer, Sergott, Shields, and Vander

Year Book of Orthopedics®: Drs Morrey, Beauchamp, Huddleston, Swiontkowski, and Trigg

Year Book of Otolaryngology-Head and Neck Surgery®: Drs Sindwani, Balough, Franco, Gapany, and Mitchell

Year Book of Pathology and Laboratory Medicine®: Drs Raab, Parwani, Bejarano, and Bissell

Year Book of Pediatrics®: Dr Stockman

Year Book of Plastic and Aesthetic Surgery™: Drs Miller, Gosain, Gurtner, Gutowski, Ruberg, Salisbury, and Smith

Year Book of Psychiatry and Applied Mental Health®: Drs Talbott, Ballenger, Buckley, Frances, Krupnick, and Mack

Year Book of Pulmonary Disease®: Drs Barker, Jones, Maurer, Raza, Tanoue, and Willsie

Year Book of Sports Medicine®: Drs Shephard, Cantu, Feldman, Jankowski, Khan, Lebrun, Nieman, Pierrynowski, and Rowland

Year Book of Surgery®: Drs Copeland, Behrns, Daly, Eberlein, Fahey, Huber, Jones, Mozingo, and Pruett

Year Book of Urology®: Drs Andriole and Coplen

Year Book of Vascular Surgery®: Drs Moneta, Gillespie, Starnes, and Watkins

2011

The Year Book of PATHOLOGY AND LABORATORY MEDICINE®

Editors-in-Chief

Stephen S. Raab, MD
Vice Chair of Quality and Director of Anatomic Pathology, Department of Pathology, University of Colorado, Denver Health Science Center, Anschutz Medical Campus, Aurora, Colorado

Anil V. Parwani, MD, PhD
Director, Division of Pathology Informatics, University of Pittsburgh School of Medicine, Staff Pathologist, University of Pittsburgh Medical Center Shadyside, Pittsburgh, Pennsylvania

Editor

Pablo A. Bejarano, MD
Professor of Clinical Pathology, Director of Surgical Pathology, Director of Histology Laboratory, University of Miami Leonard M. Miller School of Medicine; Pathologist, Jackson Memorial Hospital, Miami, Florida

Editor-in-Chief, Laboratory Medicine

Michael G. Bissell, MD, PhD, MPH
Professor of Pathology, Ohio State University Medical Center, Columbus, Ohio

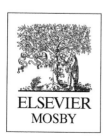

ELSEVIER
MOSBY

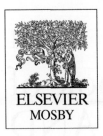

ELSEVIER
MOSBY

Vice President, Continuity: Kimberly Murphy
Editor: Katie Hartner
Supervisor, Electronic Year Books: Donna M. Skelton
Electronic Article Manager: Emily Ogle
Illustrations and Permissions Coordinator: Dawn Vohsen

Composition by TNQ Books and Journals Pvt Ltd, India

Editorial Office:
Elsevier
Suite 1800
1600 John F. Kennedy Blvd.
Philadelphia, PA 19103-2899

International Standard Serial Number: 1077-9108
International Standard Book Number: 978-0-323-08424-6

Printed and bound by CPI Group (UK) Ltd, Croydon, CR0 4YY

Transferred to Digital Print 2011

Contributing Editors

Miriam D. Post, MD
Assistant Professor, Department of Pathology, University of Colorado School of Medicine, Aurora, Colorado

M. Sherif Said, MD, PhD
Associate Professor, Director of Head and Neck Pathology, Department of Pathology, University of Colorado School of Medicine, Aurora, Colorado

Sharon B. Sams, MD
Assistant Professor, Department of Pathology, University of Colorado School of Medicine, Aurora, Colorado

Jeffrey T. Schowinsky, MD
Assistant Professor, Department of Pathology, University of Colorado School of Medicine, Aurora, Colorado

Maxwell L. Smith, MD
Assistant Professor, Director of Liver and Transplant Pathology, Department of Pathology, University of Colorado School of Medicine, Aurora, Colorado

Joshua Wisell, MD
Assistant Professor, Department of Pathology, University of Colorado School of Medicine, Aurora, Colorado

Contributing Editors

Miriam D. Post, MD
Assistant Professor, Department of Pathology, University of Colorado School of Medicine, Aurora, Colorado

M. Sherif Said, MD, PhD
Associate Professor, Director of Head and Neck Pathology, Department of Pathology, University of Colorado School of Medicine, Aurora, Colorado

Sharon B. Sams, MD
Assistant Professor, Department of Pathology, University of Colorado School of Medicine, Aurora, Colorado

Jeffrey T. Schowinsky, MD
Assistant Professor, Department of Pathology, University of Colorado School of Medicine, Aurora, Colorado

Maxwell L. Smith, MD

Table of Contents

Journals Represented

Journals represented in this YEAR BOOK are listed below.

Academic Medicine
Acta Otolaryngol
American Journal of Clinical Pathology
American Journal of Gastroenterology
American Journal of Infection Control
American Journal of Medicine
American Journal of Pathology
American Journal of Preventive Medicine
American Journal of Surgical Pathology
American Journal of Transplantation
Annals of Internal Medicine
Annals of Oncology
Annals of Surgical Oncology
Archives of Internal Medicine
Archives of Pathology & Laboratory Medicine
British Journal of Anaesthesia
British Journal of Urology International
British Medical Journal
Cancer
Cancer Cytopathology
Cancer Journal for Clinicians
Cardiovascular Pathology
Clinical Cancer Research
Clinical Chemistry
Clinical Toxicology
Critical Care Medicine
CytoJournal
Cytopathology
European Urology
Fertility and Sterility
Gastroenterology
Gut
Heart
Hepatology
Histopathology
Human Pathology
International Journal of Cancer
International Journal of Gynecology & Pathology
International Journal of Surgical Pathology
Journal of Cellular Physiology
Journal of Clinical Endocrinology & Metabolism
Journal of Clinical Microbiology
Journal of Clinical Pathology
Journal of Cutaneous Pathology
Journal of Heart and Lung Transplantation
Journal of Infectious Diseases
Journal of Lower Genital Tract Disease

Journal of Molecular Diagnostics
Journal of Pathology
Journal of the American Society of Nephrology
Journal of Urology
Kidney International
Medical Care
Modern Pathology
Nephrology (Carlton)
New England Journal of Medicine
Oral Oncology
Otol Neurotol
Pediatric Radiology
Pediatrics
Social Science & Medicine
Transfusion
Transplantation
Urology

STANDARD ABBREVIATIONS

The following terms are abbreviated in this edition: acquired immunodeficiency syndrome (AIDS), cardiopulmonary resuscitation (CPR), central nervous system (CNS), cerebrospinal fluid (CSF), computed tomography (CT), deoxyribonucleic acid (DNA), electrocardiography (ECG), health maintenance organization (HMO), human immunodeficiency virus (HIV), intensive care unit (ICU), intramuscular (IM), intravenous (IV), magnetic resonance (MR) imaging (MRI), ribonucleic acid (RNA), ultrasound (US), and ultraviolet (UV).

NOTE

The YEAR BOOK OF PATHOLOGY AND LABORATORY MEDICINE is a literature survey service providing abstracts of articles published in the professional literature. Every effort is made to assure the accuracy of the information presented in these pages. Neither the editors nor the publisher of the YEAR BOOK OF PATHOLOGY AND LABORATORY MEDICINE can be responsible for errors in the original materials. The editors' comments are their own opinions. Mention of specific products within this publication does not constitute endorsement.

To facilitate the use of the YEAR BOOK OF PATHOLOGY AND LABORATORY MEDICINE as a reference tool, all illustrations and tables included in this publication are now identified as they appear in the original article. This change is meant to help the reader recognize that any illustration or table appearing in the YEAR BOOK OF PATHOLOGY AND LABORATORY MEDICINE may be only one of many in the original article. For this reason, figure and table numbers will often appear to be out of sequence within the YEAR BOOK OF PATHOLOGY AND LABORATORY MEDICINE.

Introduction

Welcome to the 2011 YEAR BOOK OF PATHOLOGY AND LABORATORY MEDICINE! The 2011 YEAR BOOK has an online format, eClips Consult (eclips.consult.com), as well as the printed hard-bound edition. The online site provides the reader with up-to-date abstracts, commentary, and suggested readings by the expert panel of reviewers. The 2011 YEAR BOOK continues to emphasize timely articles with critiques of current practice for the busy pathologist in both anatomic and clinical pathology. Several important articles were published in the past year, and the 2011 YEAR BOOK highlights these articles with exemplary commentary and views on how these data affect your practice.

The editors of the current YEAR BOOK are: Stephen S. Raab, Anil V. Parwani, Michael G. Bissell, Maxwell L. Smith, Sharon B. Sams, M. Sherif Said, Jeffrey T. Schowinsky, Miriam D. Post, Joshua Wisell, and Pablo A. Bejarano.

Please feel free to provide either of us with feedback. Thank you and please enjoy the 2011 YEAR BOOK!

Stephen S. Raab, MD

Anil V. Parwani, MD, PhD

ANATOMIC PATHOLOGY

1 Outcomes Analysis

Association of Interruptions With an Increased Risk and Severity of Medication Administration Errors
Westbrook JI, Woods A, Rob MI, et al (Univ of Sydney, Australia; et al)
Arch Intern Med 170:683-690, 2010

Background.—Interruptions have been implicated as a cause of clinical errors, yet, to our knowledge, no empirical studies of this relationship exist. We tested the hypothesis that interruptions during medication administration increase errors.

Methods.—We performed an observational study of nurses preparing and administering medications in 6 wards at 2 major teaching hospitals in Sydney, Australia. Procedural failures and interruptions were recorded during direct observation. Clinical errors were identified by comparing observational data with patients' medication charts. A volunteer sample of 98 nurses (representing a participation rate of 82%) were observed preparing and administering 4271 medications to 720 patients over 505 hours from September 2006 through March 2008. Associations between procedural failures (10 indicators; eg, aseptic technique) and clinical errors (12 indicators; eg, wrong dose) and interruptions, and between interruptions and potential severity of failures and errors were the main outcome measures.

Results.—Each interruption was associated with a 12.1% increase in procedural failures and a 12.7% increase in clinical errors. The association between interruptions and clinical errors was independent of hospital and nurse characteristics. Interruptions occurred in 53.1% of administrations (95% confidence interval [CI], 51.6%-54.6%). Of total drug administrations, 74.4% (n = 3177) had at least 1 procedural failure (95% CI, 73.1%-75.7%). Administrations with no interruptions (n = 2005) had a procedural failure rate of 69.6% (n = 1395; 95% CI, 67.6%-71.6%), which increased to 84.6% (n = 148; 95% CI, 79.2%-89.9%) with 3 interruptions. Overall, 25.0% (n = 1067; 95% CI, 23.7%-26.3%) of administrations had at least 1 clinical error. Those with no interruptions had a rate of 25.3% (n = 507; 95% CI, 23.4%-27.2%), whereas those with 3 interruptions had a rate of 38.9% (n = 68; 95% CI, 31.6%-46.1%). Nurse experience provided no protection against making a clinical error and was associated with higher procedural failure rates. Error severity increased with interruption frequency. Without interruption, the estimated risk of a major error was 2.3%; with 4 interruptions this risk doubled to 4.7% (95% CI, 2.9%-7.4%; $P < .001$).

Conclusion.—Among nurses at 2 hospitals, the occurrence and frequency of interruptions were significantly associated with the incidence of procedural failures and clinical errors.

▶ Studies suggest that interruptions produce a negative impact on memory by requiring individuals to switch attention from one task to another. Returning to the disrupted task requires completion of the interrupted task and then regaining the context of the original task. Anatomic pathologists are frequently interrupted in their tasks of sign-out, gross tissue examination, and intraoperative consultation. I find the work by Westbrook et al highly informative and translatable to pathology practice. Because pathologists are interrupted in their daily activities, I believe that errors, similar to the clinical errors observed in nursing work interrupted practice, are manifested as errors in reporting and/or diagnosis. If the error frequency in pathology practice as a result of interrupted work is as high as reported by Westbrook et al, then our field needs to seriously redesign workflow to prevent these interruptions. Some pathology groups have redesigned aspects of their work, such as assigning pathologists to specific tasks (eg, not combining daily tasks of intraoperative consultation with daily sign-out practice) as a means to reduce interruptions.[1,2] However, many pathologists continue to work in practices where interruptions are commonplace. It would be useful for a similar study to be conducted in pathology practice to see the effects of interruptions as well as determine whether pathology practice could be redesigned in an effective manner.

S. S. Raab, MD

References

1. Rogers RD, Monsell S. Costs of a predictable switch between simple cognitive tasks. *J Exp Psychol Gen.* 1995;124:207-231.
2. Bailey BP, Konstan JA. On the need for attention-aware systems: measuring effects of interruption on task performance, error rate and effective state. *Comput Human Behav.* 2006;22:685-708.

Residents' and Attending Physicians' Handoffs: A Systematic Review of the Literature
Riesenberg LA, Leitzsch J, Massucci JL, et al (Christiana Care Health System, Newark, Delaware; et al)
Acad Med 84:1775-1787, 2009

Purpose.—Effective communication is central to patient safety. There is abundant evidence of negative consequences of poor communication and inadequate handoffs. The purpose of the current study was to conduct a systematic review of articles focused on physicians' handoffs, conduct a qualitative review of barriers and strategies, and identify features of structured handoffs that have been effective.

TABLE 1.—Barriers and Strategies Identified in Articles on U.S. Residents' and Attending Physicians' Handoffs in the English-Language Literature, 1987 to June 2008

Categories	Frequency
Barrier categories	
Communication barriers (hierarchy, language, general communication)	
General communication problems[49,51,53,58,60–62,64,67,70,81]*	14
Hierarchy/social barriers[38,51,56,59,61,62,80,82]	8
Language/ethnic barriers[56,59,62]	3
Communication style[38,56,59]	3
Lack of standard system/requirement (no tool, no requirements, no system)	
No standardization or structure[42,51,57,59,61,65,75]	8
No requirements[52,59,61,80]	5
Lack of a tool/protocol[54,73]	2
Lack of training (training, education)	
Lack of education[62,65,70,75,81]	7
Lack of training[44,47,57,60,75]	6
Missing information (omitted information, incorrect information)	
Incomplete/missing information[41,42,49,60,65,69,71,80,83]	9
Errors in information[43,65,71,80]	4
Physical barriers (lighting, location, noise, interruptions)	
Interruptions/distractions[43,47,62,83]	5
Chaotic environment[47,53,80]	3
Lack of time	
Time-consuming processes[48,52,62,69]	4
Time constraints[38,47,83]	3
Difficulties due to complexity/high numbers	
Complexity[51,81]	3
Large number of patients[52,64]	2
Cross-coverage[53,60]	2
Strategy categories	
Standardization	
Standardized process[47,62,65,73]	4
Specific techniques[45,47,51,56,57,61,79,81,83]	15
Preparation[47,51,60,61,69,79]	9
Face-to-face communication[44,47,51,60,62]	5
Read-back[47,57]	2
Standardized content/template[41,42,44,51,56,57,61,65,66,72,81]	14
Mnemonics[38,40,44,56,57,59,60,63,75,80,81]	13
Technology[45–48,50,52,55,57,62,64,69,71,72,74,76–79,81,83]	23
Communication skills (hierarchy, language, general communication)	
General communication skills[38,45,49,51,57,62,80]	13
Limit hierarchy[38,79,82]	3
Training/education[41,44,45,57,60–62,69,70,73,75,80,81]	14
Evaluate the process[40,42,45,61,65,80,81]	10
Physical environment (lighting, location, noise, interruptions)	
Location[57,61,62]	3
Limit interruptions[47,83]	2
Address physical environment[38,83]	3
Recognize transfer of responsibility/accountability[45,56,58,60]	7

*Note: Some articles mentioned a barrier or strategy more than once in different sections of the article, using different descriptions. When these seemed to fit the same category but expressed a different aspect of the category, they were counted as separate barriers or strategies. Thus, some frequencies are greater than the number of references.

Method.—The authors conducted a thorough, systematic review of English-language articles, indexed in PubMed, published between 1987 and June 2008, and focused on physicians' handoffs in the United States. The search strategy yielded 2,590 articles. After title review, 401 were obtained for further review by trained abstractors.

Results.—Forty-six articles met inclusion criteria, 33 (71.7%) of which were published between 2005 and 2008. Content analysis yielded 91 handoffs barriers in eight major categories and 140 handoffs strategies in seven major categories. Eighteen articles involved research on handoffs. Quality assessment scores for research studies ranged from 1 to 13 (possible range 1–16). One third of the reviewed research studies obtained quality scores at or below 8, and only one achieved a score of 13. Only six studies included any measure of handoff effectiveness.

Conclusions.—Despite the negative consequences of inadequate physicians' handoffs, very little research has been done to identify best practices. Many of the existing peer-reviewed studies had design or reporting flaws. There is remarkable consistency in the anecdotally suggested strategies; however, there remains a paucity of evidence to support these strategies. Overall, there is a great need for high-quality handoff outcomes studies focused on systems factors, human performance, and the effectiveness of structured protocols and interventions (Table 1).

▶ This review by Riesenberg et al provides an excellent overview of handoffs in medicine that provides insight into pathology laboratory handoffs, including handoffs involving residents and other laboratory personnel. A handoff is the transfer of patient care from 1 health care provider to another, and handoffs are vulnerable to communication failures. In previous studies,[1,2] handoffs were a contributing factor in up to 24% of medical errors. Handoffs occur at multiple steps in diagnostic testing services and involve the passage of patient specimen material from 1 person to another. For example, handoffs in anatomic pathology occur between gross room personnel and histopathologists, clinicians providing adequate clinical information to pathologists, and pathologists ordering immunohistochemical stains. Riesenberg et al identified 91 barriers to effective handoffs with communication issues being reported most frequently (30.8%). However, barriers also included hierarchy and social barriers that resulted in effective handoffs and communication. Table 1 identifies barriers and strategies for improvement and the relevant articles in the medical literature (as listed by reference number) in the reference section of the article by Riesenberg et al. The appendix to the article also is worth browsing. As reported by Riesenberg et al, little work has been performed evaluating the effectiveness of the implementation strategies to improve the quality of handoffs and best practices in laboratories are an excellent place to start.

S. S. Raab, MD

References

1. Donchin Y, Gopher D, Olin M, et al. A look into the nature and causes of human errors in the intensive care unit. *Qual Saf Health Care*. 2003;12:143-147.
2. White AA, Wright SW, Blanco R, et al. Cause-and-effect analysis of risk management files to assess patient care in the emergency department. *Acad Emerg Med*. 2004;11:1035-1041.

Adequacy of Surgical Pathology Reporting of Cancer: A College of American Pathologists Q-Probes Study of 86 Institutions

Idowu MO, Bekeris LG, Raab S, et al (Virginia Commonwealth Univ Health System, Richmond; Phoenixville Hosp, PA; Univ of Colorado Denver, Aurora; et al)
Arch Pathol Lab Med 134:969-974, 2010

Context.—Inclusion of all scientifically validated elements in surgical pathology cancer reports is needed for optimal patient care.

Objective.—To evaluate the frequency with which surgical pathology cancer reports contain all the scientifically validated elements required by the American College of Surgery (ACS) Commission on Cancer (CoC), the extent to which checklists are used, and the effects that the use of checklists have on the completeness of cancer reports.

Design.—Participants in the College of American Pathologists voluntary Q-Probes program reviewed 25 consecutive surgical pathology reports to include cancer reports from breast, colon, rectum, and prostate cancer specimens. For each report, the type and total number of missing required elements, deemed essential by the ACS CoC, was recorded.

Results.—A total of 2125 cancer reports were reviewed in 86 institutions; 68.8% of all surgical pathology cancer reports included all the required elements. Institutions in which checklists were routinely used reported all required elements at a higher rate than those that did not use checklists (88% versus 34%), and institutions that had a system in place to track errors also reported all required elements at a higher rate when compared to those that did not have such a system in place (88% versus 68%). The missing mandated elements, common to cancer reports of all tumor types, were extent of invasion and status of the resection margin.

Conclusions.—This study demonstrates that about 30% of cancer reports do not have all the scientifically validated elements required by the ACS CoC. Pathology departments in which checklists are not routinely used have a substantially lower rate of reports that include all the required elements.

▶ The article by Idowu et al highlights the utility of medical checklists as a method of error prevention, which is nicely discussed in Atul Gawande's[1] book. All areas of medicine are complex, and physicians make thousands of decisions a day; checklists are useful decision-making tools for memory and organization. For pathologists, if one considers all the questions involved in the diagnostic interpretation and reporting steps in anatomic pathology, checklists are invaluable for step completion. These questions involve determining if the appropriate histologic sections were obtained and processed, a specimen mix-up has not occurred, the proper diagnoses have been considered, the appropriate number and type of immunohistochemical stains have been obtained, the appropriate consultations have been obtained, and the report is complete and accurate.[2] Many checklists are internalized in our training and practice, but external checklists are of assistance in tasks where many different elements are required. Idowu and colleagues show that checklists are helpful in reporting data elements in cancer cases. Checklists could also be of immense importance for other steps (such as ordering the correct immunohistochemical stains) outlined above.

S. S. Raab, MD

References

1. Gawande A. *The Checklist Manifesto: How to Get Things Right.* New York: Henry Holt and Company; 2009.
2. Leslie KO, Rosai J. Standardization of the surgical pathology report: formats, templates and synoptic reports. *Semin Diagn Pathol.* 1994;11:253-257.

Objective Criteria for the Grading of Venous Invasion in Colorectal Cancer
Sato T, Ueno H, Mochizuki H, et al (Natl Defense Med College, Tokorozawa, Japan)
Am J Surg Pathol 34:454-462, 2010

Purpose.—To establish an objective histologic grading system of venous invasion.

Methods.—A total of 229 patients with pT3 and pT4 colorectal cancer who underwent curative surgery with lymph node dissection were retrospectively analyzed. Potential prognosis-related characteristics of venous invasion, including the number of venous invasion, morphologic type of venous invasion, maximum size of veins invaded, and location of venous vessel involved were evaluated on elastica van Gieson stained sections.

Results.—The relapse-free survival curves between the venous-invasion-positive group and the negative group were significantly different (5 y survival rates were 73.4% and 92.2%, respectively, $P = 0.001$). When patients were divided into 3 groups according to the average number of venous invasions observed in a glass slide [G0 (none), G1 (positive but <4), and G2 (4 or more)], there was a significant difference in the survival rate among the 3 groups [5 y survival rates were 92.2%, 77.8%, and 56.4%, respectively, $P = 0.008$ (G0 vs. G1), $P = 0.017$ (G1 vs. G2)]. The postoperative recurrence rate was 10.8% in the G0 patients, whereas it was 32.5% in the G1 and 51.7% in the G2 patients [$P = 0.0007$ (G0 vs. G1), $P = 0.047$ (G1 vs. G2)]. Multivariate analysis showed the number of venous invasions [hazard ratio (HR) 2.72, $P = 0.027$], depth of invasion (HR 2.26, $P = 0.014$), and lymph node metastasis (HR 2.43, $P = 0.008$) were independent prognostic factors.

Conclusions.—Three ranked tumor grading system based on the number of venous invasion in a glass slide with elastica van Gieson staining could be an objective and important treatment index for colorectal cancer patients.

▶ In the past decade, the study and reporting of pathologic prognostic indicators, such as morphologic characteristics and ancillary test features, has increased. The presence of venous invasion is considered an important prognostic indicator for many tumor types, such as colorectal cancer,[1] and has been associated with an increased risk of recurrence and decreased overall survival. Objective criteria for grading and reporting venous invasion in colorectal tumors are lacking.[2] Saito et al reported that the most important characteristic of venous invasion is the number of invasions in a glass slide, which required the use of an elastic tissue stain. These study findings will need to be further evaluated in terms of pathologist reproducibility and association with patient outcome prior to becoming widely used. However, studies like this one indicate that pathologist reporting will become increasingly focused on the evaluation of specific morphologic details, such as counting foci of invasion using special stains, in addition to reporting basic tumor details (eg, tumor type, differentiation, depth of invasion, etc). These details are already being incorporated in synoptic reports, although the specific grading systems will need to be listed and learned.

S. S. Raab, MD

References

1. Minsky B, Mies C. The clinical significance of vascular invasion in colorectal cancer. *Dis Colon Rectum.* 1989;32:794-803.
2. Sternberg A, Amar M, Alfici R, Groisman G. Conclusions from a study of venous invasion in stage IV colorectal cancer. *J Clin Pathol.* 2002;55:17-21.

Measuring and Comparing Safety Climate in Intensive Care Units
France DJ, Greevy RA Jr, Liu X, et al (Ctr for Perioperative Res in Quality, Nashville, TN; Vanderbilt Univ School of Medicine, Nashville, TN; et al)
Med Care 48:279-284, 2010

Background.—Learning about the factors that influence safety climate and improving the methods for assessing relative performance among hospital or units would improve decision-making for clinical improvement.

Objectives.—To measure safety climate in intensive care units (ICU) owned by a large for-profit integrated health delivery system; identify specific provider, ICU, and hospital factors that influence safety climate; and improve the reporting of safety climate data for comparison and benchmarking.

Research Design.—We administered the Safety Attitudes Questionnaire (SAQ) to clinicians, staff, and administrators in 110 ICUs from 61 hospitals.

Subjects.—A total of 1502 surveys (43% response) from physicians, nurses, respiratory therapists, pharmacists, managers, and other ancillary providers.

Measures.—The survey measured safety climate across 6 domains: teamwork climate; safety climate; perceptions of management; job satisfaction; working conditions; and stress recognition. Percentage of positive scores, mean scores, unadjusted random effects, and covariate-adjusted random effect were used to rank ICU performance.

Results.—The cohort was characterized by a positive safety climate. Respondents scored perceptions of management and working conditions significantly lower than the other domains of safety climate. Respondent job type was significantly associated with safety climate and domain scores. There was modest agreement between ranking methodologies using raw scores and random effects.

Conclusions.—The relative proportion of job type must be considered before comparing safety climate results across organizational units. Ranking methodologies based on raw scores and random effects are viable for feedback reports. The use of covariate-adjusted random effects is recommended for hospital decision-making.

▶ There has been little formal study of patient safety climates in laboratories, although the methods to study safety climates have been relatively well developed. This article by France et al illustrates the use of a survey method to evaluate 6 domains of a safety climate in intensive care units (ICUs), and the results are informative for areas outside ICUs. The 2 domains that generally were ranked lower for safety were management and working conditions. These domains might seem obvious to frontline workers but often may not be known by laboratory directors and/or pathologists. I believe that the same findings would hold true in laboratories where a domain, such as teamwork, is well incorporated into a safety culture, but other domains, such as management, are not fully evaluated or understood. Laboratories in the United States are organized in a variety of ways such that pathologists may not have immediate supervisory authority over laboratory personnel. This may limit the ability of pathologists to improve patient safety conditions for laboratory workers. Another important finding was that physicians and nonphysicians have a different perception of the level of patient safety. Individuals not embedded in frontline work often do not fully grasp the factors that affect a quality and safety culture. This point argues that a specific organizational structure (ie, a system in which management is knowledgeable and participatory in day-to-day safety activities) would improve patient safety in laboratories and in other health care settings.[1,2]

S. S. Raab, MD

References

1. Sexton JB, Helmreich RL, Neilands TB, et al. The Safety Attitudes Questionnaire: psychometric properties, benchmarking data, and emerging research. *BMC Health Serv Res.* 2006;6:44.

2. Rowan K, Brady A, Vella K, Boyden J, Sexton J. Teamwork and safety attitudes among staff in critical care units and the relationship to patient mortality. *Crit Care*. 2004;8:341.

Quality in Cancer Diagnosis

Raab SS, Grzybicki DM (Univ of Colorado–Denver, Aurora; Rocky Vista Univ School of Osteopathic Medicine, Parker, CO)
CA Cancer J Clin 60:139-165, 2010

Improving the quality of oncologic pathology diagnosis is immensely important as the overwhelming majority of the approximately 1.6 million patients who will be diagnosed with cancer in 2010 have their diagnoses established through the pathologic interpretation of a tissue sample. Millions more patients have tissue samples obtained to rule out cancer and do not have cancer. The majority of studies on the quality of oncologic pathology diagnoses have focused on patient safety and have documented a variety of causes of error that occur in the clinical and pathology laboratory testing phases of diagnostic testing. The reported frequency of a diagnostic error made by oncologic pathology depends on several factors, such as definitions and detection methods, and ranges from 1% to 15%. The large majority of diagnostic errors do not result in severe harm, although mild to moderate harm in the form of additional testing or diagnostic delays occurs in up to 50% of errors. Clinical practitioners play an essential role in error reduction through several avenues such as effective test ordering, providing accurate and pertinent clinical information, procuring high-quality specimens, providing timely follow-up on test results, effectively communicating on potentially discrepant diagnoses, and advocating second opinions on the pathology diagnosis in specific situations (Table 4).

▶ Problems and errors occur in all steps of the total testing process, which is a system-based framework for examining all possible interactions and activities that affect the quality of laboratory tests. Pathologists are quite familiar with errors that occur in the analytic steps of oncologic diagnostic testing, and this article discusses these errors as well as errors occurring in the preanalytic and postanalytic processes. Pathologists are aware of the errors that occur outside of the pathology laboratory but may not know the extent to which these errors affect anatomic pathology laboratory services. Raab and Grzybicki provide a summary of interinstitutional slide reviews for cases involving a cancer diagnosis (please see Table 4). The overall mean discrepant case rate in these 41 studies was 11.4%, and the major discrepant rate was 4.7%. Although the original studies varied markedly in design, definitions, and methods, these overall means indicate the level of precision in oncologic cancer diagnosis. Many of these discrepancies represent differences in the standardization of diagnoses, rather than missed cancers. Standardizing diagnoses is a challenge because the effort to achieve this task depends on a larger national endeavor, rather

TABLE 4.—Interinstitutional Pathology Slide Review Studies

Year	Authors	Area	Total Cases Reviewed	Total Discrepancy (%)	Major Discrepancy (%)
2009	Wayment[199]	Urologic surgical pathology	213	22 (10.3)	18 (8.5)
2009	Thway[200]	Soft tissue surgical pathology	349	93 (26.6)	38 (10.9)
2009	Bomeisl[201]	Fine needle aspiration cytopathology	742	201 (27.1)	69 (9.3)
2009	Lueck[202]	Cytopathology	499	92 (18.4)	37 (7.4)
2008	Manion[10]	Surgical pathology	5,629	639 (11.3)	132 (2.3)
2007	Tan[203]	Thyroid fine needle aspiration cytopathology	147	27 (18.4)	8 (5.6)
2007	Thomas[204]	Prostate surgical pathology	1,323	334 (25.2)	196 (14.8)
2005	Raab[13]	Surgical pathology and cytopathology	1,069	92 (8.6)	8 (0.7)
2005	Hamady[205]	Thyroid cancer surgical pathology	66	12 (18.2)	5 (7.6)
2004	Tsung[206]	Surgical pathology	715	42 (5.9)	16 (2.2)
2004	Ngyuen[207]	Prostate surgical pathology (Gleason scoring)	602	265 (44)	55 (9.1)
1999	Kronz[223]	Prostate needle biopsy	3,251	87 (2.7)	15 (0.5)
2003	Weir[209]	Surgical pathology and cytopathology	1,522	68 (6.8)	37 (2.4)
2002	McGinnis[210]	Dermatopathology (pigmented lesions)	5,136	559 (10.9)	120 (2.3)
2002	Wetherington[211]	Surgical pathology	6,678	213 (3.2)	213 (3.2)
2002	Staradub[212]	Breast cancer	346	278 (80)	27 (7.8)
2002	Vivino[213]	Labial salivary gland	60	32 (53.3)	32 (53.3)
2002	Layfield[214]	Cytopathology	146	24 (16.4)	11 (7.5)
2002	Westra[215]	Head and neck surgical pathology	814	54 (6.6)	21 (2.6)
2001	Arbiser[216]	Soft tissue surgical pathology	266	85 (31.9)	65 (24.4)
2001	Coblentz[217]	Bladder biopsy and transurethral resections	131	24 (18.3)	24 (18.3)
2001	Hahm[218]	Gastrointestinal and hepatic surgical pathology	194	50 (25.8)	14 (7.2)
2001	Baloch[219]	Cytopathology	183	110 (60.1)	28 (15.3)
2001	Murphy[220]	Urologic surgical pathology	150	29 (19.3)	14 (9.3)
2000	Chafe[221]	Gynecologic surgical pathology	599	200 (33.3)	63 (10.5)
2000	Aldape[222]	Neuropathology	457	105 (23.0)	17 (3.7)
1999	Kronz[223]	Surgical pathology	6,171	86 (1.4)	86 (1.4)
1999	Selman[224]	Gynecologic surgical pathology	295	50 (16.9)	14 (4.8)
1999	Lee[225]	Testicular surgical pathology	208	-	12 (5.8)
1999	Chan[226]	Gynecologic surgical pathology and cytopathology	569	108 (19.0)	37 (6.5)
1998	Wurzer[227]	Prostate biopsies (Gleason scoring)	538	212 (39.4)	69 (12.8)
1998	Jacques[228]	Gynecologic surgical pathology (endometrial curettings and biopsy)	182	43 (23.6)	43 (23.6)
1998	Jacques[229]	Gynecologic surgical pathology (hysterectomy)	76	24 (31.6)	24 (31.6)
1998	Santoso[230]	Gynecologic surgical pathology	720	119 (16.5)	15 (2.1)
1997	Sharkey[231]	Urologic surgical pathology and cytopathology	376	133 (35.3)	133 (35.3)
1997	Bruner[232]	Neuropathology	500	214 (42.8)	140 (28.0)
1996	Epstein[233]	Prostate surgical pathology	535	7 (1.3)	7 (1.3)
1995	Prescott[234]	Surgical pathology	227	53 (23.3)	19 (8.3)
1995	Abt[235]	Surgical pathology and cytopathology	777	71 (9.1)	45 (5.8)
1995	Scott[236]	Neuropathology	680	74 (10.9)	74 (10.9)
1993	Segelov[237]	Testicular surgical pathology	87	28 (32.0)	10 (11.4)

Editor's Note: Please refer to original journal article for full references.

than local education, which is the means by which diagnostic terminology is currently learned.[1,2,3]

S. S. Raab, MD

References

1. Kohn LT, Corrigan JM, Donaldson MS. *To Err is Human: Building a Safer Health System.* Washington, DC: National Academy Press; 1999.
2. Berwick DM. A user's manual for the IOM's 'Quality Chasm' report. *Health Aff (Millwood).* 2002;21:80-90.
3. Committee on Quality and Health Care in America. *Crossing the Quality Chasm: A New Health System for the 21st Century.* Washington, DC: National Academy Press; 2001.

Pathology Reporting of Neuroendocrine Tumors: Application of the Delphic Consensus Process to the Development of a Minimum Pathology Data Set

Klimstra DS, Modlin IR, Adsay NV, et al (Memorial Sloan-Kettering Cancer Ctr, NY; Yale Univ School of Medicine, New Haven, CT; Emory Univ, Atlanta, GA; et al)

Am J Surg Pathol 34:300-313, 2010

Epithelial neuroendocrine tumors (NETs) have been the subject of much debate regarding their optimal classification. Although multiple systems of nomenclature, grading, and staging have been proposed, none has achieved universal acceptance. To help define the underlying common features of these classification systems and to identify the minimal pathology data that should be reported to ensure consistent clinical management and reproducibility of data from therapeutic trials, a multidisciplinary team of physicians interested in NETs was assembled. At a group meeting, the participants discussed a series of "yes" or "no" questions related to the pathology of NETs and the minimal data to be included in the reports. After discussion, anonymous votes were taken, using the Delphic principle that 80% agreement on a vote of either yes or no would define a consensus. Questions that failed to achieve a consensus were rephrased once or twice and discussed, and additional votes were taken. Of 108 questions, 91 were answerable either yes or no by more than 80% of the participants. There was agreement about the importance of proliferation rate for tumor grading, the landmarks to use for staging, the prognostic factors assessable by routine histology that should be reported, the potential for tumors to progress biologically with metastasis, and the current status of advanced immunohistochemical and molecular testing for treatment-related biomarkers. The lack of utility of a variety of immunohistochemical stains and pathologic findings was also agreed upon. A consensus could not be reached for the remaining 17 questions, which included both minor points related to extent of disease assessment and some major areas such as terminology, routine immunohistochemical staining for general neuroendocrine markers, use of Ki67 staining to assess proliferation, and the relationship of tumor grade to degree of differentiation. On the basis of the results of the Delphic voting, a minimum pathology data set was developed. Although there remains disagreement among experts about the specific classification system that should be used, there is agreement about the fundamental pathology data that should be reported. Examination of the areas of disagreement reveals significant opportunities for collaborative study to resolve unanswered questions.

▶ One source of variability in anatomic pathology is the absence of standardization of diagnostic reports.[1] For a variety of tumors arising in different organ systems, there is variability in classification systems, grading, staging, reporting, and use of immunohistochemical tests. The article by Klimstra and coauthors is a first attempt to standardize reporting for neuroendocrine tumors. A Delphi approach is used when there is a general lack of published data linking process to outcome and is a form of consensus building based on expert opinion, which is a relatively low level of evidence for medical decision making. Klimstra et al wrote that a number of data elements are important for neuroendocrine tumor reporting and for some of these elements, most pathologists already report (eg, anatomic site of tumor, size in resection specimens).[2] Other elements, such as the use of immunohistochemical stains, are more controversial, and it appears that the number and types of immunohistochemical stains vary among experts. Experts agree that the use of immunohistochemistry is recommended for diagnostic purposes in most cases, including biopsy tissues of metastatic disease. The group recommended that 2 stains be routinely ordered (chromogranin A and synaptophysin), although the use of other neuroendocrine markers was controversial. Recommendations based on expert opinion should be followed up with formal investigations to determine if factors such as number and type of immunohistochemical stain actually affect patient outcome.

S. S. Raab, MD

References

1. Fink A, Kosecoff J, Chassin M, Brook RH. Consensus methods: characteristics and guidelines for use. *Am J Public Health.* 1984;74:979-983.
2. Oberg K, Jelic S. Neuroendocrine gastroenteropancreatic tumors: ESMO clinical recommendations for diagnosis, treatment and follow-up. *Ann Oncol.* 2008;19: ii104-ii105.

A problem shared...? Teamwork, autonomy and error in assisted conception
Kerr A (Univ of Leeds, UK)
Soc Sci Med 69:1741-1749, 2009

This paper explores the benefits and drawbacks of new team-based approaches to error management in medicine through a case study of teamwork, double witnessing and incident reporting in assisted conception clinics in the UK. This is based upon the analysis of a series of semi-structured interviews with people working in assisted conception clinics and two periods of ethnography in clinics, conducted between 2004 and 2007, as part of an ESRC-funded study on the ethics of assisted conception and embryo research. In common with other studies of practitioners' management of error, I identify a series of tensions around individual and collective autonomy in identifying and preventing error, for the assisted conception team as a whole, and for particular groups within it, notably consultants and embryologists. I found that team-based approaches could create the conditions for error to occur when it undermined independent thinking, responsibility or concentration. There was also a danger that teamwork could come to be associated with particular 'technical' practices or occupational groups, diminishing its relevance and value in clinical settings. I, therefore, conclude that team-based approaches and professional autonomy have their 'dark' as well as their 'light' sides (Vaughan, D. (1999). The dark side of organisations: mistake, misconduct, and disaster. *Annual Review of Sociology*, 25, 271–305). Errors cannot be prevented in their entirety, but they can be well managed when teamwork and autonomy are complementary. Drawing on Reason (Reason, J. [2004]. Beyond the organisational accident: the need for "error wisdom" on the frontline. *Quality Safety in Health Care*, 12, ii28–ii33), I argue that informed vigilance and intelligent wariness is a necessary compliment to systems-based approaches to error management in assisted conception in particular, and medicine in general.

▶ Kerr outlines the tensions between teamwork and autonomy in patient safety practice. The use of teamwork, evidence-based medicine practices, clinical guidelines, and protocols (eg, standardized reports) have been introduced on a wide scale in medicine and in laboratory settings to reduce medical error and improve quality.[1] An effort to reduce errors in the United States has been the development of cross-boundary teams including practitioners within and outside of laboratories. Kerr cautions against the overreliance on a team-based approach and eschewing the individualistic approach to reduce medical error. This article focuses on conception (in the field of reproductive medicine) but equally could be applied to laboratory testing. For James Reason,[2] informed vigilance and intelligence wariness are complements to systems-based approaches to error management. Organizations need to be receptive to the messages from frontline staff in order for the benefits of error wisdom to be realized. Kerr argues that systems already have error reduction practices that are hidden from view in the rush to compare and contrast errors that rise to the surface. This contrast is important for laboratory personnel to have in mind as they implement error reduction strategies or choose quality improvement programs.

S. S. Raab, MD

References

1. Mizrahi T. Managing medical mistakes: ideology, insularity, and accountability among internists-in-training. *Soc Sci Med.* 1984;19:135-146.
2. Reason J. Beyond the organisational accident: the need for "error wisdom" on the frontline. *Qual Saf Health Care.* 2004;13:ii28-ii33.

False positive endoscopic ultrasound fine needle aspiration cytology: incidence and risk factors

Gleeson FC, Kipp BR, Caudill JL, et al (Mayo Clinic College of Medicine, Rochester, MN)
Gut 59:586-594, 2010

Objective.—It is broadly accepted that the false positive (FP) rate for endoscopic ultrasound fine needle aspiration (EUS FNA) is 0–1%. It was hypothesised that the FP and false suspicious (FS) rates for EUS FNA are greater than reported. A study was undertaken to establish the rate and root cause of discordant interpretation.

Design.—Using a prospectively maintained endoscopic database, cyto-histological discordant EUS FNA examinations from 30 July 1996 to 31 December 2008 were identified retrospectively.

Setting.—Tertiary referral centre.

Main Outcome Measures.—Discordant FNA was defined by positive or suspicious FNA cytology in the absence of malignancy or neoplasm in the subsequent surgical pathology specimen, specifically in the absence of neo-adjuvant therapy. Three cytopathologists conducted a blinded review of randomised discordant and matched specimens.

Results.—FNA was performed in 5667/18 066 (31.4%) patients under-going EUS, of whom 2547 had cytology results interpreted as 'positive' or 'suspicious' or 'atypical' for malignancy or neoplasm. Subsequent surgical resection without prior neoadjuvant therapy was performed in 377 patients with positive or suspicious cytology. The FP rate was 20/377 (5.3%) and increased to 27/377 (7.2%) when FS cases were included. The incidence of discordance was consistent over time (1996–2002: 10/118 (8.6%) vs 2003–2008: 17/259 (6.6%); p=0.5) and was higher in non-pancreatic FNA (15%) than pancreatic FNA (2.2%; p=0.0001). Two-thirds of the non-pancreatic FP cases involved sampling of perioesophageal or perirectal nodes in patients with luminal neoplasms or Barrett's oesophagus. Following pathological re-review, discordance was attributed to translocated cell contamination/sampling error (50%) or cytopathologist interpretive error (50%).

TABLE 1.—Data for Non-Pancreatic Parenchymal FNA

	EUS FNA Lymph Node Site	EUS FNA Cytology Result	Surgical Technique Performed	Surgical Pathology Findings	No of Nodes at Surgery	Consensus Pathology Re-Review	Explanation for Discordance
1	Perioesophageal	Positive	Ivor Lewis oesophagectomy	Adenocarcinoma, Barrett's oesophagus (T1N0)	8	Positive	EUS contamination/sampling error
2	Perioesophageal	Positive	Ivor Lewis oesophagectomy	Adenocarcinoma without Barrett's oesophagus (T1N0)	14	Negative	Pathology misinterpretation
3	Perioesophageal	Positive	Ivor Lewis oesophagectomy	Adenocarcinoma, Barrett's oesophagus (T1N0)	17	Negative	Pathology misinterpretation
4	Perioesophageal	Positive	Ivor Lewis oesophagectomy	Adenocarcinoma without Barrett's oesophagus (T1N0)	17	Negative	Pathology misinterpretation
5	Perioesophageal	Positive	Ivor Lewis oesophagectomy	Barrett's oesophagus with low-grade dysplasia	26	Specimen unavailable	Specimen not available
6	Perioesophageal	Positive	Ivor Lewis oesophagectomy	Adenocarcinoma, Barrett's oesophagus (T1N0)	8	Positive	EUS contamination/sampling error
7	Perioesophageal	Positive	Ivor Lewis oesophagectomy	Adenocarcinoma without Barrett's oesophagus (T3N0)	25	Positive	EUS contamination/sampling error
8	Perioesophageal	Positive	Ivor Lewis oesophagectomy	Adenocarcinoma, Barrett's oesophagus (T1N0)	33	Atypical	EUS contamination/sampling error
9	Perioesophageal	Suspicious	Ivor Lewis oesophagectomy	Barrett's oesophagus with high-grade dysplasia	17	Negative	Pathology misinterpretation
10	Perioesophageal	Suspicious	Ivor Lewis oesophagectomy	Adenocarcinoma, Barrett's oesophagus (T2N0)	15	Atypical	EUS contamination/sampling error
11	Perioesophageal	Suspicious	Mediastinoscopy and thoracotomy	Lung adenocarcinoma (T2N0)	27	Negative	Pathology misinterpretation
12	Peripancreatic	Positive	Exploratory laparotomy	Neuroendocrine tumour (jejunal)	7	Atypical	EUS contamination/sampling error
13	Peripancreatic	Positive	Whipple procedure	Pancreatic adenocarcinoma (T2N0)	6	Negative	EUS contamination/sampling error
14	Peripancreatic	Positive	Whipple procedure	Chronic pancreatitis (without neoplasia)	7	Negative	Pathology misinterpretation
15	Peripancreatic	Positive	Extended distal pancreatectomy	Pancreatic adenocarcinoma (T2N0)	8	Positive	EUS contamination/sampling error
16	Perigastric	Positive	Subtotal gastrectomy	Reactive gastropathy	10	Positive	EUS contamination/sampling error

(Continued)

TABLE 1. (*continued*)

	EUS FNA Lymph Node Site	EUS FNA Cytology Result	Surgical Technique Performed	Surgical Pathology Findings	No of Nodes at Surgery	Consensus Pathology Re-Review	Explanation for Discordance
17	Perigastric	Positive	Exploratory laparotomy	Autoimmune pancreatitis	Not reported	Negative	Pathology misinterpretation
18	Perirectal	Positive	Abdominoperineal resection	Rectal cancer (T2N0)	14	Positive	EUS contamination/sampling error
19	Perirectal	Positive	Abdominoperineal resection	Rectal cancer (T2N0)	4	Suspicious	EUS contamination/sampling error
20	Perirectal	Positive	Low anterior resection	Rectal cancer (T1N0)	30	Positive	EUS contamination/sampling error
21	Perirectal	Positive	Low anterior resection	Rectal cancer (T3N0)	30	Positive	EUS contamination/sampling error
22	Liver parenchyma	Suspicious	Whipple, wedge liver biopsy	Sclerosing haemangioma	34	Negative	Pathology misinterpretation

EUS, endoscopic ultrasound; FNA, fine needle aspiration.

Conclusions.—These findings refute the accepted paradigm that FP cytology rarely occurs with EUS FNA. Further investigation revealed that FP FNA developed secondary to endosonographer technique or initial cytological misinterpretation, and is particularly likely when perioesophageal or perirectal nodes are aspirated in the setting of a luminal neoplasm or Barrett's oesophagus. Further study is needed to determine the significance of these findings and potential impact on the performance of FNA and patient outcomes (Table 1).

▶ Depending on the clinical setting, false-positive diagnoses may lead to unnecessary surgery or other forms of treatment and patient harm.[1,2] Gleeson and colleagues report the root cause analytic findings of false-positive (including cases interpreted as suspicious) diagnoses. For the practicing cytopathologist, Gleeson et al detail several factors that should be assessed prior to making a final interpretation of neoplastic or suspicious diagnoses: (1) consider if the glandular cells in a lymph node aspirate are contaminants from the gastrointestinal tract rather than metastatic disease (see Table 1 for nonpancreatic aspirate data); (2) make sure that definitively malignant cells in a lymph node aspirate were not obtained by the needle passing through a luminal tumor; (3) do not overcall cancer in pancreatic aspirates that contain inflammation and rare atypical cells; and (4) do not overcall atypical histiocytes as malignant. Of course, being overly cautious may lead to false-negative diagnoses, as the root cause analytic data must be used in consideration of a specific prospective case.

S. S. Raab, MD

References

1. Mishra G. DNA analysis of cells obtained from endoscopic ultrasound-fine needle aspiration in pancreatic adenocarcinoma: Fool's Gold, Pandora's Box, or Holy Grail? *Am J Gastroenterol.* 2006;101:2501-2503.
2. Wiersema MJ, Vilmann P, Giovannini M, Chang KJ, Wiersema LM. Endosonography-guided fine-needle aspiration biopsy: diagnostic accuracy and complication assessment. *Gastroenterology.* 1997;112:1087-1095.

Patient Record Review of the Incidence, Consequences, and Causes of Diagnostic Adverse Events
Zwaan L, de Bruijne M, Wagner C, et al (EMGO Inst for Health and Care Res, Amsterdam, the Netherlands; et al)
Arch Intern Med 170:1015-1021, 2010

Background.—Diagnostic errors often result in patient harm. Previous studies have shown that there is large variability in results in different medical specialties. The present study explored diagnostic adverse events (DAEs) across all medical specialties to determine their incidence and to gain insight into their causes and consequences by comparing them with other AE types.

Methods.—A structured review study of 7926 patient records was conducted. Randomly selected records were reviewed by trained physicians in 21 hospitals across the Netherlands. The method used in this study was based on the well-known protocol developed by the Harvard Medical Practice Study. All AEs with diagnostic error as the main category were selected for analysis and were compared with other AE types.

Results.—Diagnostic AEs occurred in 0.4% of hospital admissions and represented 6.4% of all AEs. Of the DAEs, 83.3% were judged to be preventable. Human failure was identified as the main cause (96.3%), although organizational-and patient-related factors also contributed (25.0% and 30.0%, respectively). The consequences of DAEs were more severe (higher mortality rate) than for other AEs (29.1% vs 7.4%).

Conclusions.—Diagnostic AEs represent an important error type, and the consequences of DAEs are severe. The causes of DAEs were mostly human, with the main causes being knowledge-based mistakes and information transfer problems. Prevention strategies should focus on training physicians and on the organization of knowledge and information transfer.

▶ In this article, Zwaan et al examine the consequences and causes of diagnostic errors associated with adverse events. For the most part, Zwaan and colleagues collect diagnostic errors in nonpathology fields, such as internal medicine, surgery, and pediatrics. However, I think adverse events in pathology have similar causes and consequences. It is intuitive, as Zwaan et al conclude, that most diagnostic adverse events are caused by human failings that are usually knowledge-based failures or mistakes. However, I think that the conclusions by Zwaan et al also are misleading, as most knowledge-based mistakes are in turn caused by antecedent failures—at least in the field of anatomic pathology. For example, in anatomic pathology, some diagnostic adverse events consist of the over- or underinterpretation of poor clinical samples.[1,2] Although an anatomic pathologist may make a knowledge-based mistake in this scenario, educating that pathologist to deal more appropriately with over- or underinterpretation is only part of the overall solution. Clinicians also must be trained to obtain better samples, or technical staff must be trained to improve specimen preparation techniques. As all steps in the diagnostic process are connected, the entire process of diagnostic testing (or a diagnostic workup for the purposes of the article by Zwaan et al) needs to be reexamined for improvement opportunities, rather than simply examining cognitive failures of the pathologist.

S. S. Raab, MD

References

1. Ghandi TH, Kachalia A, Thomas EJ, et al. Missed and delayed diagnoses in the ambulatory setting: a study of closed malpractice claims. *Ann Intern Med.* 2006;145:488-496.
2. Redelmeier DA. Improving patient care: the cognitive psychology of missed diagnoses. *Ann Intern Med.* 2005;142:115-120.

Safety coaches in radiology: decreasing human error and minimizing patient harm

Dickerson JM, Koch BL, Adams JM, et al (Cincinnati Children's Hosp Med Ctr, OH)

Pediatr Radiol 40:1545-1551, 2010

Successful programs to improve patient safety require a component aimed at improving safety culture and environment, resulting in a reduced number of human errors that could lead to patient harm. Safety coaching provides peer accountability. It involves observing for safety behaviors and use of error prevention techniques and provides immediate feedback. For more than a decade, behavior-based safety coaching has been a successful strategy for reducing error within the context of occupational safety in industry. We describe the use of safety coaches in radiology. Safety coaches are an important component of our comprehensive patient safety program.

▶ In industry, safety coaching has been shown to reduce workforce injury, risk behaviors, and workplace error. Dickerson et al discuss safety coaching in radiology although the concepts may be equally applied to pathology laboratories. Safety coaching provides peer accountability by observing for safety behaviors and use of error prevention techniques and providing immediate feedback. Dickerson et al discuss the use of safety coaches in radiology practice by training individuals to perform observations of actual practice. In the Toyota Production System model, these observers are similar to team leaders who observe behaviors and provide feedback on practices that may lead to error. Some laboratories have experimented with the use of team leaders although the cost of funding these individuals often is an issue. The manner with which observers work with frontline personnel also may be problematic; unless these individuals are accepted, frontline personnel may feel picked on or have a negative view of the observational process. In my experience, the use of coaches or observers needs to be adopted into a quality management system and become full-time positions. Such a quality system needs to periodically check on the effectiveness of coaches/observers by using specific metrics. This last practice has not uniformly been adopted along with the embedding of observers in practice.[1,2]

S. S. Raab, MD

References

1. Geller ES. Behavior-based safety in industry: realizing the large-scale potential of psychology to promote human welfare. *Appl Prev Psychol.* 2001;10:87-105.
2. Kahlon PS. Patient safety: a collaborative, blame-free, team approach. *Radiol Manage.* 2006;28:47-50.

Patient safety: latent risk factors
van Beuzekom M, Boer F, Akerboom S, et al (Leiden Univ Med Centre, The Netherlands; Leiden Univ, The Netherlands)
Br J Anaesth 105:52-59, 2010

The *person-centred* analysis and prevention approach has long dominated proposals to improve patient safety in healthcare. In this approach, the focus is on the individual responsible for making an error. An alternative is the *systems-centred* approach, in which attention is paid to the organizational factors that create precursors for individual errors. This approach assumes that since humans are fallible, systems must be designed to prevent humans from making errors or to be tolerant to those errors. The questions raised by this approach might, for example, include asking *why* an individual had specific gaps in their knowledge, experience, or ability. The systems approach focuses on working conditions rather than on errors of individuals, as the likelihood of specific errors increases with unfavourable conditions. Since the factors that promote errors are not directly visible in the working environment, they are described as latent risk factors (LRFs). Safety failures in anaesthesia, in particular, and medicine, in general, result from *multiple* unfavourable LRFs, so we propose that effective interventions require that attention is paid to interactions between multiple factors and actors. Understanding how LRFs affect safety can enable us to design more effective control measures that will impact significantly on both individual performance and patient outcomes.

▶ Latent risk factors often are talked about but rarely examined in detail when performing root cause analysis in anatomic pathology. I think 2 reasons are the lack of expertise in performing latent risk root cause analysis and the general inability to effect changes that would reduce these risks. The article by van Beuzekom et al is a good review article of latent risk factor and is similar to the Eindhoven method of root cause analysis reported for transfusion medicine. Multiple latent risk factors may combine to result in errors. Contrast this view of risk and root cause analysis to the one traditionally used in the cytologic-histologic correlation method. In the typical way of performing correlation, the root cause generally is attributed to a cytologic or a histologic failure, secondarily attributable to interpretation or clinical sampling. The latent risk factors leading to these causes are almost never examined and therefore rarely corrected. This is why correlation error frequencies generally do not change over time, unless the system changes (eg, a new technology is introduced or a new pathologist begins work). Imagine if correlation were performed with an analysis of latent risk factors. Possible causes of noncorrelation could be linked to inadequate training, lack of experience, insufficient staffing, or failures in communication. These causes of error could be addressed differently than addressing an error caused by sampling. As safety science evolves in pathology, quality improvement will be based on incorporating concepts such as latent error into actual practice redesign.[1,2]

S. S. Raab, MD

References

1. Shappell S, Detwiler C, Holcomb K, Hackworth C, Boquet A, Wiegmann DA. Human error and commercial aviation accidents: an analysis using the human factors analysis and classification system. *Hum Factors.* 2007;49:227-242.
2. Wagenaar WA, Hudson PTW, Reason JT. Cognitive failures and accidents. *Appl Cogn Psychol.* 1990;4:273-294.

2 Breast

American Society of Clinical Oncology/College of American Pathologists Guideline Recommendations for Immunohistochemical Testing of Estrogen and Progesterone Receptors in Breast Cancer (Unabridged Version)
Hammond MEH, Hayes DF, Dowsett M, et al (Univ of Utah School of Medicine, Salt Lake City; Washington Univ School of Medicine, St Louis, MO; American Society of Clinical Oncology, Alexandria, VA; et al)
Arch Pathol Lab Med 134:e48-e72, 2010

Purpose.—To develop a guideline to improve the accuracy of immuno-histochemical (IHC) estrogen receptor (ER) and progesterone receptor (PgR) testing in breast cancer and the utility of these receptors as predictive markers.

Methods.—The American Society of Clinical Oncology and the College of American Pathologists convened an international Expert Panel that conducted a systematic review and evaluation of the literature in partnership with Cancer Care Ontario and developed recommendations for optimal IHC ER/PgR testing performance.

Results.—Up to 20% of current IHC determinations of ER and PgR testing worldwide may be inaccurate (false negative or false positive). Most of the issues with testing have occurred because of variation in pre-analytic variables, thresholds for positivity, and interpretation criteria.

Recommendations.—The Panel recommends that ER and PgR status be determined on all invasive breast cancers and breast cancer recurrences. A testing algorithm that relies on accurate, reproducible assay performance is proposed. Elements to reliably reduce assay variation are specified. It is recommended that ER and PgR assays be considered positive if there are at least 1% positive tumor nuclei in the sample on testing in the presence of expected reactivity of internal (normal epithelial elements) and external controls. The absence of benefit from endocrine therapy for women with ER-negative invasive breast cancers has been confirmed in large overviews of randomized clinical trials.

▶ Accurate determination of estrogen receptor (ER) and progesterone receptor (PR) status in mammary carcinoma is imperative as a prognostic factor and a guide to treatment decisions including the use of endocrine therapy. Recent well-publicized research has identified significant variation in ER and PR positivity rates performed by immunohistochemical analysis across multiple laboratories. Given the clinical significance of ER and PR analysis, the American

Society of Clinical Oncology and the College of American Pathologists convened an expert panel to produce these guideline recommendations that address some of the specific etiologies behind the discordance in receptor status reporting. The guidelines set standardized parameters for the preanalytic phase of specimen handling, the testing phase, including validation and the postanalytic phase of test reporting. Most importantly, while in the process of developing these guidelines, the panel maintained their focus on the implication for patient care and patient outcomes. These guideline recommendations are a must read for any pathologist or laboratory director who is handling breast specimens.

S. B. Sams, MD

Clinical Importance of Histologic Grading of Lobular Carcinoma In Situ in Breast Core Needle Biopsy Specimens: Current Issues and Controversies

Gao F, Carter G, Tseng G, et al (Univ of Pittsburgh Med Ctr, PA)
Am J Clin Pathol 133:767-771, 2010

Lobular carcinoma in situ (LCIS) is considered a risk factor for development of invasive carcinoma (IC). Many variants of LCIS have been described based on pathologic features such as nuclear grade, pleomorphism, and necrosis, but little is known about the biology of these variants. The proposed 3-tier grading system for LCIS has not been validated or endorsed across laboratories. We found significant upstaging of pure pleomorphic LCIS (LCIS with nuclear grade [NG] 3), up to 25% in core needle biopsy (CNB) specimens, in an earlier study. The aim of the current study was to address the importance of pure classical LCIS (NGs 1 and 2) in CNB specimens along with clinicopathologic follow-up. In follow-up resection specimens, IC or ductal carcinoma in situ was seen in 18% (7/39), a high incidence of residual LCIS was seen in 69% (27/39), and other high-risk lesions, such as atypical ductal hyperplasia, were seen in 36% (14/39) of LCIS NG 2 cases. Our study illustrates the importance of grading LCIS; we recommend follow-up excision in LCIS NG 2 cases owing to a high incidence of residual LCIS and the likelihood of identifying other high-risk lesions.

▶ With the recent recognition of pleomorphic lobular neoplasia as a distinct variant, it was only a matter of time before advocating for additional grading of lobular neoplasia in a manner similar to ductal neoplasia. The argument for the distinction of pleomorphic lobular neoplasia is its more aggressive nature that warrants a treatment similar to ductal neoplasia. By logical conclusion, we would expect lobular neoplasia to have a continuum of differentiation that is directly related to its behavior. Rakha et al[1] demonstrated that indeed the higher histologic grade of invasive lobular carcinoma is associated with an increased risk of occurrence and increased distant metastasis and is an independent predictor for shorter survival and disease-free survival. The authors turn their attention to lobular carcinoma in situ (LCIS), and in a previous study demonstrate that pleomorphic LCIS, diagnosed on core needle biopsy, is upstaged to a more significant lesion on resection in up to 25% of cases.[2] In this study, they compare the clinical outcome of patients diagnosed with low nuclear grade (NG) 1 and intermediate NG 2 classical LCIS. Their findings, in conjunction with their previous study, support a correlation between the histologic grade of LCIS and subsequent risk of upstaging to a more significant lesion on resection. This study is an important step toward the validation of a 3-tiered grading system of LCIS prior to its use in directing therapy.

S. B. Sams, MD

References

1. Rakha EA, El-Sayed ME, Menon S, Green AR, Lee AH, Ellis IO. Histologic grading is an independent prognostic factor in invasive lobular carcinoma of the breast. *Breast Cancer Res Treat.* 2008;111:121-127.
2. Chivukula M, Haynik DM, Brufsky A, Carter G, Dabbs DJ. Pleomorphic lobular carcinoma in situ (PLCIS) on breast core needle biopsies: clinical significance and immunoprofile. *Am J Surg Pathol.* 2008;32:1721-1726.

EGFR and HER-2/neu expression in invasive apocrine carcinoma of the breast

Vranic S, Tawfik O, Palazzo J, et al (Creighton Univ Med Ctr, Omaha, NE; Univ of Kansas Med Ctr; Thomas Jefferson Univ Hosp, Philadelphia, PA; et al)
Mod Pathol 23:644-653, 2010

This study was undertaken to investigate epidermal growth factor receptor (EGFR) and human epidermal growth factor receptor 2 (HER-2)/neu expression in a cohort of apocrine carcinomas of the breast with emphasis on the classification of the breast tumors with apocrine morphology. In total, 55 breast carcinomas morphologically diagnosed as apocrine were evaluated for the steroid receptor expression profile characteristic of normal apocrine epithelium (androgen receptor positive/estrogen receptor (ER) negative/progesterone receptor (PR) negative), and for the expression of EGFR and Her-2/neu proteins, and the copy number ratios of the genes *EGFR/CEP7* and *HER-2/CEP17*. On the basis of the results of steroid receptors expression, 38 (69%) cases were classified as pure apocrine carcinoma (androgen receptor positive/ER negative/PR negative), whereas 17 (31%) were re-classified as apocrine-like carcinomas because they did not have the characteristic steroid receptor expression profile. Her-2/neu overexpression was observed in 54% of the cases (57% pure apocrine carcinomas *vs* 47% apocrine-like carcinomas). *HER-2/neu* gene amplification was demonstrated in 52% of all cases (54% pure apocrine carcinomas *vs* 46% apocrine-like carcinomas). EGFR protein (scores 1 to 3+) was detected in 62% of all cases and was expressed in a higher proportion of pure apocrine carcinomas than in the apocrine-like carcinomas group (76 *vs* 29%, $P = 0.006$). In the pure apocrine carcinoma group, Her-2/neu and EGFR protein expression were inversely correlated ($P = 0.006$, $r = -0.499$). EGFR gene amplification was observed in two pure apocrine carcinomas and one apocrine-like carcinoma. Polysomy 7 was commonly present in pure apocrine carcinomas (61 vs 27% of apocrine-like carcinomas; $P = 0.083$) and showed a weak positive correlation with EGFR protein expression ($P = 0.025$, $r = 0.326$). Our study showed that apocrine breast carcinomas are a molecularly diverse group of carcinomas. Strictly defined pure apocrine carcinomas are either HER-2-overexpressing breast carcinomas or triple-negative breast carcinomas, whereas apocrine-like carcinomas predominantly belong to the luminal phenotype. Pure apocrine carcinomas show consistent overexpression of either EGFR or HER-2/neu, which could have significant therapeutic implications.

▶ Apocrine carcinoma of the breast is a rare subtype of carcinoma with characteristic histopathologic features of apocrine differentiation and a distinct molecular gene expression profile of increased androgen receptor (AR) and human epidermal growth factor receptor 2 (Her2/neu) signaling. The immunophenotypic criteria of pure apocrine carcinoma show positive expression for AR and lacks expression for estrogen receptor and progesterone receptor. The authors of this study examine this distinction between pure apocrine and apocrine-like carcinoma in this retrospective review of 55 cases previously diagnosed by morphology as apocrine carcinoma. Their results support the evidence that if the criteria for steroid receptor expression profile are applied stringently, pure apocrine carcinoma is a distinct subgroup defined by its molecular classification. In particular, the authors note a statistically significant inverse correlation between epidermal growth factor (EGRF) and Her2/neu overexpression in pure apocrine carcinomas. This strict definition is clinically relevant, given the prognostic significance and treatment modalities directed at carcinomas with EGRF receptors.

S. B. Sams, MD

Flat epithelial atypia is a common subtype of B3 breast lesions and is associated with noninvasive cancer but not with invasive cancer in final excision histology
Noske A, Pahl S, Fallenberg E, et al (Universitätsmedizin Charité Berlin, Germany)
Hum Pathol 41:522-527, 2010

The biological behavior and the optimal management of benign breast lesions with uncertain malignant potential, the so-called B3 lesions, found in breast needle core biopsies is still under debate. We addressed this study to compare histologic findings in B3 needle core biopsies with final excision specimens to determine associated rates of malignancy. Consecutive needle core biopsies were performed in a 3-year period (January 1, 2006-December 31, 2008). Biopsies were image-guided

(31 by ultrasound, 85 stereotactic vacuum-assisted, 6 unknown) for evaluation of breast abnormalities. We reviewed 122 needle core biopsies with B3 lesions of 91 symptomatic patients and 31 screen-detected women and compared the B3 histologic subtypes with the final excision histology. A total of 1845 needle core biopsies were performed and B3 lesions comprised 6.6% of all B categories. The most common histologic subtype in biopsies was flat epithelia atypia in 35.2%, followed by papillary lesions in 21% and atypical ductal hyperplasia in 20%. Reports on excision specimens were available in 66% (81 patients). Final excision histology was benign in 73 (90.2%) and malignant in 8 (9.8%) patients (2 invasive cancer, 6 ductal carcinoma in situ). Of all B3 subtypes, atypical ductal hyperplasia and flat epithelial atypia were associated with malignancy, whereas only atypical ductal hyperplasia was accompanied by invasive cancer. Of all lesions, flat epithelial atypia was most frequently found in excision specimens (18%). In our study, flat epithelial atypia and atypical ductal hyperplasia are common lesions of the B3 category in needle core biopsies of the breast. Both lesions are associated with malignancy, whereas only atypical ductal hyperplasia was related to invasive cancer. We conclude that an excision biopsy after diagnosis of flat epithelial atypia is recommended depending on clinical and radiologic findings.

▶ Flat epithelial atypia (FEA), an entity with recently increasing recognition in breast pathology, is problematic because of unclear clinical significance. Whereas ductal carcinoma in situ (DCIS) and atypical ductal hyperplasia (ADH) have a well established 4- to 5-fold increase in risk for invasive cancer, the risk associated with FEA is still unknown. Some authors have noted the concurrent presence of FEA in the background of higher grade lesions and speculate on its significance as either an indicator or precursor lesion. Subsequently, the management of isolated FEA in the absence of a higher grade lesion remains controversial, ranging from close follow-up evaluation to systematic surgical excision.

The authors address this issue with a correlation study of core needle biopsies and final excisional histology. Malignant lesions were identified in 6.6% (2 of 30 cases) of excisions for isolated flat atypia and identified in 35% (5 of 14 cases) of excisions for ADH. Of note, 2 of the 5 malignant cases identified by ADH were invasive, whereas both cases identified with FEA were in situ. These findings seem to support the suggestion of a lower risk for progression of FEA versus ADH. However, given the still inconsistent terminology regarding FEA and the risk of sampling error, the authors maintain that individual biopsies with isolated FEA should be managed via a multidisciplinary team approach that considers the associated clinical and radiological findings.

S. B. Sams, MD

Pleomorphic Ductal Carcinoma of the Breast: Predictors of Decreased Overall Survival

Nguyen CV, Falcón-Escobedo R, Hunt KK, et al (Univ of Texas M.D. Anderson Cancer Ctr, Houston; Med School of the Autonomous Univ of San Luis Potosí, Mexico)

Am J Surg Pathol 34:486-493, 2010

The World Health Organization classification of tumors of the breast includes a rare variant of invasive ductal carcinoma termed pleomorphic carcinoma. This variant has marked nuclear pleomorphism (>6-fold variation in nuclear size by definition, but often >10-fold) and characteristically contains multinucleated tumor giant cells. Approximately one-third of the cases in the initial series contained a focal spindle cell metaplastic component. The tumors are reported to have an aggressive behavior, but because some contain a spindle cell metaplastic component, it is unclear whether the metaplastic component or other clinicopathologic features account for the poor clinical outcome. We identified 37 cases of pleomorphic carcinoma of the breast and evaluated the association between clinical outcome and multiple clinicopathologic features. Patients with invasive pleomorphic lobular carcinoma and those without at least a tissue biopsy before chemotherapy were excluded. Patients ranged in age from 23 to 78 years (median, 49 y). Tumor size was >5 cm in 12 cases and <5 cm in 22. A focal spindle cell component (<25% of the tumor) was present in 14 tumors (38%). Clinical follow-up was available for 36 patients (median, 17 mo). In multivariate analysis, when the 2 stage-IV patients were excluded, the presence of a spindle cell component and tumor size >5 cm were each independently associated with decreased overall survival. The actuarial 5-year overall survival for patients with and without a metaplastic spindle cell component was 38% ± 15% and 89% ± 7%, respectively. Poor clinical outcome, therefore, is associated with the subset of pleomorphic carcinomas with a spindle cell metaplastic component. As the morphologic features of pleomorphic carcinoma can be seen in primary tumors from other sites, it is important to recognize this tumor as a rare variant of invasive breast carcinoma.

▶ Similar to other sites, tumors with marked pleomorphism and associated giant cells have been identified in the breast and have been associated with a particularly poor prognosis.[1] This study is the largest series of these uncommon breast tumors to date. The investigators performed univariate and multivariate analyses on several clinicopathologic features. Two features proved to be independently significant: the presence of a spindle cell component and a tumor size greater than 5 cm. The World Health Organization Classification for breast tumors has classified this tumor as a subtype of invasive ductal carcinoma.[2] Though apart from this entity, breast tumors with a spindle cell component are generally included in the somewhat heterogenous group of metaplastic carcinomas. While this could be considered a minor taxonomic discrepancy, the presence or absence of this spindle cell component in these tumors was found to have a dramatic difference in survival, 38% versus 89% 5-year survival, respectively (Fig 2A from the original article). Thus, regardless of how this entity should be placed in the broader classification of breast neoplasia, the findings of this study assert that the identification of a spindle cell component within these lesions should be noted.

J. Wisell, MD

References

1. Silver SA, Tavassoli FA. Pleomorphic carcinoma of the breast: clinicopathological analysis of 26 cases of an unusual high-grade phenotype of ductal carcinoma. *Histopathology.* 2000;36:505-514.
2. Tavassoli FA, Devilee P, eds.. World Health Organization Classification of Tumours: Pathology and Genetics of Tumours of the Breast and Female Genital Organs. Lyon, France: IARC Press; 2003.

Initial Margin Status for Invasive Ductal Carcinoma of the Breast and Subsequent Identification of Carcinoma in Reexcision Specimens
Skripenova S, Layfield LJ (Univ of Utah School of Medicine, Salt Lake City)
Arch Pathol Lab Med 134:109-114, 2010

Context.—Margin status of lumpectomy specimens is related to frequency of local recurrence. Optimal surgical technique requires microscopic margins free of carcinoma by at least 2 mm. Recurrence following lumpectomy is associated with residual carcinoma secondary to inadequate resection.

Objective.—To review our series of breast excisions to determine the frequency of residual carcinoma for positive, close, and negative margins.

Design.—We reviewed lumpectomies and excisional biopsies for invasive ductal carcinoma that had subsequent reexcisions. Margin status of specimens was recorded as positive, less than 1 mm, 1 to 2 mm, or greater than 2 mm.

Results.—A total of 123 lumpectomies and excisional biopsies of invasive ductal carcinoma with reexcision were reviewed. Residual invasive carcinoma was found in 44% (17), 25% (6), 28% (8), and 16% (5) of cases with positive, less than 1 mm, 1 to 2 mm, and greater than 2 mm margins, respectively. Residual invasive carcinomas were found in 57% (8), 100% (5), 67% (2), and 100% (2) of mastectomies with positive, less than 1 mm, 1 to 2 mm, and greater than 2 mm margins, respectively, in the initial lumpectomy or excisional biopsy.

Conclusions.—Frequency of residual invasive carcinoma was related to margin status of the original lumpectomy/biopsy. Even when margins were positive, most reexcisions were free of carcinoma. Residual invasive carcinoma was found in greater than 25% of patients with margins less than 2 mm, supporting reexcision for patients with margins of less than 2 mm. Sixteen percent of cases with margins greater than 2 mm harbored residual invasive carcinoma. Evaluation of margin status was complicated by tissue distortion and fragmentation.

▶ Although breast-conserving surgery is currently the standard of care for early-stage carcinoma of the breast, the ideal method of determining a negative surgical margin and the proximity of the surgical margins is still open to debate. The current practice at many institutions is to consider negative margins as the absence of tumor cells within a fixed distance of the surgical edge, typically ranging from 1 mm to 5 mm. The importance of defining this margin is illustrated by the near consensus among published studies that the pathologic margin status is the most important factor in determining risk of local recurrence[1]; however, widespread agreement on the appropriate distance has yet to be determined.

This study evaluates the frequency of residual carcinoma in re-excision and mastectomy specimens and correlates the percentage of residual carcinoma with initial margin status. The methods and results of this study highlight some major barriers encountered in both this area of research and the daily practice of breast pathology. The absence of residual invasive carcinoma in approximately one-half and one-quarter of specimens with initial positive and less than 1 mm margins, respectively, is perhaps the most interesting finding within this study. These numbers clearly reflect the relationship between a defined distance to margin and the risk of residual carcinoma. Of interest, previous studies by Gage et al[2] and Park et al[3] found that the rates of 5- and 8-year ipsilateral breast cancer recurrence were similar in patients with a negative margin and those with a close margin, defined as within 1 mm. Further investigation is needed to untangle these seemingly contradictory findings.

The authors then identify the percentage of residual carcinoma in cases with margins of 1 to 2 mm and margins greater than 2 mm within numerous subsets including lumpectomies with delayed re-excision, lumpectomies with concurrent cavity margins, and lumpectomies with subsequent mastectomies. Because the current standard of care is to not re-excise negative margins, as reflected by the small number of cases in these subsets, the determination of a percentage of residual carcinoma is markedly skewed by the numerous nonexcised cases with an unknown residual carcinoma status. One can speculate that additional clinical factors, notably not addressed by the authors, drove the decision to re-excise or perform a mastectomy in many of these cases. Perhaps such cases with negative margins are better assessed by long-term studies of recurrence and morbidity.

S. B. Sams, MD

References

1. Swanson GP, Rynearson K, Symmonds R. Significance of margins of excision of breast cancer recurrence. *Am J Clin Oncol.* 2002;25:438-441.
2. Gage I, Schnitt SJ, Nixon AJ, et al. Pathologic margin involvement and the risk of recurrence in patients treated with breast-conserving therapy. *Cancer.* 1996;78: 1921-1928.

3. Park CC, Mitsumori M, Nixon A, et al. Outcome at 8 years after breast-conserving surgery and radiation therapy for invasive breast cancer: influence of margin status and systemic therapy on local recurrence. *J Clin Oncol.* 2000;18: 1668-1675.

Triple Negative Breast Cancer: Outcome Correlation With Immunohistochemical Detection of Basal Markers

Thike AA, Iqbal J, Cheok PY, et al (Singapore General Hosp; et al)
Am J Surg Pathol 34:956-964, 2010

We earlier evaluated the relationship of 653 triple negative breast cancers (TNBC) with basal immunophenotypic expression by using antibodies to basal cytokeratins (CK5/6, CK14, CK17, 34βE12), p63, smooth muscle actin (SMA), epidermal growth factor receptor, and CD117, and found that a triple panel of CK14, 34βE12 and epidermal growth factor receptor determined 84% of our cases to be basal-like. Women with basal-like TNBC tended to be younger ($P = 0.04$), have histologically higher-grade tumors ($P = 0.047$), with positive nodal status ($P = 0.047$), than those whose tumors were nonbasal-like. Using univariate Cox regression analysis, tumor size ($P = 0.003$), histologic grade ($P = 0.006$), and nodal status ($P = 0.017$) were significant factors for disease-free survival (DFS) among TNBC, whereas age ($P = 0.004$), tumor size ($P = 0.001$), histologic grade ($P < 0.001$), nodal status ($P = 0.011$), lymphovascular invasion ($P = 0.032$), and pushing borders ($P = 0.042$) were important for overall survival (OS). On multivariate analysis, age was statistically significant for both DFS and OS ($P = 0.033$, 0.001 respectively), whereas histologic grade was important for OS ($P < 0.001$). Kaplan Meier curves showed CK17 positivity to impact adversely on DFS ($P = 0.003$) and OS ($P = 0.014$), whereas CD117 positive staining was accompanied by diminished OS ($P = 0.036$). SMA expression in TNBC however, revealed a trend for improved DFS ($P = 0.05$). Our findings indicate that basal-like TNBC are associated with adverse clinicopathologic parameters, and that individual biologic markers of CK17, CD117, and SMA have prognostic implications on survival. Possibilities exist for future targeted therapy for this challenging group of breast cancers.

▶ Molecular analysis over the last decade has provided further opportunities for the classification of breast carcinoma.[1] One of the tumor subtypes to be identified from this work is basal-like carcinoma (BLC). These tumors typically do not express hormone receptors (estrogen receptor and progesterone receptor) and do not overexpress HER2, a so called triple-negative pattern. Other tumors may also have a triple-negative pattern but not the other gene expression characteristics and thus are not classified as BLC. Both BLC and tumors with a triple-negative pattern have been associated with a worse prognosis than other subtypes. This study adds to an increasing collection of BLC data and correlates specific markers that have been associated with the BLC phenotype, including the high-molecular weight cytokeratin 17 (CK17), CD117, and smooth muscle actin (SMA). They find that both CK17 and CD117 expression carried a worse overall survival. The CK17, although indicating basal cell differentiation, is interesting as it may have some prognostic value regardless of the classification. CD117 always generates interest when identified in tumors as it provides a potential opportunity for directed treatment. Lastly, they note an improved survival with SMA expression, raising the possibility of a subset of myoepithelial-leaning BLC with unique features. The practical point of the study is that all 3 markers are readily performed in virtually all modern pathology practices, allowing for straightforward confirmation of their findings and relatively swift integration into routine evaluation of breast tumors should these markers ultimately prove clinically valuable.

J. Wisell, MD

Reference

1. Perou CM, Sørlie T, Eisen MB, et al. Molecular portraits of human breast tumours. *Nature*. 2000;406:747-752.

Performance of Common Genetic Variants in Breast-Cancer Risk Models

Wacholder S, Hartge P, Prentice R, et al (Natl Cancer Inst, Bethesda, MD; Fred Hutchinson Cancer Res Ctr, Seattle, WA; et al)
N Engl J Med 362:986-993, 2010

Background.—Genomewide association studies have identified multiple genetic variants associated with breast cancer. The extent to which these variants add to existing risk-assessment models is unknown.

Methods.—We used information on traditional risk factors and 10 common genetic variants associated with breast cancer in 5590 case subjects and 5998 control subjects, 50 to 79 years of age, from four U.S. cohort studies and one case–control study from Poland to fit models of the absolute risk of breast cancer. With the use of receiver-operating-characteristic curve analysis, we calculated the area under the curve (AUC) as a measure of discrimination. By definition, random classification of case and control subjects provides an AUC of 50%; perfect classification provides an AUC of 100%. We calculated the fraction of case subjects in quintiles of estimated absolute risk after the addition of genetic variants to the traditional risk model.

Results.—The AUC for a risk model with age, study and entry year, and four traditional risk factors was 58.0%; with the addition of 10 genetic variants, the AUC was 61.8%. About half the case subjects (47.2%) were in the same quintile of risk as in a model without genetic variants; 32.5% were in a higher quintile, and 20.4% were in a lower quintile.

Conclusions.—The inclusion of newly discovered genetic factors modestly improved the performance of risk models for breast cancer.

The level of predicted breast-cancer risk among most women changed little after the addition of currently available genetic information.

▶ The genome-wide association studies identified 14 single-nucleotide polymorphisms (SNPs) that are associated with increased risk of breast cancer. A recent study by Reeves et al[1] estimated the per allele odds ratio for individual SNPs in relation to a polygenic risk score by tumor subtype and determined a strong association, particularly in estrogen receptor-positive breast cancers. The authors of this study examine the practical application of integrating 10 known genetic variants with an increased breast cancer risk into a breast cancer screening model. Indeed, the authors find modest improvements in discrimination and prediction models applicable to a clinical setting. Of note, the improvement was greatest among the women with the lowest absolute risk and negligible among those with the highest estimated risk. As pointed out by the authors themselves, in this era of limited medical resources, this modest increase in detection is precluded by the substantial cost of obtaining genetic information. The analyses of SNPs are valuable in the research setting regarding the molecular pathways of developing breast cancers, but with the current cost structure, clinically we should continue to rely on the traditional screening models.

S. B. Sams, MD

Reference

1. Reeves GK, Travis RC, Green J, et al. Incidence of breast cancer and its subtypes in relation to individual and multiple low-penetrance genetic susceptibility loci. *JAMA*. 2010;304:426-434.

Predicting the Likelihood of Additional Nodal Metastases in Breast Carcinoma Patients With Positive Sentinel Node Biopsy
Mustać E, Matušan-Ilijaš K, Marijić B, et al (Univ of Rijeka, Croatia)
Int J Surg Pathol 18:36-41, 2010

Axillary lymph node dissection (ALND) is an important procedure in the staging of breast cancer patients. However, it is associated with a significant morbidity rate. In addition, using early diagnosis a high number of cases with negative lymph nodes can be identified. A lymph node defined as sentinel lymph node (SLN) would be the first to receive tumoral drainage. A less morbid but accurate staining procedure using mapping and SLN biopsy has been introduced. The aim of this study was to estimate the likelihood of additional disease in the axilla after SLN analysis. A total of 259 breast carcinomas and SLN biopsies followed by ALND were examined. The patient median age was 59 years, approximately 75% of them postmenopausal. Tumor size was 1.4 ± 0.8 cm (almost 80% in pT1). SLNs were positive in 59 of 259 (22.8%) carcinomas, 30 (11.6%) with micrometastases (<2.0 mm) and 29 (11.2%) with metastases. Tumor size ($P = .004$) and presence of lymphovascular invasion (LVI; $P = .034$) were found to be significant predictors of pathologically positive SLN. Following ALND, positive non-SLNs were present mostly in patients with metastasis >2 mm in SLN ($P = .003$), in carcinoma with higher nuclear grade ($P = .044$), decreased estrogen receptor (ER; $P = .042$), and progesterone receptor (PR; $P = .042$). Finally, lymph node status (pN) following SLN and ALND was found to be significantly associated with tumor size ($P = .006$), LVI ($P = .037$), PR ($P = .023$), and Her-2 status ($P < .001$). These results point to detailed analysis of primary tumor and SLN that may increase the precision of patient selection for further axillary surgery or radiotherapy.

▶ Sentinel lymph node (SLN) biopsy with histological examination has in recent years been adopted as the standard of care in patients with early-stage breast cancer (T1 or T2) and clinically negative axillary nodes. Numerous studies demonstrate that the SLN is typically the initial axillary node involved by metastatic tumor, has significant staging and prognostic implications, and meets the surgical goal of reduction of morbidity that may result from a complete axillary dissection.[1] Given the low incidence of subsequent metastases to remaining axillary lymph nodes following a negative sentinel node biopsy, there is a consensus that patients with a negative result typically need no further treatment. However, numerous questions remain regarding the extent and manner of additional treatment for patients with positive sentinel node biopsies, particularly in patients in whom the perceived risk of additional disease is low.

In this study, the authors attempt to identify factors associated with additional metastatic axillary disease in the setting of a positive SLN, presumably with the goal of guiding further medical management for individual patients. It has already been shown that approximately 50% of patients with positive SLNs have additional disease and that the size of the metastasis positively correlates with the increased likelihood of additional metastasis.[2] Macrometastases, defined as greater than 2 mm in diameter, are typically treated with additional axillary lymph node dissection, as the incidence of additional involvement is greatest. Submicrometastases or isolated tumor cells, defined as less than 0.2 mm, are most commonly found via immunohistochemical analysis and to date show no significant correlation with residual metastases, regardless of primary tumor characteristics. Thus, the identification of submicrometastases can be clinically ignored and brings into question the practice of routine immunohistochemical analysis in the absence of findings on hematoxylin and eosin-stained slides. It is the prognostic significance and subsequent therapy of micrometastases (0.2-2 mm in size) that is still under debate, and presumably, the identification of additional associated factors can guide treatment in this nonspecific group. In this study, nuclear grade, estrogen receptor status, and progesterone receptor status in addition to the size of metastasis were found to be statistically significantly associated with non-SLN disease. These are interesting results but with a total number of 59 patients with a positive node and a total number of 56 patients with correlating axillary dissections, the strength of this study is not enough to act upon. Of note, the American

College of Surgeons Oncology Group has currently enrolled over 5000 patients in the Z0010 and Z0011 trials, which aim to examine the efficacy, safety, and morbidity in patients who undergo sentinel node dissection as well as the prognostic significance of SLN micrometastases. We eagerly await the results.

S. B. Sams, MD

References

1. Schwartz GF, Giuliano AE, Veronesi U. Proceedings of the consensus conference on the role of sentinel lymph node biopsy in carcinoma of the breast, April 19 to 22, 2001, Philadelphia, Pennsylvania. *Hum Pathol.* 2002;33:579-589.
2. Cserni G, Bianchi S, Vezzosi V, et al. Sentinel lymph node biopsy in staging small (up to 15 mm) breast carcinomas. Results from a European multi-institutional study. *Pathol Oncol Res.* 2007;13:5-14.

Variable Specimen Handling Affects Hormone Receptor Test Results in Women With Breast Cancer: A Large Multihospital Retrospective Study
Nkoy FL, Hammond MEH, Rees W, et al (Intermountain Healthcare, Salt Lake City, UT)
Arch Pathol Lab Med 134:606-612, 2010

Context.—Intermountain Healthcare hospitals use a single, standardized laboratory and automated testing process for estrogen receptor/progesterone receptor (ER/PR) tests to minimize testing errors.

Objectives.—To test the (1) variability in ER/PR negativity among hospitals and (2) association between specimen handling conditions and ER/PR negativity.

Design.—Retrospective study of women who had breast cancer surgery at 7 Intermountain hospitals and ER/PR tests ordered between 1997 and 2003. Data were extracted from cancer registry. Frequency of ER/PR negativity was calculated for each surgery day and compared among hospitals and between 2 groups: regular (specimens obtained Sunday through Thursday, more likely to be tested within 24 hours of surgery) and prolonged (specimens obtained on Friday and Saturday, more likely to be tested more than 24 hours after surgery) specimen handling conditions.

Results.—Five thousand seventy-seven women were tested for ER/PR. The frequency of ER and PR negativity was 20.9% and 27.9%, respectively. It increased with each day of the week for both ER ($P = .03$) and PR ($P = .059$) and tended to be higher for prolonged specimens for ER (23.6% versus 20.4%; $P = .03$) and for PR (30.1% versus 27.4%; $P = .11$) compared with regular specimens. After controlling for age and tumor size, both ER ($P = .02$) and PR ($P = .02$) negativity was significantly different among the hospitals and was associated with prolonged specimens for ER ($P = .04$) but not for PR ($P = .09$).

Conclusions.—Estrogen receptor and PR negativity remained highly variable among hospitals despite use of a single laboratory and tended to be significantly associated with prolonged specimen handling. More studies are needed to confirm these findings.

▶ Accurate assessment of estrogen/progesterone receptor (ER/PR) expression in breast cancer is crucial as both an important prognostic indicator and a directive for hormonal therapy. In recent years, there has been a focus on variability in testing and false-negative results leading to the 2008 consensus recommendations for the standardization of preanalytical, analytical, and postanalytical variables in ER testing.[1] The results of this study, a large multihospital retrospective review of frequency of ER/PR negativity, highlight the logistical difficulties encountered in standardized procedure yet emphasize the need for such standardized practice. The authors conclude that despite the use of a single standardized laboratory for testing (ie, a standardized analytical phase), there is significant variability in ER/PR negativity between the 7 associated hospitals, which the authors attribute to the nonstandardized preanalytical phase. The limitations of a retrospective study include an inability to tease out which specific factors in the preanalytic phase, such as source of surgical specimen, specimen handling, and fixation time, are critical for reliable and precise immunohistochemical analysis. And although the authors propose the day of the week of surgery as a marker for fixation time, additional studies that specifically address these questions are warranted. We can expect to see results of such studies in the near future, as the reporting of fixation intervals is now standard process. The next step is determining optimal and feasible standards for specimen handling in both the academic and community hospital setting.

S. B. Sams, MD

Reference

1. Yaziji H, Taylor C, Goldstein NS, et al. Consensus recommendations on estrogen receptor testing in breast cancer by immunohistochemistry. *Appl Immunohistochem Mol Morphol.* 2008;16:513-520.

3 Gastrointestinal System

Appendiceal Mucinous Neoplasms: Clinicopathologic Study of 116 Cases With Analysis of Factors Predicting Recurrence
Pai RK, Beck AH, Norton JA, et al (Stanford Univ, CA)
Am J Surg Pathol 33:1425-1439, 2009

The classification and nomenclature of appendiceal mucinous neoplasms are controversial. To determine the outcome for patients with appendiceal mucinous neoplasms and further evaluate whether they can be stratified into groups that provide prognostic information, the clinicopathologic features of 116 patients (66 with clinical follow-up) with appendiceal mucinous neoplasms were studied. From a wide variety of histopathologic features assessed, the important predictors that emerged on univariate statistical analysis were presence of extra-appendiceal neoplastic epithelium ($P = 0.01$), high-grade cytology ($P < 0.0001$), architectural complexity ($P < 0.001$), and invasion ($P < 0.001$). Stratification using a combination of these predictors resulted in a 4-tiered classification scheme. All 16 patients with mucinous neoplasms confined to the appendix and lacking high-grade cytology, architectural complexity, and invasion were alive with no recurrences at median 59 months follow-up (= mucinous adenoma). One of 14 patients with low-grade cytology and acellular peritoneal mucin deposits developed recurrent tumor within the peritoneum at 45 months with no patient deaths to date (median, 48-mo follow-up) (= low-grade mucinous neoplasm with low risk of recurrence). None of the 2 patients with acellular peritoneal mucinous deposits outside of the right lower quadrant developed recurrence at 163 and 206 months. Twenty-seven patients with low-grade mucinous neoplasms with extra-appendiceal neoplastic epithelium had 1-year, 3-year, 5-year, and 10-year overall survival rates of 96%, 91%, 79%, and 46%, respectively, at median 53 months follow-up (= low-grade mucinous neoplasm with high risk of recurrence). Three of the 4 patients with extra appendiceal epithelium limited to the right lower quadrant developed full-blown peritoneal disease at 6, 41, and 99 months follow-up and 1 patient eventually died of disease. Nine patients with appendiceal neoplasms with invasion or high-grade cytology and follow-up showed 1-year, 3-year, and 5-year overall survival rates of 86%, 57%, and 28% (= mucinous adenocarcinoma). At 10 years, all patients with mucinous adenocarcinoma were either dead or lost to follow-up. Appendiceal mucinous neoplasms can be stratified into 4 distinct risk groups on the basis of a careful histopathologic assessment of cytoarchitectural features and extent of disease at presentation.

▶ For decades extensive observational research has been carried out and literature has been published on the topic of pseudomyxoma peritonei. However, each time that acellular mucin is found in a specimen in the vicinity of the appendix, pathologists and clinicians do not seem to know what the true meaning of the finding is. Appendiceal mucinous tumors are an enigma in many aspects as there is no consensus on the use of diagnosis terminology and the lack of criteria to predict the behavior of these tumors with certainty. In fact, there is still controversy regarding what to call acellular mucin or the presence of bland strips of epithelium in the peritoneal cavity accompanying mucin. There are authors who consider these findings as adenocarcinoma, whereas others argue that it is an extreme term as these proliferations do not metastasize to lymph nodes or routinely produce destructive metastasis to visceral organs. The importance of this article is based on the long follow-up in many of the patients studied. Also, it reviews not only the histopathological features, but also takes in consideration the localization of the lesions in the abdominal cavity. The article is long and may be complex to comprehend initially because of the statistical analysis; however, in the end, it leaves the reader with a classification scheme that is easy to grasp. Tumors are divided in 4 categories, and it is emphasized that when a mucinous lesion is encountered the entire appendix should be submitted for microscopic examination. The purpose of complete examination is to rule out the presence of high-grade cytological features of the epithelial lining, architectural complexity, presence or absence of invasion, extra-appendiceal cellular or acellular mucin, and to assess the margin of excision. These are the features that should be informed to the clinician regardless of the classification. For the surgeon, the message is that if mucin is encountered in the pelvis, a search for an appendiceal tumor should ensue. The term benign mucinous tumor of the appendix is not to be used unless the entire appendix is examined and no severe features other than adenoma are found and margins are free of adenoma.

P. A. Bejarano, MD

Beta-catenin Nuclear Labeling is a Common Feature of Sessile Serrated Adenomas and Correlates With Early Neoplastic Progression After *BRAF* Activation
Yachida S, Mudali S, Martin SA, et al (Johns Hopkins Med Institutions, Baltimore, MD)
Am J Surg Pathol 33:1823-1832, 2009

Recent observations indicate that some sessile serrated adenomas (SSAs) have aberrant β-catenin nuclear labeling, implicating the Wnt pathway in the molecular progression of SSAs to colorectal carcinoma. We sought to expand upon this finding by characterizing β-catenin expression in the full spectrum of serrated colorectal polyps, and correlating these findings with the genetic status of *BRAF, KRAS* and *CTNNB1*. Immunolabeling for β-catenin confirmed the presence of abnormal nuclear accumulation in SSAs, with 35/54 (67%) SSAs showing nuclear labeling compared with 0/12 hyperplastic polyps. Abnormal nuclear labeling was also identified in 4/11 (36%) traditional serrated adenomas (TSAs) ($P = 0.00001$). When SSAs were further analyzed with respect to the presence or absence of conventional epithelial dysplasia, nuclear β-catenin labeling was seen in 8/27 (29%) SSAs without dysplasia (SSA) but in 27/27 (100%) of SSAs with dysplasia ($P = 0.000001$). Sequencing of genomic DNA extracted from a subset of hyperplastic polyps, SSAs, SSAs with dysplasia, TSAs and tubular adenomas failed to identify any *CTNNB1* mutations to account for abnormal β-catenin nuclear labeling. However, abnormal nuclear labeling always occurred in the setting of a *BRAF* V600E mutation, indicating aberrant nuclear labeling occurs on a background of *BRAF* activation. Of interest, all 6 TSAs contained a *KRAS* mutation confirming that SSAs and TSAs are genetically distinct entities. These findings validate previous reports implicating activation of the Wnt signaling pathway in SSAs, and further indicate that Wnt pathway activation plays a role in the neoplastic progression of SSAs and TSAs to colonic carcinoma by mechanisms independent of *CTNNB1* mutation.

▶ Examination of large intestine polyps is no longer a simple task as it was in the past when general pathologists had to determine if a given polyp was hyperplastic, a tubular adenoma, or a tubulovillous adenoma. This article increases the awareness that further morphological discrimination among the serrated polyps is necessary. In addition to hyperplastic polyps (HP), there are 2 more players in the serrated category. They include sessile serrated adenoma (SSA) and traditional serrated adenoma (TSA). The TSA should not create much struggle among pathologists as this polyp has features of both, HP and tubular adenoma. What appears to create difficulty is distinguishing between a large HP and a SSA. The distinction is important because HP lacks neoplastic potential and should not prompt close follow-up other than the routine screening. On the other hand, a SSA has the potential to give rise to an adenocarcinoma. Most of the SSAs are located in the right side of the colon. It appears that the sequence of events that lead to carcinoma in SSAs is related to early *BRAF* mutations followed by methylation that eventually will lead to silencing of *MLH1* in advanced lesions with high levels of microsatellite instability in the frank adenocarcinomas. This is in contrast to the classical adenoma-carcinoma pathway in which there is accumulation of mutations in key genes, such as *KRAS* and *p53*, leading to chromosomal instability. Molecular studies, including this one, show that HPs and SSAs are also distinct entities. Importantly, the identification of nuclear beta-catenin stain by immunohistochemistry may identify SSAs with neoplastic potential that have not yet lost *MLHI* expression.

P. A. Bejarano, MD

Esophagitis Dissecans Superficialis ("Sloughing esophagitis"): A Clinicopathologic Study of 12 Cases
Carmack SW, Vemulapalli R, Spechler SJ, et al (The Univ of Texas Southwestern Med Ctr, Dallas)
Am J Surg Pathol 33:1789-1794, 2009

Esophagitis Dissecans Superficialis (EDS) is a term applied to a rare endoscopic finding characterized by sloughing of large fragments of the esophageal squamous mucosa that may be coughed up or vomited. Although EDS has been reported in association with certain medications and esophageal strictures, most cases remain unexplained and the histopathologic features of EDS are inadequately described. We undertook this study to define useful diagnostic criteria based on the examination of a series of well-characterized cases of EDS. To identify patients with EDS, we searched our endoscopy and pathology databases, reviewed the esophageal biopsy specimens from candidate cases, and correlated them with pertinent clinical information. Twelve patients (11 men and 1 woman) had endoscopic and histologic findings of EDS and 9 had the histologic features without the endoscopic correlates. Biopsies from confirmed EDS patients showed sloughing and flaking of superficial squamous epithelium with occasional bullous separation of the layers, parakeratosis, and varying degrees of acute or chronic inflammation. Fungal elements were identified in 3 patients, but were not associated with acute inflammation. None of the EDS patients were on bisphosphonate therapy or had bullous skin disorders. Follow-up endoscopy in 5 patients showed complete resolution of the esophageal abnormalities in 4 and mild esophagitis in one. In spite of its sometimes, dramatic presentation, EDS is a benign condition that resolves without lasting esophageal pathology. Although an association with medications, skin conditions, heavy smoking, and physical trauma has been reported, the pathogenesis of EDS remains unexplained.

▶ This endoscopic finding was first described in the 1950s. The gross striking appearance is that of white strips or streaks of peeling esophageal mucosa resembling pseudomembranes. Despite the dramatic finding, the symptoms are nonspecific and most patients resolve the injury favorably. Some patients are helped with the use of proton pump inhibitors. Interestingly, the literature is sparse on this subject. The entity is described as esophagitis dissecans superficialis (EDS) or sloughing esophagitis with about 35 cases reported in peer-reviewed journals. However, other 24 cases appear in abstract form only. However, the authors found 21 cases in a period of 8 years at their institution, which suggests that it is not that uncommon and that it may be underrecognized, underreported, or both. Pathologists often observed detached strips of squamous epithelium in esophageal biopsies for other conditions, and therefore, this finding alone should not be diagnostic of EDS. In fact, each of the individual features of EDS is not diagnostic for it. However, the constellation of features in aggregate should raise the possibility of EDS and thus clinical correlation would be needed. The individual features of EDS such as parakeratosis, orthokeratosis, intraepithelial bullae, epithelial detachment, necrosis, inflammation, and spongiosis can be seen in entities, including esophageal strictures, infection, pemphigo, Steven-Johnson syndrome, the intake of drugs for osteoporosis, and reflux esophagitis. In fact, EDS has been associated to inflammatory skin conditions, heavy smoking, immunosuppression, and physical trauma. It is being postulated that EDS may be a type of topical allergic response akin to contact dermatitis. However, the true pathogenesis has not been identified. This article increases the awareness of this entity among pathologists and gastroenterologists.

P. A. Bejarano, MD

Molecular markers and biological targeted therapies in metastatic colorectal cancer: expert opinion and recommendations derived from the 11th ESMO/World Congress on Gastrointestinal Cancer, Barcelona, 2009

Van Cutsem E, Dicato M, Arber N, et al (Univ Hosp Gasthuisberg, Leuven, Belgium; Centre Hospitalier de Luxembourg; Tel Aviv Sourasky Med Ctr and Sackler Faculty of Medicine, Israel; et al)
Ann Oncol 21:vi1-vi10, 2010

The article summarizes the expert discussion and recommendations on the use of molecular markers and of biological targeted therapies in metastatic colorectal cancer (mCRC), as well as a proposed treatment decision strategy for mCRC treatment. The meeting was conducted during the 11th ESMO/World Gastrointestinal Cancer Congress (WGICC) in Barcelona in June 2009. The manuscript describes the outcome of an expert discussion leading to an expert recommendation. The increasing knowledge on clinical and molecular markers and the availability of biological targeted therapies have major implications in the optimal management in mCRC.

▶ This is a consensus document released by a panel of international experts that discussed the current status of the molecular markers in colorectal adenocarcinoma. They provide recommendations on the management of these patients. Most of the points stated in this article are directed to oncologists. However, today's therapy of colorectal cancer requires a multidisciplinary approach, and therefore, pathologists need to be strongly involved. There has been progress in the survival of patients, with the medial survival of patients with metastatic cancer participating in clinical trials improving from 6 months to 2 years. This is in part because of the use of new cytotoxic drug and the involvement of specialists from various disciplines including surgeons whose role is the removal of metastatic foci. Also, the developments of targeted agents have improved survival and broadened the therapeutic options. One of the strongest prognostic factors is the stage of the disease as it appears in the American Joint Committee on Cancer. A colonic primary tumor is a positive prognostic marker compared with a rectal tumor. A mucinous histology has a negative effect. Metachronous metastases have a better outcome compared with synchronous metastases. Metastatic tumor confined to the liver is better that having multiple organs involved. However, patients with liver metastases have a shorter survival than those with pulmonary metastases. Peritoneal metastases carry a worse outcome. Of importance for pathologists as well is to know that 2 molecular markers have a consistent prognostic value. One is microsatellite instability (MSI). Those patients with high MSI have a survival advantage regardless of stage. The second is *BRAF* mutation, which as associated with a significantly high cancer-specific mortality. Regarding predictive markers, patients with the presence of *KRAS* mutation in 40% of colorectal cancers will have no benefit from antiepidermal growth factor receptor agents such as cetuximab or panitumumab. This is so consistent that the use of these agents requires testing for *KRAS* before the administration. Other markers include *ERCC1*. The presence of this nucleotide excision repair molecule results in resistance to platinum-derived drugs. In summary, the panel recommends *KRAS* and *BRAF* to guide the treatment. It also recommends MSI testing in young patients as part of a genetic evaluation and predisposition of family members for the development of colon cancer. This testing, however, is not to be used currently to guide treatment. This consensus implies the proactive role that pathologists should play in the care of patients with metastatic colorectal carcinoma.

P. A. Bejarano, MD

The Clinical Significance of Incidental Chronic Colitis: A Study of 17 Cases
Deshpande V, Hsu M, Kumarasinghe MP, et al (Massachusetts General Hosp and Harvard Med School, Boston; Univ of Western Australia, Nedlands Perth, Australia)
Am J Surg Pathol 34:463-469, 2010

Introduction.—A histologic diagnosis of chronic colitis raises a relatively limited differential diagnosis that includes inflammatory bowel disease, long-standing infections, and chronic ischemia. In routine clinical practice, inflammatory bowel disease accounts for the majority of cases of chronic colitis. Although a variety of drug-induced injury patterns in the colon have been recognized, there are few well-documented examples of drug-induced chronic colitis. In this study, we report the clinical, histologic, and follow-up data on 17 cases of histologically documented cases of chronic colitis in which a definitive etiologic factor could not be identified.

Methods.—Using our electronic databases we recorded all cases of chronic colitis in adults over an 8-year period. Patients with a history (prior or subsequent) of inflammatory bowel disease were excluded. Cases showing histologic features of ischemic, pseudomembranous, or granulomatous colitis were excluded. The biopsies were evaluated and semiquantitatively scored for established histologic features of activity and chronicity. The clinical, endoscopic, and follow-up data, including drug usage, was recorded.

Results.—There were 10 males and 7 females and the mean age was 59 years. The majority of cases involved the cecum or ascending colon (16 of 17 cases). A majority of patients were asymptomatic (n = 11), and in others, indications for colonoscopy were occult blood (n = 3), hematochezia (n = 2), and melena (n = 1). The most common mucosal abnormality was erythema (n = 10), ulcers (n = 3), congestion (n = 3), and edematous mucosa (n = 1). All cases showed histologic features of chronicity and showed either basal plasmacytosis (94%) or crypt architectural distortion (94%). Eight (47%) patients reported nonsteroidal anti-inflammatory drugs (NSAID) use. Withdrawal of NSAIDs in 2 cases resulted in normalization of the colonic mucosa. On follow-up, all 17 patients were asymptomatic (median follow-up 42.8 mo) and did not progress to inflammatory bowel disease.

Conclusions.—We report a series of 17 histologically documented cases of incidental chronic colitis without a conventional etiology. However, both the frequent usage of NSAIDs, and normalization of mucosal changes after withdrawal of this drug suggest that NSAIDs may account for this cecal-based chronic colitis. The awareness of this histologically dramatic but clinically innocuous form of chronic colitis may avoid errors in mucosal biopsy diagnosis.

▶ The presence of glandular architectural distortion accompanied by lympho-plasmacytosis of the lamina propria in colonic biopsy tissues raises the possibility of chronic colitis. Quiescent inflammatory bowel disease characterizes those features in the absence of acute epithelial damage, that is, active disease in the form of cryptitis, crypt abscess, or ulceration. However, it can be seen in long-standing infection, chronic ischemia, immunodeficiency states, and drug-induced colitis. Acute effects of nonsteroidal anti-inflammatory drugs (NSAIDs) are known and include ulceration, focal active colitis, ischemia, strictures, and perforation. We have heard for several years now that NSAIDs may cause intestinal changes that mimic chronic inflammatory bowel disease. However, those cases may have been labeled as right-sided colitis or may have been classified as asymptomatic inflammatory bowel disease. This article is one of the first to link the effects of NSAIDs to chronic colitis of the right colon. The authors describe cases of chronic changes in the right side of the colon with no features of acute active disease, granulomas, collagenous colitis, lymphocytic colitis, chronic ischemia, or pseudomembranous colitis. It is postulated that the low gravity of the cecum helps with the accumulation of the drug components at this site. However, a systemic effect has not been ruled out as NSAIDs disrupt the cytoprotective effect of prostaglandins on the gastrointestinal tract. The main differential diagnoses are ulcerative colitis and Crohn disease. However, the isolated involvement of the cecum is not typical of ulcerative colitis. The lack of granulomas with no ileum involvement in asymptomatic individuals would argue against Crohn disease.

P. A. Bejarano, MD

4 Hepatobiliary System and Pancreas

Both Fibrous Capsule Formation and Extracapsular Penetration Are Powerful Predictors of Poor Survival in Human Hepatocellular Carcinoma: A Histological Assessment of 365 Patients in Japan
Iguchi T, Aishima S, Sanefuji K, et al (Kyushu Univ, Fukuoka, Japan; et al)
Ann Surg Oncol 16:2539-2546, 2009

Background.—A new definition of infiltration to the capsule (fc-inf) has been proposed as a novel marker for predicting the prognosis of 88 patients with hepatocellular carcinoma (HCC). The current aim was to present evidence to develop the fibrous capsule and fc-inf, from the Japanese histological findings for HCC, and to validate their biological significances and predictive power of survival in a large series.

Methods.—A total of 365 HCCs were divided into HCCs without the fibrous capsule (NC type; $n = 135$) and HCCs with the fibrous capsule (FC type; $n = 230$). Then, FC type was subclassified into two types: extracapsular infiltrating (EC) type ($n = 125$), in which cancer cells penetrated outside the fibrous capsule, and intracapsular (IC) type ($n = 105$), in which the infiltrating cancer cells stayed inside the fibrous capsule.

Results.—The proportion of less histological differentiation and portal venous invasion was higher in FC type than in NC type. The fibrous capsule came to be observed according to the increase of tumor size ($P < 0.0001$). FC type had significantly poorer outcome for overall survival than NC type ($P = 0.0022$). EC type showed more intrahepatic metastasis than IC type. The macroscopic subclassifications were significantly affected the presence of fc-inf. EC type had significantly poorer outcome for disease-free survival than IC type ($P = 0.0132$) and was an independent prognostic factor for disease-free survival ($P = 0.0482$).

Conclusions.—Fc-inf defined as extracapsular penetration was verified to be a novel marker for predicting prognosis, and presence of fc-inf might be predicted by tumor gross features.

▶ The incidence of hepatocellular carcinoma continues to increase in the United States and Europe. Unfortunately, it still is a lethal disease in most cases. It is interesting that there are macroscopic and microscopic variables that are not considered in the routine practice of surgical pathology, and thus they are not addressed in the pathology reports. Some of these features may have predictive and prognostic implications. One of them is the presence or absence of capsules surrounding a tumor in the liver. This study from Japan addresses this issue in resected tumors. The authors send the message that evaluation of a capsule surrounding a hepatocellular carcinoma is important. The capsule may be complete or partial. It may be confined to a tumor or may be bridged, allowing for extracapsular extension, the latter conveying a more aggressive behavior. There are, however, several aspects that this article did not address. For instance, there is no discussion on the distinction between multifocality of hepatocellular carcinoma and intrahepatic metastasis. Another issue is that this study is limited to resected tumors without considering the value of capsules in biopsies or in organs that have been removed for transplantation and that contains hepatocellular carcinoma. It would be interesting to know what it is that causes some tumors to have a capsule whereas others lack it altogether. It is also unknown what properties make a fibrous capsule interfere with growth and invasion. This study may be followed by further research using radiological methods to evaluate the potential of therapeutic approaches alternative to surgery depending on the presence or absence of a capsule.

P. A. Bejarano, MD

Biobanking of Human Pancreas Cancer Tissue: Impact of Ex-Vivo Procurement Times on RNA Quality
Rudloff U, Bhanot U, Gerald W, et al (Memorial Sloan-Kettering Cancer Ctr, NY)
Ann Surg Oncol 17:2229-2236, 2010

Background.—Tissue banking has become a major initiative at many oncology centers. The influence of warm ex-vivo ischemia times, storage times, and biobanking protocols on RNA integrity and subsequent microarray data is not well documented.

Methods.—A prospective institutional review board–approved protocol for the banking of abdominal neoplasms was initiated at Memorial Sloan-Kettering Cancer Center in 2001. Sixty-four representative pancreas cancer specimens snap-frozen at various ex-vivo procurement times (≤10 min, 11–30 min, 31–60 min, >1 h) and banked during three time periods (2001–2004, 2004–2006, 2006–2008) were processed. RNA integrity was determined by microcapillary electrophoresis using the RNA integrity number (RIN) algorithm and by results of laser-capture microdissection (LCM).

Results.—Overall, 42% of human pancreas cancer specimens banked under a dedicated protocol yielded RNA with a RIN of ≥7. Limited warm ex-vivo ischemia times did not negatively impact RNA quality (percentage of tissue with total RNA with RIN of ≥7 for ≤10 min, 42%; 11–30 min, 58%; 31–60 min, 33%; >60 min, 42%), and long-term storage of banked pancreas cancer biospecimens did not negatively

**Percent of Pancreas
Tumor Biospecimens Collected**

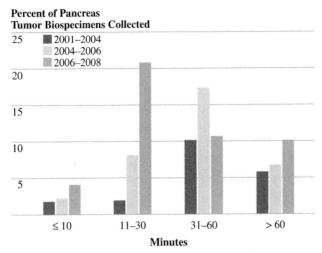

FIGURE 1.—Relation between ex-vivo procurement times (in minutes, from excision to cryopreservation) and time periods 2006–2008, 2004–2006, and 2001–2004. (With kind permission from Springer Science+Business Media: Annals of Surgical Oncology, Rudloff U, Bhanot U, Gerald W, et al. Biobanking of human pancreas cancer tissue: impact of ex-vivo procurement times on RNA quality. *Ann Surg Oncol.* 2010;17:2229-2236.)

**Percent of Total
RNA with RIN ≥ 7**

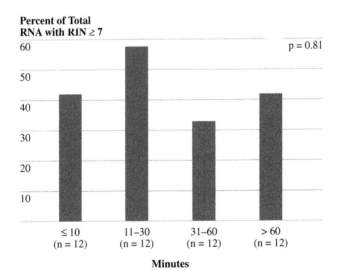

FIGURE 3.—Percentage of samples suitable for gene expression arrays (RNA integrity number [RIN] of ≥7) at different ex-vivo procurement times (time from surgical removal to cryopreservation) for a ≤10 min, b 11–30 min, c 31–60 min, and d >1 h. For each group, total RNA from 12 fresh-frozen tissue blocks (total of 48) was extracted and RIN determined after electropherogram and analysis on Agilent 2100 Bioanalyzer. (With kind permission from Springer Science+Business Media: Annals of Surgical Oncology, Rudloff U, Bhanot U, Gerald W, et al. Biobanking of human pancreas cancer tissue: impact of ex-vivo procurement times on RNA quality. *Ann Surg Oncol.* 2010;17:2229-2236.)

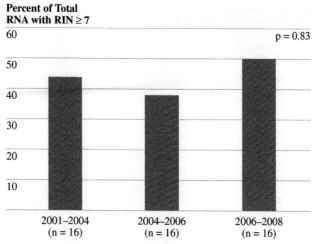

**Percent of Total
RNA with RIN ≥ 7**

FIGURE 4.—Impact of procurement period on RNA degradation. a 2001–2004. b 2004–2006. c 2006–2008. Percentage of cases with RNA integrity numbers (RINs) of ≥7 for each group is shown. (With kind permission from Springer Science+Business Media: Annals of Surgical Oncology, Rudloff U, Bhanot U, Gerald W, et al. Biobanking of human pancreas cancer tissue: impact of ex-vivo procurement times on RNA quality. *Ann Surg Oncol.* 2010;17:2229-2236.)

influence RNA quality (total RNA with RIN of ≥7 banked 2001–2004, 44%; 2004–2006, 38%; 2006–2008, 50%). RNA retrieved from pancreatic cancer samples with RIN of ≥7 subject to LCM yielded RNA suitable for further downstream applications.

Conclusions.—Fresh-frozen pancreas tissue banked within a standardized research protocol yields high-quality RNA in approximately 50% of specimens and can be used for enrichment by LCM. Quality of tissues of the biobank were not adversely impacted by limited variations of warm ischemia times or different storage periods. This study shows the challenges and investments required to initiate and maintain high-quality tissue repositories (Figs 1, 3, and 4).

▶ Biobanking surgical material is quickly becoming more common but is fairly costly in time and resources. Biobanked material is useful only if it was correctly selected to contain the lesional tissue of interest and if it was procured in a manner so as to preserve the molecular elements required for study. Procurement methodology is only now being tested for optimal performance. This article addresses some of the variables, including ex vivo ischemic times and specimen age. It is interesting that as the center gained experience with tissue banking, the speed of sample acquisition decreased (Fig 1). Ex vivo procurement times (Fig 3) and age of specimen/procurement period (Fig 4) did not appear to affect RNA isolation. However, only 42% of specimens yielded RNA of high enough quality for gene expression microarray analysis. While the authors attribute this to factors beyond their control, a process where more than 50% of the banked material is not suitable for analysis is not optimal and adds to the cost per acceptable specimen. Further studies are required to identify factors that may influence RNA viability in vivo and during the time of the surgery.

M. L. Smith, MD

5 Dermatopathology

CD10, p63 and CD99 expression in the differential diagnosis of atypical fibroxanthoma, spindle cell squamous cell carcinoma and desmoplastic melanoma

Kanner WA, Brill LB II, Patterson JW, et al (Univ of Virginia Health System, Charlottesville)
J Cutan Pathol 37:744-750, 2010

Background.—Atypical fibroxanthoma (AFX) is a pleomorphic spindle cell lesion of the skin; it is considered in the differential diagnosis with spindle cell malignant melanoma (MM) and sarcomatoid carcinoma/spindle cell squamous cell carcinoma (SCC). An optimum approach has yet to fully emerge with respect to the immunohistochemical discrimination of these lesions.

Methods.—Departmental archives from 1978 onwards were searched for clinicopathologically confirmed cases of AFX, MM and SCC. Immunostains for CD10, CD99 and p63 were performed in each case. Scored staining results were analyzed using Fisher's Exact Test.

Results.—Twenty-seven of 31 cases of AFX were positive for CD10, as compared with 3 of 22 SCCs and 0 of 20 MMs. CD10 positivity was preferentially associated with the diagnosis of AFX (p < 0.001). p63 reactivity was observed in 15/22 cases of SCCs, 5/31 AFXs and 1/20 MMs. CD99 reactivity was observed in 3/31 cases of AFX, 2/22 SCCs and 3/20 MMs.

Conclusion.—CD10 positivity is relatively specific in this context for the diagnosis of AFX. Its utility is enhanced when only strong, diffuse membranocytoplasmic staining is considered as a positive result. In contrast to prior reports, p63 was not found to be highly sensitive for SCC. Similarly, CD99 showed no preferential staining of any single diagnostic group of lesions.

▶ Though not a comprehensive histologic differential diagnosis, the presence of a spindled malignant-appearing neoplasm in the dermis primarily raises 3 possibilities: squamous cell carcinoma, spindled cell melanoma, and the occasionally elusive atypical fibroxanthoma (AFX). All these conditions are often ooon in a similar age group on sun-exposed skin, increasing the likelihood for potential misclassification. The morphologic features du differ between the lesions, but because significant histologic overlap exists, pathologists routinely rely on immunohistochemical studies to establish the correct diagnosis. Spindle cell melanoma reliably labels with S100, though S100-negative cases do exist. Squamous cell carcinoma routinely labels with cytokeratin, but with an increasing degree of spindle cell morphology, and thus an increasing degree of morphologic similarity to an AFX, cytokeratin studies become less reliable. The AFX, however, is left without a similarly trusted and specific differentiating marker. Given the aforementioned caveats with the melanoma and squamous cell carcinoma markers, this leaves a gap in the immunohistochemical evaluation of these lesions. Enter this study, which examines 2 purported markers for AFX (CD10 and CD99) and a marker increasingly used for squamous cell carcinomas (p63). As in prior studies, these authors find CD10, in this context, to be a fairly useful marker. Importantly, however, they note that 3 (14%) of their spindled squamous cell carcinoma cases also label with CD10. Of the other markers, this group found p63 to be a less reliable marker than previous studies. In fact, other observers have found nearly all spindled squamous cell carcinomas labeling with p63. Hopefully the discordance between this and other studies will prompt further investigation into the value of p63 labeling; an additional marker for squamous differentiation is quite useful, particularly in spindle cell lesions. Prior to this study, CD99 has been evaluated in fewer cases than the other markers but has shown promise in these earlier studies. This case series found this to be a poor differential marker for AFX, indeed, their spindle cell melanoma cases were positive more frequently (15%). As this is the largest case series evaluating CD99 in AFX, these findings raise serious concerns for the use of this marker in this setting. Given the relatively large number of cases evaluated in this study, their findings add significant evidence toward the use of CD10, suggest caution in the use of p63, and question the validity of using CD99 at all.

J. Wisell, MD

The diagnostic utility of immunohistochemistry in distinguishing primary skin adnexal carcinomas from metastatic adenocarcinoma to skin: an immunohistochemical reappraisal using cytokeratin 15, nestin, p63, D2-40, and calretinin

Mahalingam M, Nguyen LP, Richards JE, et al (Boston Univ School of Medicine, MA; et al)
Mod Pathol 23:713-719, 2010

Often the distinction of primary adnexal carcinoma from metastatic adenocarcinoma to skin from breast, lung, and other sites can be a diagnostic dilemma. Current markers purportedly of utility as diagnostic adjuncts include p63 and D2-40; however, their expression has been demonstrated in 11–22% and 5% of metastatic cutaneous metastases, respectively. Both cytokeratin (CK) 15 and nestin have been reported as follicular stem cell markers. We performed CK15 and nestin, as well as previously reported stains (such as p63, D2-40, and calretinin) on 113 cases (59 primary adnexal carcinomas and 54 cutaneous metastases). Expressions of p63, CK15, nestin, D2-40, and calretinin were observed in 91, 40, 37, 44, and 14% of primary adnexal carcinoma, respectively, and in 8, 2, 8, 4, and 10% of cutaneous metastases, respectively.

p63 appeared to be the most sensitive marker (with a sensitivity of 91%) in detecting primary adnexal carcinomas. CK15 appeared to be the most specific marker with a specificity of 98%. Using χ^2 analysis, statistically significant *P*-values (<0.05) were observed for p63, CK15, nestin, and D2-40 in the distinction of primary adnexal carcinoma *versus* cutaneous metastases. In logistic regression and stepwise selection for predicting a primary adnexal carcinoma, statistical significance was observed for p63, CK15, and D2-40 (*P*-values: <0.001, 0.0275, and 0.0298, respectively) but not for nestin (*P*-value = 0.4573). Our study indicates that diagnostic sensitivity and specificity are significantly improved using a selected panel of immunohistochemical markers, including p63, CK15, and D2-40. Positive staining with all three markers argues in favor of a primary cutaneous adnexal neoplasm.

▶ Differentiating metastatic carcinoma to skin from a primary cutaneous adenocarcinoma is not necessarily a frequent task of the practicing dermatopathologist or pathologist, but it is often a memorable one. This occasionally difficult discrimination has increasingly relied on immunohistochemical (IHC) studies to confirm a diagnosis and even help to point toward the primary location of a previously undiscovered carcinoma. A principal difficulty associated with the use of IHC studies in this differential diagnosis relates to the divergent differentiation of cutaneous adnexal tumors and to the variety of possible metastatic tumors, each with differing IHC properties. Hence the chief limitation of this study, as it treats skin metastases and primary tumors as homogenous groups, with the results greatly influenced by the makeup of each group's constituent tumor types. The numbers of cases for some of the tumor types are low—2 cases each for ovary, endometrium, and stomach. For example, both of the ovarian tumors in this study were positive for D2-40, unlike every other type of extracutaneous tumor in their study. Thus, the degree of statistical significance for each marker depends in large part on the specific types of tumors included in the study; if a few more ovarian metastases were included, this would have decreased the specificity for D2-40. This is not to say that the study is not useful. In practice, the possible subtype of cutaneous adnexal carcinoma is often not clear, and similarly, the primary site of a possible metastasis may not be known; thus, the pathologist initially may begin with the query of primary versus malignant, precisely what this study addresses. Finding basic common trends or patterns of expression in types of tumors can be quite helpful when working up a case. Knowing that skin tumors, as a group, generally express a specific set of markers can point one in the right direction. Another helpful feature of this study is the effort toward developing a panel of markers. Most importantly, however, this study adds useful data to the increasing body of knowledge of IHC studies, particularly the role of p63 and potential role of cytokeratin 15 in cutaneous lesions. Expansion of these findings both in number of cases and with additional markers would be quite welcome to the daily practice of pathology.

J. Wisell, MD

Comparative genome hybridization analysis of laser-capture microdissected *in situ* melanoma
Vincek V, Xu S, Fan Y-S (Univ of Florida College of Medicine, Gainesville; Univ of Miami, FL)
J Cutan Pathol 37:3-7, 2010

Background.—The progression of melanoma occurs through discrete stages with known clinical and histologic features. Although many molecular events that occur during the progression of invasive and metastatic melanomas have been elucidated, there is limited knowledge of genetic changes that occur in the earliest stages of melanoma development. In this pilot study, we investigated genetic changes that happen in *in situ* melanoma so that we can better understand early melanoma development.

Materials and Methods.—DNA was extracted from five laser-capture microdissected Clark's level III melanomas, five *in situ* melanomas and five compound nevi all from sun exposed skin. Array-based comparative genomic hybridization was performed using Agilent 44 K platform.

Results.—The group of Clark's level III melanomas was characterized with multiple large deletions and duplications. In the group of *in situ* melanoma, deletions and duplications were limited in size. Deletions in *in situ* melanomas were present only on chromosomes 13q and 16q. Compound nevi did not show any significant chromosomal aberrations.

Conclusion.—*In situ* melanomas show characteristic chromosomal aberrations that are limited compared to melanomas that invade the dermis. Deletion of 13q found in *in situ* melanomas, which encompass the Rb1 tumor suppressor gene, might be one of the first events in the development of melanoma.

▶ In recent years, several studies have considered the comprehensive genetic alterations in melanoma using comparative genomic hybridization and gene expression profiling.[1] These studies have enlightened concepts about pathogenesis and even challenged the current histologic classification.[2] What have been lacking thus far are similar studies on the earliest melanoma lesions, believed to often be the necessary precursors of the invasive malignant tumors. Studying these early tumors can be technically challenging, as melanoma in situ (MIS) lesions contain a relatively small volume of tumor cells; indeed, when arising in association with benign nevi, the malignant cells may be dwarfed by the benign lesion. This study attempts this type of whole-genome evaluation of these early lesions by using laser-capture microdissection techniques to isolate the specific cells of interest from the hematoxylin and eosin–stained slides. The obvious criticism is that only 2 cases of MIS were able to produce usable data (out of a total of 5 attempted), highlighting the difficulty of studying these lesions. However, these 2 cases did show restricted changes when compared with cases of superficially invasive melanoma, implying progressive changes with tumor development. Included in the more limited changes seen in the MIS lesions were deletions of 13q where the important tumor suppressor gene, retinoblastoma (*Rb1*), resides. While these techniques and concepts will clearly require further corroboration and expansion, the possibility of finding consistent early genetic alterations in melanoma, such as deletion of *Rb1*, is exciting and provides hope that it could lead to a more complete understating of the disease and its progression.

J. Wisell, MD

References

1. Bittner M, Meltzer P, Chen Y, et al. Molecular classification of cutaneous malignant melanoma by gene expression profiling. *Nature.* 2000;406:536-540.
2. Curtin JA, Fridlyand J, Kageshita T, et al. Distinct sets of genetic alterations in melanoma. *N Engl J Med.* 2005;353:2135-2147.

Immunohistochemical detection of lymphovascular invasion with D2-40 in melanoma correlates with sentinel lymph node status, metastasis and survival

Petersson F, Diwan AH, Ivan D, et al (Karolinska Univ Hosp, Stockholm, Sweden; Univ of Texas, Houston)
J Cutan Pathol 36:1157-1163, 2009

Using immunohistochemistry with anti-D2-40 for the detection of lymphovascular invasion (LVI-IHC) in 74 cases of invasive melanoma, we found LVI in 23% (16/74) of the tumors. Data on sentinel lymph node (SLN) biopsy were available for 36 patients. Sixty-seven percent (6/9) of patients with LVI-IHC and 19% (5/27) without LVI-IHC had positive SLN. Follow-up data were available for 60 patients. Data on recurrence/ metastasis were available for 60 patients. Twenty-five percent (15/60) had LVI with immunohistochemistry. Fifty-three percent (8/15) of these patients had "distant" metastasis or regional recurrence compared with 11% (5/45) in those without LVI-IHC. Overall and disease-specific survival was shorter for patients with LVI. In both the univariate and multivariate Cox proportional hazards regression models, LVI-IHC in addition to ulceration was statistically significant with respect to overall survival. Specifically, in the reduced multivariate model, compared with patients with no LVI, patients with intratumoral LVI had a hazard ratio (HR) of 5.4 (95% CI 1.6–18.4), while patients with peritumoral LVI had a HR of 3.8 (95% CI 0.7–20.9). In addition, patients with ulceration had an increased hazard of 4.4 (95% CI 1.2–16.8).

For the first time, we herein show a positive correlation with LVI in melanoma detected with immunohistochemistry and distant metastasis, overall survival and disease-free survival.

▶ Studies have indicated that lymphovascular invasion (LVI) by melanoma correlates independently with worsened overall survival.[1] While these findings may make intuitive sense to many of us, other studies have not been able to conclusively corroborate this association.[2] This study adds to this discussion by using the increasingly popular D2-40 immunohistochemical (IHC) study to assist in the detection of LVI and, importantly, uses clinical outcome to investigate the significance of their findings. Similar to previous studies, they found the D2-40 IHC study to be quite useful in identifying LVI, though this point is neither controversial nor particularly surprising. As their Fig 4 in the original article illustrates, confidently identifying LVI in a melanoma case on routine hematoxilyn and eosin–stained sections is not always easy. More important than simply being able to visualize the LVI, these investigators' findings provide evidence that the presence of LVI, as identified with IHC studies, correlates with sentinel lymph node status and imparts an independently significant worse overall prognosis. While the presence of LVI is not currently used in the most recent American Joint Committee on Cancer staging system,[3] this study helps to make the case for routinely reporting this feature in diagnostic pathology reports.

J. Wisell, MD

References

1. Straume O, Akslen LA. Independent prognostic importance of vascular invasion in nodular melanomas. *Cancer.* 1996;78:1211-1219.
2. Sahni D, Robson A, Orchard G, Szydlo R, Evans AV, Russell-Jones R. The use of LYVE-1 antibody for detecting lymphatic involvement in patients with malignant melanoma of known sentinel node status. *J Clin Pathol.* 2005;58:715-721.
3. . Edge SB, Byrd DR, Carducci MA, Compton CA, eds. AJCC Cancer Staging Manual. 7th ed. New York, NY: Springer; 2009.

Outcome of Patients with a Positive Sentinel Lymph Node who do not Undergo Completion Lymphadenectomy
Kingham TP, Panageas KS, Ariyan CE, et al (Memorial Sloan-Kettering Cancer Ctr, NY)
Ann Surg Oncol 17:514-520, 2010

Background.—Completion lymph node dissection (CLND), although considered a standard approach for patients with melanoma and a positive sentinel lymph node (SLN), is not performed in as many as 50% of indicated cases. This study evaluates the outcome of patients who had a positive SLN but did not undergo CLND at Memorial Sloan-Kettering Cancer Center.

Methods.—A prospective database was used to identify all patients with a positive SLN from 1992 to 2008. Patient and tumor characteristics, number of positive SLNs, recurrence pattern, reason for not performing a CLND, and current status were evaluated.

Results.—There were 2269 patients who underwent SLN biopsy. Three hundred thirteen had a positive SLN, of whom 271 (87%) had a CLND and 42 (13%) did not. Patients in the no-CLND group were older (median age 70 vs. 56 years, $P < .01$), and had a trend toward thicker melanomas (3.5 vs. 2.8 mm, $P < .06$). A significantly higher percentage of no- CLND patients had lower-extremity melanomas (40% vs. 13% CLND;

$P < .01$). The most common reason for not performing a CLND was patient refusal (45%). There were similar rates and patterns of recurrence between the two groups. Recurrence-free survival and disease-specific survival were also similar between the groups.

Conclusions.—It remains unclear whether CLND must be performed in all melanoma patients with a positive SLN. For selected informed patients who choose not to participate in the Multicenter Selective Lymphadenectomy Trial II trial, or in centers where the trial is not available, nodal observation may be an acceptable option.

▶ The practice of performing a sentinel node (SLN) biopsy following the diagnosis of melanoma has gained popularity over the previous 2 decades. However, the subsequent management of patients based on the information obtained from this procedure remains controversial. Involvement of the SLN by metastatic disease almost certainly has significant prognostic value,[1] but if SLN metastasis compels it, a subsequent completion lymph node dissection remains controversial with no consensus that such a procedure confers a survival advantage. This study reviews 16 years of SLN experience at the Memorial Sloan-Kettering Cancer Center and focuses on patients with an SLN positive for metastatic melanoma. Some of these patients (13%) ultimately chose not to pursue a completion lymph node dissection immediately following their positive SLN diagnosis. Surprisingly, however, the authors find that the patients who chose not to pursue removal of the remaining lymph nodes in the affected area experienced a nearly identical median time to recurrence as those who had the lymph nodes removed (14 and 13 months, respectively). It is important to note that this is a retrospective review and that the 2 groups were not randomized. For a randomized, controlled, prospective trial addressing this question, we will have to wait until 2022 when the results of the Multicenter Selective Lymphadenectomy Trial II are complete. Though far from definitive, this study does call into question the compulsory need for completion lymph node dissections in all positive SLN patients. The authors also sought some understanding as to why these patients did not pursue completion lymph node dissection and found that the most common reason (45%) for not having the remaining lymph nodes removed was patient refusal.

J. Wisell, MD

Reference

1. Morton DL, Thompson JF, Cochran AJ, et al. Sentinel-node biopsy or nodal observation in melanoma. *N Engl J Med.* 2006;355:1307-1317.

The use of elastin immunostain improves the evaluation of melanomas associated with nevi

Kamino H, Tam S, Tapia B, et al (New York Univ School of Medicine; Caris Cohen Dx, Newton, MA; et al)

J Cutan Pathol 36:845-852, 2009

Background.—Twenty to 30% of malignant melanomas are associated with melanocytic nevi; however, sometimes it is difficult to distinguish the melanoma from the nevus by routine histology. We have previously described distinctive patterns of elastic fibers in nevi and in melanomas.

Methods.—We analyzed elastic fiber patterns using elastin immunostain and elastic van Gieson (EVG) stain in 30 cases of invasive melanomas associated with nevi, 12 control melanocytic nevi and 14 control invasive melanomas.

Results.—Elastin immunostain was superior to EVG in showing the elastic fiber patterns. In nevi, the elastic fibers were preserved between nests and often around individual melanocytes. In contrast, melanomas had markedly decreased elastic fibers in the stroma and within the nests of melanocytes. The melanoma pushed down the pre-existing thin elastic fibers of the papillary dermis, forming a compressed layer at its base, which separated the melanoma from the nevus. On sun-damaged skin, the solar elastosis had similar elastin and EVG patterns. In three cases with dense inflammation, the layer of elastic fibers between melanoma and nevus was still present but less evident.

Conclusions.—The distinctive patterns of elastic fibers, best shown by the elastin immunostain, were helpful in evaluating melanomas associated with melanocytic nevi.

▶ While receiving less attention than the cellular constituents of melanocytic lesions, the stromal changes surrounding melanocytic lesions have also been previously investigated. This study adds to earlier work examining the changes in elastic fibers by the same group. The authors sought to exploit alteration of dermal elastic fibers in melanoma to deal with the occasional difficulty that arises in determining exactly where a melanoma starts and an adjacent nevus ends. This can be a critical distinction as tumor thickness is generally considered to be the most important prognostic factor to be gleaned from the examination of primary melanomas. The tumor thickness is also often used to make a determination for doing a sentinel lymph node procedure. With images from their cases the authors nicely demonstrate how evaluating for changes in the elastic fibers can clarify the nevus/melanoma interface (Fig 10 in the original article). As those who have had to make this distinction are aware, having an objective feature to aid in this distinction could occasionally prove useful. It is not surprising that the authors did not find marked differences in the depth between the original hematoxylin and eosin–based measurement and the measurement aided by elastic fiber evaluation from their 30 cases. From experience, it seems that in many cases one can identify nevus cells apart from melanoma cells reasonably well. There are, however, those less common cases where the distinction is more difficult. Of these less frequent cases, the change in thickness may still not be large, but given the amount of attention tumor thickness receives, having as accurate and reproducible measurements as possible allays concerns of arbitrariness. This study also adds to the more general ideas about how melanomas grow and the stromal interactions that take place during tumor development.

J. Wisell, MD

Atypical neurofibroma of the skin and subcutaneous tissue: clinicopathologic analysis of 11 cases
Jokinen CH, Argenyi ZB (Univ of Washington, Seattle)
J Cutan Pathol 37:35-42, 2010

Background.—Neurofibroma (NF) is a relatively common cutaneous tumor, which typically presents little diagnostic difficulty. Occasionally, however, pleomorphic cells may be present in NF raising consideration of other neoplasms like malignant peripheral nerve sheath tumor (MPNST).

Methods.—This study examines the clinicopathologic and immunohistochemical features of 11 dermal and subcutaneous 'atypical' NF.

Results.—9/11 (82%) atypical NF were from females, aged 8–70 years. One patient had neurofibromatosis-1. Most presented on the extremities or trunk. The atypical cells had large hyperchromatic, irregular nuclei, and were arranged in a distinct lamellar or fibrillar pattern. Some tumors were hypercellular, but marked density characteristic of MPNST was not observed. All were nonplexiform. Mitoses were mostly absent. The pleomorphic cells expressed S-100 protein. All were negative for p53. MIB-1 was negative in 7/10 (70%) and stained only rare cells in 3 (30%). Epithelial membrane antigen (EMA) and p16 expression were variable. Of six patients with available follow-up, no tumor recurred and none developed malignancy (range 6–63, mean 33 months).

Conclusions.—Superficial atypical NF, while morphologically unusual, has no apparent association with neurofibromatosis-1 or short-term risk of recurrence or malignant transformation. Awareness of this variant is important in order to avoid misdiagnosis of a more aggressive neoplasm.

▶ Recognizing unusual variants of common tumors is a familiar task of the astute pathologist. Neurofibromas are among the more common stromal tumors encountered in routine evaluation of skin biopsies, usually requiring minimal time or concern. However, occasionally these tumors harbor scattered atypical cells and an occasional mitotic figure, raising concern for a more ominous process but still falling short of a malignant diagnosis. This phenomenon is not unique to neurofibromas and in fact is quite well known to occur in the closely related schwannoma, where these changes are often termed degenerative atypia or ancient change. While the inclination may be to extrapolate that these changes in neurofibromas are as equally incidental, only a few cases examining the issue have been reported in the literature. The largest case series evaluating this phenomenon is almost exclusively from neurofibromatosis type 1 patients (NF1),[1,2] leaving this study and the study by Lin et al in 1997, which had a series of 6 patients.[3] The study by Lin et al included 3 patients with NF1 and, despite follow-up as long as 6 years, did not find any recurrence or development of associated malignancy. This earlier study also evaluated the role of immunohistochemical studies, finding that p53 and Ki-67 may help in distinguishing atypia from outright malignancy. This study includes more patients (11), a similar short to medium length of follow-up, and also no evidence of recurrence or malignancy in any of the tumors. In addition to corroborating the 1997 study's potentially helpful findings of p53 and Ki-67 patterns in these cases, this study also adds p16 to the discussion; they found this marker to be less telling of malignancy as many of the atypical cells showed loss of expression similar to the common loss of expression seen in malignant peripheral nerve sheath tumors. This study adds welcome reassurance that the troublesome findings of scattered atypical cells or occasional mitotic figures in neurofibromas are not necessarily harbingers of soon-to-be outright malignant transformation and may just be incidental findings. As suggested in the study by Lin et al, the findings of this study do not provide any evidence that more than conservative treatment of these lesions is indicated.

J. Wisell, MD

References

1. Valeyrie-Allanore L, Ortonne N, Lantieri L, et al. Histopathologically dysplastic neurofibromas in neurofibromatosis 1: diagnostic criteria, prevalence and clinical significance. *Br J Dermatol.* 2008;158:1008-1012.
2. McCarron KF, Goldblum JR. Plexiform neurofibroma with and without associated malignant peripheral nerve sheath tumor: a clinicopathologic and immunohisto-chemical analysis of 54 cases. *Mod Pathol.* 1998;11:612-617.
3. Lin BT, Weiss LM, Medeiros LJ. Neurofibroma and cellular neurofibroma with atypia: a report of 14 tumors. *Am J Surg Pathol.* 1997;21:1443-1449.

HRAS-mutated Spitz Tumors: A Subtype of Spitz Tumors With Distinct Features

van Engen-van Grunsven ACH, van Dijk MCRF, Ruiter DJ, et al (Radboud Univ Nijmegen Med Ctr, The Netherlands; Univ Med Ctr Groningen, The Netherlands; et al)
Am J Surg Pathol 34:1436-1441, 2010

It is often very difficult to confidently distinguish benign and malignant Spitz lesions, and a diagnosis of Spitz tumor of unknown malignant potential (STUMP) is rendered. To address this problem, we performed molecular genetic analysis in a large group of Spitz tumors (93 Spitz nevi and 77 STUMPs) and identified a subgroup of 24 lesions harboring a *HRAS* mutation. This subgroup lay predominantly in the dermis, had a relatively low cellularity, showed desmoplasia (with single cells interspersed between the collagen bundles), and had an infiltrating base. In 7 of these 24 cases (29%) melanoma had been the initial diagnosis, or an important differential diagnostic consideration, mainly based on the presence of multiple or deeply located mitotic figures, especially in adult patients. In our series none of the patients with the *HRAS*-mutated lesions developed recurrences or metastases (mean and median follow-up: 10.5 y). This was in accordance with the literature: review showed that no *HRAS* mutations had so far been reported in Spitzoid melanomas. We therefore conclude that *HRAS* mutation analysis may be a useful diagnostic tool to help differentiate between Spitz nevus and Spitzoid melanoma, thereby reducing the frequency of overdiagnosis of melanoma, and to help predict the biological behavior of a STUMP. Moreover, this might be a first step toward a more reproducible classification of Spitz tumors combining histological and genetic data.

▶ The increasing use of molecular studies in clinical practice has provided another avenue for classification of entities beyond histomorphology and immunohistochemistry. One area that desperately needs additional input for optimal classification is the group of melanocytic lesions commonly labeled with the moniker Spitz. Originally described by Dr Spitz as "juvenile melanoma," she noted that unlike their adult counterparts, they only rarely metastasize[1]; this lesion has come to be known commonly as Spitz nevus. Similar histologic features have been noted in a minority of melanomas, referred to by some as Spitzoid melanomas. Further blurring the distinction between benign and malignant, those lesions with intermediate features have been labeled as Spitzoid tumor of unknown malignant potential. The authors of this article add their experience evaluating for *HRAS* mutations in Spitz lesions. They, along with previous studies, note a subgroup of Spitz lesions that contain a mutation in the *HRAS* oncogene. They have found that all 24 of their patients with Spitz lesions containing an *HRAS* mutation have no evidence of disease recurrence; the significance of their findings is supported by an impressive 10.5-year average follow-up. Thus despite being a mutation in an oncogene, this finding appears to portend a good prognosis and lends support for the diagnosis of a Spitz nevus in these cases. It has been estimated that only 10% to 20% of Spitz nevi carry this genetic alteration, somewhat limiting its use.[2,3] However, the authors note that of their 24 cases of *HRAS*-related Spitz nevi, 7 initially either carried the diagnosis of melanoma or included melanoma in the differential diagnosis, indicating an important role for *HRAS* testing in some cases. Bringing it all together, the authors of the study delineate certain morphologic features that tend to characterize *HRAS*-related Spitz nevi. This study also illustrates how molecular studies will likely aid the future histopathologist in making more meaningful tumor classifications.

J. Wisell, MD

References

1. Spitz S. Melanomas of childhood. *Am J Pathol.* 1948;24:591-609.
2. van Dijk MC, Bernsen MR, Ruiter DJ. Analysis of mutations in B-RAF, N-RAS, and H-RAS genes in the differential diagnosis of Spitz nevus and spitzoid melanoma. *Am J Surg Pathol.* 2005;29:1145-1151.
3. Bastian BC, LeBoit PE, Pinkel D. Mutations and copy number increase of HRAS in Spitz nevi with distinctive histopathological features. *Am J Pathol.* 2000;157: 967-972.

Indolent CD8+ lymphoid proliferation of the ear: A phenotypic variant of the small-medium pleomorphic cutaneous T-cell lymphoma?

Beltraminelli H, Müllegger R, Cerroni L, et al (Med Univ of Graz, Austria; Hosp of Wiener Neustadt, Austria)
J Cutan Pathol 37:81-84, 2010

Background.—Recently, Petrella et al. described four patients with an unusual CD8+ lymphoid proliferation arising on the ear. These cases do not correspond clearly to any recognized category of cutaneous T-cell lymphoma (CTCL) described in the World Health Organization (WHO)/European Organization for Research and Treatment of Cancer (EORTC) 2005 classification.

Methods and Results.—Three patients (all men; median age 64; range: 61-69) presented with plaques or small tumors localized on the ears. All lesions showed histopathologically a dense, diffuse infiltration of lymphocytes within the entire dermis without epidermotropism. Cytomorphology revealed predominance of medium-sized pleomorphic lymphocytes. Immunohistochemistry showed a cytotoxic phenotype (CD3+ /CD4−/CD8+). Polymerase chain reaction (PCR) analysis of the T-cell receptor (TCR)-gamma gene revealed a monoclonal rearrangement in two of three patients. Follow-up data of two patients were available; one is alive without skin or systemic manifestations of the disease after 28 months, whereas the other is alive with persistent skin disease after 7 months.

Conclusions.—Our observation confirms that some patients present with a peculiar lymphoid proliferation of small-medium pleomorphic cytotoxic lymphocytes located on the ear, probably representing a phenotypic variant of the cutaneous small/medium pleomorphic T-cell lymphoma (CSMPTCL). These cases should not be misinterpreted as a high-grade cytotoxic lymphoma.

▶ Classification of cutaneous lymphomas continues to evolve, particularly the nonmycoses fungoides (non-MF) T-cell lymphomas. Two of the provisional diagnoses included in the 2005 World Health Organization/European Organization for Research and Treatment of Cancer[1] classification are primary cutaneous aggressive epidermotropic CD8 T-cell lymphoma (CE8TL) and primary cutaneous CD4 small/medium-sized pleomorphic T-cell lymphoma

(CSMPTCL). These 2 entities represent attempts to better clarify the heterogeneous group of unspecified primary cutaneous peripheral T-cell lymphomas. CE8TL is proving to be an important entity because of its typically aggressive clinical course with a median survival of less than 2 years. CSMPTCL may be important to consider as a distinct entity for the opposite reason; these patient's tend to follow a better, but still guarded, prognosis, with a 5-year survival above 60%. Enter the interesting cases reported in this article. These 3 cases add to a 2007 report.[2] In total, all 7 of these patients have features of both CE8TL and CSMPTCL. They have a cytotoxic (CD8) phenotype but no epidermotropism. Though follow-up information is extremely limited, the reports show a relatively favorable clinical course. These features, in addition to the localization on the ear, indicate a possible role for classifying these cases as a separate entity. The authors of this more recent case series, however, have taken more of a lumping approach than a splitting approach and suggest that these cases could be considered CD8 variants of CSMPTCL; similar to the CD8 phenotypic variation recognized in MF. The classification of such lesions may experience continued debate, but whether one recognizes these as entities in their own right or as subtypes of another entity, the important element is that we are recognizing them. As additional follow-up data are accumulated, we will hopefully make clearer sense of the non-MF group of cutaneous lymphomas. For the practicing pathologist or dermatologist, these cases also help to illustrate the features and differences among the different proposed entities within the "primary cutaneous peripheral T-cell lymphoma, unspecified," as information accumulates and our understanding evolves.

J. Wisell, MD

References

1. Willemze R, Jaffe ES, Burg G, et al. WHO-EORTC classification for cutaneous lymphomas. *Blood*. 2005;105:3768-3785. PMID: 15692063.
2. Petrella T, Maubec E, Cornillet-Lefebvre P, et al. Indolent CD8-positive lymphoid proliferation of the ear: a distinct primary cutaneous T-cell lymphoma? *Am J Surg Pathol*. 2007;31:1887-1892.

6 Lung and Mediastinum

Comprehensive Histologic Assessment Helps to Differentiate Multiple Lung Primary Nonsmall Cell Carcinomas From Metastases
Girard N, Deshpande C, Lau C, et al (Memorial Sloan-Kettering Cancer Ctr, NY; et al)
Am J Surg Pathol 33:1752-1764, 2009

The pathologic classification of nonsmall cell lung cancer (NSCLC) is evolving. Lung adenocarcinoma is morphologically heterogeneous, with mixtures of acinar, papillary, bronchioloalveolar, and solid patterns in more than 80% of cases. In case of synchronous or metachronous multiple NSCLC, the distinction of intrapulmonary metastases from independent primary tumors is of great clinical importance as it influences staging and potentially the therapeutic strategy. Here we took advantage of a cohort of 20 patients with 42 multiple NSCLC tumors (24 potential pair comparisons) that were annotated molecularly using genomic and mutational profiling to evaluate the value of comprehensive histologic assessment in this setting. Using the Martini-Melamed criteria, paired tumors were characterized as multiple primary NSCLCs in 21 cases and as intrapulmonary metastases in 3 cases. Genomic and mutational data led to a diagnosis of multiple primaries in 14 cases and of metastases in 8 cases; 2 cases could not be assessed. This molecular characterization contradicted the Martini-Melamed diagnosis in 7 (32%) of the 22 assessable comparisons. Adenocarcinoma was found in 32 (76%) of the 42 tumors. After review in a blinded fashion, semiquantitative comprehensive histologic assessment of paired tumors was different in 16 and similar in 8 paired tumors. We found that comparing adenocarcinomas is a complex issue that requires assessment not only of percentages of the histologic subtypes, but also the recording of additional histologic details such as cytologic features, patterns of stroma, necrosis, discrete nodularity versus miliary growth and variants such as clear cell, signet ring, mucinous, and fetal patterns. We also found that paired squamous cell carcinomas could be compared based on histologic subtyping in addition to cytologic and stromal characteristics. Considering histologically different tumors as multiple primaries, and similar tumors as metastases, comprehensive histologic subtyping was consistent with the molecular characterization in 20 (91%) of the 22 pairs comparisons. In summary, based on a well characterized cohort with detailed clinical, pathologic and molecular data, we found comprehensive histologic assessment is a powerful tool that seems to be a promising way to determine whether multiple lung adenocarcinomas or squamous cell carcinomas are metastatic or multiple primaries. This has great clinical implications for staging and therapeutic management of lung cancer patients with multiple tumors. Given its high correlation with molecular characterization of such tumors, it may provide a much cheaper and faster method to address this problem.

▶ This article discusses a very frequent issue that occurs when an oncologist requests from pathologists to compare a current lung tumor with a previous one in a given patient. This may be a rewarding or frustrating exercise as it may be difficult to determine with certainty whether one is dealing with a metastasis or different primary tumors, either synchronously or metachronously. The authors of this article shake the old parameters established in the 1970s based on the 1967 WHO classification of pulmonary nonsmall cell carcinomas. At that time, comparing 2 tumors was based on difficult features to establish, such as the presence of carcinoma in situ or tumor in shared lymphatic regions. It is interesting that we have to enter the era of molecular oncologic pathology to revise and make more emphasis in the morphologic features of lung carcinomas. The article proposes a more detailed analysis of the histological features, taking into consideration not only the epithelial features but also the characteristic features of stroma and inflammatory infiltrates to compare 2 neoplasms. For a pure morphologist, this is a welcome proposition where the classification of adenocarcinomas is now more complex than 4 decades ago. The idea of giving a percentage to the components of an adenocarcinoma for comparison purposes adds objectivity to the observations by individual pathologists. Adenocarcinomas may be acinar, papillary, bronchioloalveolar, solid, micropapillary, mucinous, fetal, colloid, signet ring, and clear cell, whereas squamous cell carcinomas may be papillary, clear cell, basaloid, or sarcomatoid. These features can be used to compare these 2 tumors. The stroma is also helpful, as one can analyze desmoplasia, necrosis, keratinization, and inflammation. Similar percentages of those components would support the possibility of metastasis, and different percentages would be features of multiple primaries. One appreciates that the data were supported by the molecular signatures of the tumors studied and, importantly, by the survival outcomes. The latter is essentially the gold standard for the conclusions based on morphology. More studies with larger series and similar conclusions are needed to feel comfortable when comparing multiple lung tumors.

P. A. Bejarano, MD

EGFR Mutation Is a Better Predictor of Response to Tyrosine Kinase Inhibitors in Non–Small Cell Lung Carcinoma Than FISH, CISH, and Immunohistochemistry

Sholl LM, Xiao Y, Joshi V, et al (Brigham and Women's Hosp, Boston, MA; Harvard Univ, Boston, MA; et al)
Am J Clin Pathol 133:922-934, 2010

About 10% of patients with non–small cell lung carcinoma (NSCLC) respond to epidermal growth factor receptor (EGFR)-targeted tyrosine kinase inhibitors (TKIs). More than 75% of "responders" have activating mutations in EGFR. However, mutation analysis is not widely available, and proposed alternatives (in situ hybridization and immunohistochemical analysis) have shown inconsistent associations with outcome. Fluorescence in situ hybridization (FISH), chromogenic in situ hybridization (CISH), immunohistochemical analysis, and DNA sequencing were compared in this study of 40 NSCLC samples from TKI-treated patients. Response rates were 12 of 19 in EGFR-mutant vs 1 of 20 EGFR wild-type tumors ($P = .0001$), 7 of 19 FISH+ vs 4 of 17 FISH− tumors (not significant [NS]), 5 of 16 CISH+ vs 6 of 21 CISH− tumors (NS), and 3 of 9 immunohistochemically positive vs 7 of 22 immunohistochemically negative tumors (NS). EGFR mutation was associated with improved progression-free survival ($P = .0004$). Increased copy number (FISH or CISH) and protein expression (immunohistochemical) did not independently predict outcome. Thus, EGFR sequence analysis was the only method useful for predicting response and progression-free survival following TKI therapy in NSCLC.

▶ This article adds knowledge and helps to lower the tone of the controversy on what method is best to guide oncologists if a decision to use tyrosine kinase inhibitors (TKIs) is made. It may be difficult to find a large series of patients in the western population whose tumors harbor the epidermal growth factor receptor (*EGFR*) mutation and respond to TKIs. The reason for this is that the mutation is infrequent. Between 10% and 15% of lung adenocarcinomas carry the mutation. Although this article intentionally gathered information on patients with mutation, the number of patients is still small. It is known that about 75% of tumors that respond to TKIs contain an activating mutation. However, it is unknown what drives the response in the remaining 25% of cases. The patients in this study had advanced adenocarcinoma, and TKIs were likely used as a second line of therapy following chemotherapy. It is not clear whether they can be used as a first line of therapy, and more studies are needed to confirm a significant improvement in patients receiving gefitinib. The comparison between the 3 methods, mutation, immunohistochemistry, and fluorescence In situ hybridization, indicates that it is likely that the mutation is the one that drives the expression and amplification of the gene; therefore, *EGFR* mutation is the test recommended to decide whether or not a patient is a candidate to receive TKIs. Eventually, identification of *EGFR* mutation may not be enough, as there are patients who do not respond despite the fact that they carry the mutation. These patients may have additional *EGFR* resistance mutations or *MET* activation or *KRAS* mutation, and these need to be identified to predict lack of response to TKIs.

P. A. Bejarano, MD

Granulomatous Reaction to *Pneumocystis jirovecii*: Clinicopathologic Review of 20 Cases
Hartel PH, Shilo K, Klassen-Fischer M, et al (Armed Forces Inst of Pathology, Washington, DC; et al)
Am J Surg Pathol 34:730-734, 2010

To better characterize the clinical and pathologic features of granulomatous reaction to *Pneumocystis jirovecii*, we reviewed 20 cases of this uncommon response. Patients included 15 males and 5 females (mean age 52 y). The most common symptom was dyspnea (5 of 14). Primary medical diagnoses included human immunodeficiency virus/acquired immunodeficiency syndrome (7 of 20), hematopoietic (6 of 20), and solid malignancies (4 of 20). Radiology findings included nodular (8 of 16) and diffuse (5 of 16) infiltrates and solitary nodules (3 of 16). Diagnostic procedures with the highest yield were open lung biopsy (13 of 20) and autopsy (5 of 20); false-negative results were most common on bronchial washings/brushings, bronchoalveolar lavage, fine needle aspiration, and transbronchial biopsy. Follow-up showed resolution of disease (6 of 13), death from disease (6 of 13), and death from unknown cause (1 of 13). Histologically, clusters of Gomori methenamine silver-positive (20 of 20) Pneumocystis organisms were identified in all cases. Organisms were identified within well (16 of 20) and poorly (4 of 20) formed necrotizing (16 of 20) and non-necrotizing (4 of 20) granulomas ranging in size from 0.1 to 2.5 cm (mean 0.5 cm); granulomas were multiple (18 of 20) or single (2 of 20). Giant cells (11 of 20), a fibrous rim (8 of 20), and eosinophils (6 of 20) were seen. Foamy eosinophilic exudates were present centrally within some granulomas (5 of 20). Cystic spaces (1 of 20) and calcification (1 of 20) were rare. Only one case demonstrated classic intra-alveolar foamy exudates containing Pneumocystis. Granulomatous *P. jirovecii* pneumonia occurs most commonly in males with human immunodeficiency virus/acquired immunodeficiency syndrome, hematopoietic, and solid malignancies. The diagnosis may be overlooked as conventional radiologic and pathologic features are absent. When suspected, open lung biopsy is most likely to yield diagnostic material. Attention to organism morphology avoids misdiagnosis as Histoplasma.

▶ Classically, infection with *Pneumocystis jirovecii* (formerly *Pneumocystis carinii*) presents histologically as intra-alveolar eosinophilic foamy exudates containing organisms that can be observed with silver stains, immunohistochemistry, and direct immunofluorescence. In our experience, the presence of granulomas in association with *Pneumocystis jirovecci* infection is based on autopsy and diagnostic biopsy material as well. Recently and coinciding with the publication of this article, we came across a patient who had undergone an intestinal transplant and whose transbronchial biopsy tissue showed abundant granulomas. The granulomas were compact and some of them contained in the center pink exudates that indeed contained pneumocystis organisms as seen with a Gomori methenamine silver (GMS) stain. The reaction of the clinical team when informed of our findings was that of incredulity. This reaction matches what the authors of the article describe, as the clinical presentation and imaging studies are not characteristic of the classical infection by *Pneumocystis jirovecci*. The clinicians may be reluctant to accept the diagnosis. However, the diagnosis is confirmed by using an immunohistochemical stain for pneumocystis. It is important not only to make the diagnosis, as mortality is high (around 50%), but also not to fall into the trap of making a call of histoplasmosis. *Histoplasma capsulatum* is similar to *Pneumocystis jirovecci*. They have 3 similarities and 3 differences. Both have thin-walled cysts and measure 2 to 5 microns, and collapsed forms are common. However, pneumocystis is spherical instead of oval, have large capsular dots, and show no budding. It is also important to keep in mind that infection with *Pneumocystis jirovecii* may show atypical histological features. These include granulomas, as shown in this article, interstitial fibrosis, absence of alveolar exudates, hyaline membranes, giant cell reaction, desquamative-like interstitial pneumonia, and interstitial lymphoid infiltrates. It is interesting that the intrinsic characteristics of the organisms associated with all those patterns of reaction are similar. This suggests that the patterns are due to host factors instead of variability in the organisms.

P. A. Bejarano, MD

7 Cardiovascular

Correlation of Donor-Specific Antibodies, Complement and Its Regulators with Graft Dysfunction in Cardiac Antibody-Mediated Rejection
Tan CD, Sokos GG, Pidwell DJ, et al (Cleveland Clinic, OH)
Am J Transplant 9:2075-2084, 2009

Antibody-mediated rejection (AMR) is an immunopathologic process in which activation of complement often results in allograft injury. This study correlates C4d and C3d with HLA serology and graft function as diagnostic criteria for AMR. Immunofluorescence staining for C4d and C3d was performed on 1511 biopsies from 330 patients as part of routine diagnostic work-up of rejection. Donor-specific antibodies were detected in 95% of those with C4d+C3d+ biopsies versus 35% in the C4d+C3d− group (p = 0.002). Allograft dysfunction was present in 84% in the C4d+C3d+ group versus 5% in the C4d+C3d− group (p < 0.0001). Combined C4d and C3d positivity had a sensitivity of 100% and specificity of 99% for the pathologic diagnosis of AMR and a mortality of

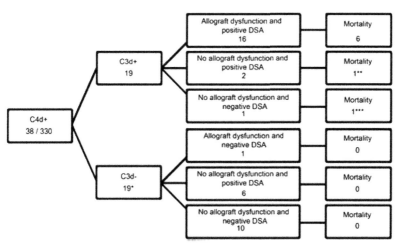

FIGURE 3.—Correlation of C4d and C3d staining with donor-specific antibodies (DSA), allograft dysfunction and survival. *Sera were not available for DSA testing in two patients of this group. **This patient died of glioblastoma multiforme. ***This patient died of coronary thrombosis. (Reprinted from Tan CD, Sokos GG, Pidwell DJ, et al. Correlation of donor-specific antibodies, complement and its regulators with graft dysfunction in cardiac antibody-mediated rejection. *Am J Transplant.* 2009;9:2075-2084.)

37%. Since activation of complement does not always result in allograft dysfunction, we correlated the expression pattern of the complement regulators CD55 and CD59 in patients with and without complement deposition. The proportion of patients with CD55 and/or CD59 staining was highest in C4d+C3d− patients without allograft dysfunction (p = 0.03). We conclude that a panel of C4d and C3d is diagnostically more useful than C4d alone in the evaluation of AMR. CD55 and CD59 may play a protective role in patients with evidence of complement activation (Fig 3).

▶ The lack of standardization and evolving understanding of antibody-mediated rejection (AMR) in cardiac allografts makes the clinical approach to diagnosis and management as well as the pathologic workup challenging. The diagnosis of AMR requires clinical, immunologic, and histologic correlation. The difficulty often arises in the definitions and cutoffs for each of these criteria. This excellent article addresses some of the more common clinicopathologic questions regarding the diagnosis of AMR. C4d is an early product of the complement cascade and binds covalently to endothelial cells and thus serves as a surrogate marker for complement activation. Likely because of its popularity in the diagnosis of AMR in renal allografts and inclusion in strict Banff criteria for renal allograft AMR, C4d is generally available at larger transplant institutions. C3d is less commonly available and is further down stream in the complement activation cascade. Pathologists who regularly screen for AMR with C4d occasionally find diffuse staining along the capillary network, but there is no clinical evidence of graft dysfunction, donor-specific antibodies (DSA), or histologic evidence of AMR (Fig 3). With the addition of C3d and staining for CD55 and CD59, this article postulates that some patients with CD55 and CD59 staining may be able to regulate the activation of complement at a point in the cascade following the generation of C4d but before the generation of C3d and the initiation of allograft dysfunction from complement activation. A strong argument is made for the addition of C3d staining in cardiac allograft workup of AMR.

M. L. Smith, MD

Heterotopic Breast Epithelial Inclusion of the Heart: Report of a Case
Sasaki K, Parwani AV, Demetris AJ, et al (Univ of Pittsburgh Med Ctr, PA)
Am J Surg Pathol 2010 [Epub ahead of print]

We report a case of heterotopic breast epithelial inclusion of the heart incidentally found on a native heart in a 73-year-old man who received orthotopic heart transplantation for ischemic cardiomyopathy. The lesion could not be recognized on gross inspection. Histologic sections from the left anterior atrium to interatrial septum showed focally microcystic ductal/tubular structures lined by a biphasic pattern of cuboidal to columnar apical epithelial cells with an outer layer of flattened basal

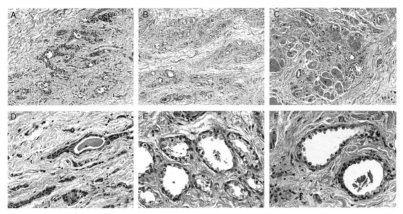

FIGURE 1.—Histologic features of the heterotopic breast epithelial inclusion of the heart, hematoxylin-eosin stain. A, Branching ductal and microcystic epithelium in collagenous stroma (20×). B, Microcystic pattern with lobular arrangement (10×). C, Microcystic structures among the cardiac myocytes showing an "infiltrative" pattern (20×). D, Elongated ductal structure containing eosinophilic secretion (40×). E, Biphasic pattern of microcystic epithelium composed of apical cells with flat and cuboidal, amphophilic granular to clear cytoplasm, and pale round nuclei surrounded by flattened basal cells with scant cytoplasm (40×). F, Microcysts with focal apical snouts formation (40×). (Reprinted from Sasaki K, Parwani AV, Demetris AJ, et al. Heterotopic breast epithelial inclusion of the heart: report of a case. *Am J Surg Pathol.* 2010 [Epub ahead of print], with permission from Lippincott Williams & Wilkins.)

cells. These glandular structures were arranged in vaguely lobular and focally infiltrative patterns in the epicardium and interstitium. No architectural or cytologic atypia or mitotic or apoptotic figures were seen. The apical epithelial cells were immunoreactive for pankeratin, cytokeratin (CK) 7, estrogen receptor, progesterone receptor, gross cystic disease fluid protein-15, and negative for CK20, calretinin, Wilms' tumor suppressor gene (WT1), CD31, suggestive of mammary epithelial differentiation. The basal cells were immunoreactive for pankeratin, CK7, CK5/6, D2-40, smooth-muscle actin and focally S100, suggestive of myoepithelial differentiation. Although the heterotopic breast tissue on the skin along the milk line is well recognized, it has not been described to involve internal organs including the heart (Fig 1, Table 1).

▶ Although this is just a single case report, it deserves mention as these findings would be highly unexpected for the vast majority of pathologists, and correct recognition and classification would be important for optimal patient care. Several different epithelial appearing inclusions have been described in the heart including an intracardiac endodermal heterotopia, mesothelial inclusions, adenomatoid tumors, metastatic epithelial tumors, and rarely epithelial components in cardiac myxoma. The benign appearance of the epithelial cells (Fig 1), presence of a myoepithelial cell layer, and immunohistochemical staining profile (Table 1) support a mammary origin of the tissue. Although reactivity for prostate-specific antigen (PSA) may raise the possibility of heterotopic prostatic tissue, PSA has been described in both benign and malignant breast tissue and prostatic cells are lined with basal cells, not myoepithelial cells as

TABLE 1.—Heterotopic Breast Epithelial Inclusion of the Heart, Immunohistochemical Expression

Antibody	Apical	Basal
	Result	
Smooth-muscle actin	Negative	Positive
S100	Negative	Occasional positive cells
p63	Negative	Positive
CK5/6	Negative	Positive
CK7	Positive	Positive
CK20	Negative	Negative
Pankeratin	Positive	Positive
Calretinin	Negative	Negative
WT1	Negative	Negative
D2-40	Negative	Positive
GCDFP-15	Positive	Negative
Mammaglobin	Negative	Negative
ER	Positive	Positive
PR	Occasional weakly positive cells	Occasional weakly positive cells
AR	Positive	Positive
PSA	Positive	Negative
PSAP	Positive	Negative
TTF-1	Negative	Negative
CD31	Negative	Negative
Ki-67	<1% positive	<1% positive

WT1 indicates Wilms' tumor suppressor gene (mesothelial marker); GCDFP- 15, gross cystic disease fluid protein-15; ER, estrogen receptor; PR, progesterone receptor; AR, androgen receptor; PSA, prostate-specific antigen; PSAP, prostate-specific acid phosphatase; TTF-1, thyroid transcription factor-1; CD31, endothelial marker; Ki-67, proliferation marker.

seen in this case. Pathologists must include heterotopic mammary tissue in the differential diagnosis of intracardiac epithelial appearing inclusions.

M. L. Smith, MD

Primary cardiac undifferentiated sarcoma: role of intraoperative imprint cytology and frozen section of two cases
Turhan N, Özgüler Z, Çağlı K, et al (Turkiye Yuksek Ihtisas Teaching and Res Hosp, Sihhiye, Ankara)
Cardiovasc Pathol 2010 [Epub ahead of print]

Primary cardiac tumors are very rare, and a vast majority of such malignant tumors are sarcomas. Associated symptoms are usually vague and nonspecific resulting in a late diagnosis and poorer prognosis. Most cardiac sarcomas have been reported in autopsy series. Although echocardiography may help make a diagnosis of a cardiac sarcoma, histopathological confirmation is quintessential. Presented here are two cases of patients who underwent successful surgery for the removal of a cardiac tumor, along with echocardiographic, cytological, and histopathological findings as well as a compact literature review. In both patients, the masses were on the surface of the mitral valve, and intraoperative evaluation of frozen sections and imprint cytology were indicative of a "probably malignant"

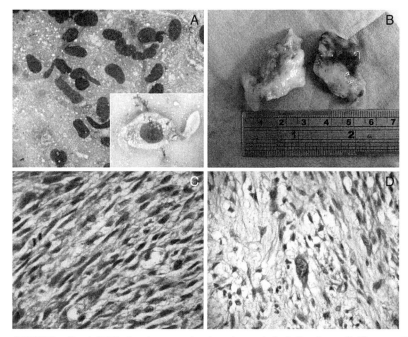

FIGURE 2.—Case 1. (A) The imprint smears show irregular, atypical spindle cells on a fibrillary myxoid background. (Inset) In between spindle cells atypical giant pleomorphic cell [May-Grunwald-Giemsa (MGG)]. (B) Macroscopically, the surgical specimen shows soft, pinkish-cream colored mass with irregular lobulated edges. (C) Microscopic examination of the undifferentiated sarcoma with hypercellular fascicular arranged spindle cells with frequent mitosis [hematoxylin and eosin (H&E)]. (D) The fibromyxoid regions are hypocellular (hypocellular regions of undifferentiated sarcoma mainly with myxoid change) (H&E). (Reprinted from Turhan N, Özgüler Z, Çağlı K, et al. Primary cardiac undifferentiated sarcoma: role of intraoperative imprint cytology and frozen section of two cases. *Cardiovasc Pathol.* 2010 [Epub ahead of print], with permission from Elsevier.)

mesenchymal tumor prompting more extensive surgical resection. Immunohistochemical staining of the resected material in both cases was only positive for vimentin, leading to a diagnosis of undifferentiated sarcoma. One of the patients died 3 months after surgery, while the other who received adjuvant chemotherapy was still alive after 4 months. Surgery remains the most definite treatment for cardiac sarcomas. The use of intraoperative frozen section and imprint cytology plays an important role in the decision to extend surgical resection (Figs 2 and 3).

▶ Frozen sections from primary tumors of the heart are markedly rare and can generate anxiety in practicing surgical pathologists. While the vast majority of cardiac lesions found to be either metastatic disease from other primary sites or benign mesenchymal tumors (myxoma), rarely primary cardiac malignancies arise. Touch preparations and frozen sections performed on 2 different cases of primary undifferentiated sarcoma of the heart showed atypical spindled-appearing cells with marked pleomorphism, high cellularity, and atypical mitotic figures (Figs 2 and 3). One case showed prominent necrosis. Preoperative

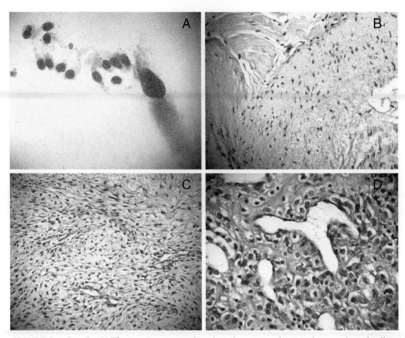

FIGURE 3.—Case 2. (A) The imprint smears show loosely connected atypical mesenchymal cells with oval hyperchromatic nuclei, undefined cytoplasmic borders, and several cytoplasmic projections. Scattered among these cells are a large bizarre cell (MGG). (B) The myocardium is infiltrated by undifferentiated sarcoma (H&E). (C) Hypocellular areas of tumoral tissue show marked myxoid degeneration (H&E). (D) In some areas, the tumor is rich in blood vessels and the cells have a polygonal epitheloid appearance with vesicular nuclei and clear cytoplasm (H&E). (Reprinted from Turhan N, Özgüler Z, Çağlı K, et al. Primary cardiac undifferentiated sarcoma: role of intraoperative imprint cytology and frozen section of two cases. *Cardiovasc Pathol.* 2010 [Epub ahead of print], with permission from Elsevier.)

transesophageal or transthoracic echocardiography can be useful in identifying tumor location, size, mobility, and attachment to adjacent structures. This information is useful in developing a preoperative plan. Intraoperative consultation can be helpful in guiding the surgical excision. When presented with primary tumors of the heart, either at frozen section or at final case sign out, undifferentiated sarcoma should always be included in the differential diagnosis.

M. L. Smith, MD

Survey of North American pathologist practices regarding antibody-mediated rejection in cardiac transplant biopsies
Kucirka LM, Maleszewski JJ, Segev DL, et al (Johns Hopkins Univ School of Medicine, Baltimore, MD; Mayo Clinic, Rochester, MN)
Cardiovasc Pathol 2010 [Epub ahead of print]

Background.—The 2004 International Society for Heart and Lung Transplantation consensus report specified an entity of histopathologic antibody-mediated rejection (hAMR) but did not define specific histologic criteria. Therefore, there is no gold standard for hAMR diagnosis.

Methods.—In May 2009 we performed a survey of pathologists from cardiac transplant centers in the United States and Canada assessing practices regarding hAMR investigation.

Results.—Of 94 centers who responded to our survey (77% response rate), 90% reported investigating for hAMR, and 80% of those reported having a defined protocol. Of centers with a defined protocol, 23% investigated all biopsies for hAMR. Of those who investigated for hAMR selectively, the most common triggers were clinical suspicion (61%) or suggestive histologic findings (36%). Sixteen different stains were used for hAMR investigation, the most common being C4d by immunofluorescence (38%), immunohistochemistry (38%) or both (21%).

Conclusions.—We found wide variation in pathologists' practices regarding hAMR diagnosis. A consensus document regarding hAMR is needed to better align our collective protocols, understand this disease process and to optimize patient care (Fig 2).

▶ This interesting article provides an overview of the collective current practice of cardiac transplant pathologists in the approach and workup of endomyocardial allograft biopsies for a histologic diagnosis of antibody-mediated rejection (AMR). Using United Network for Organ Sharing (UNOS) data, the centers involved in the survey accounted for over 80% of heart transplants in 2008. Therefore, it is a fairly comprehensive study of the current practice. Currently, 23% of centers perform C4d staining on all endomyocardial biopsies, while 10% of centers do not even investigate biopsies for AMR. Contrary to intuition,

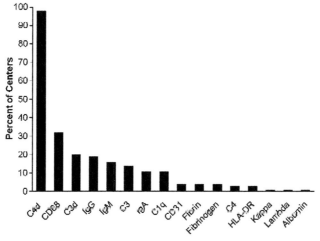

FIGURE 2.—Proteins evaluated for the investigation of hAMR. (Reprinted from Kucirka LM, Maleszewski JJ, Segev DL, et al. Survey of North American pathologist practices regarding antibody-mediated rejection in cardiac transplant biopsies. *Cardiovasc Pathol.* 2010;[Epub ahead of print], with permission from Elsevier.)

staining all biopsies for AMR did not correlate with a higher prevalence of AMR. When comparing C4d staining by immunohistochemistry and immuno-fluorescence techniques, there was a trend toward higher prevalence of AMR when using immunofluorescence. Unfortunately, both of these findings are limited by recall bias. Although recent studies have advocated for the use of C3d as a more sensitive and specific marker for AMR, only 19% of centers are currently using this stain in their protocols (Fig 2). The wide array of practice protocols is symptomatic of the lack of universally agreed upon diagnostic criteria or protocol. Even beyond histologic standardization, the incorporation of pathologic data into the overall clinical setting, similar to renal allograft AMR, is required. Additional criteria likely to be important include the presence of donor-specific antibodies and overall allograft function.

M. L. Smith, MD

The Utility of C4d, C9, and Troponin T Immunohistochemistry in Acute Myocardial Infarction
Jenkins CP, Cardona DM, Bowers JN, et al (Univ of Florida, Gainesville; et al)
Arch Pathol Lab Med 134:256-263, 2010

Context.—Full activation and involvement of the complement pathway follows acute myocardial infarction. Complement fragment C4d is a stable, covalently bound marker of complement activation. Troponin T is specific for cardiomyocytes.

Objectives.—To determine the specificity of C4d, C9, and troponin T immunoreactivity in necrotic myocytes and to establish whether they can be used to delineate acute myocardial infarction.

Design.—Twenty-six autopsy cases with a total of 54 myocardium areas of infarction were reviewed retrospectively. Immunohistochemistry for C4d, C9, and troponin T was used on paraffin sections of formalin-fixed tissue. Controls consisted of 5 cases without evidence of infarction, and histologically normal myocardium functioned as an internal control.

Results.—C4d and C9 antibodies reacted strongly and diffusely with necrotic myocytes in all samples of infarctions for up to 2 days (19 of 19; 100%). Adjacent histologically normal myocytes were nonreactive, resulting in a clear delineation between damaged and viable myocardium. Reactivity declined with increased duration and was absent in scars. Troponin T showed loss of staining in preinflammatory lesions (8 of 13; 62%); however, nonspecific patchy loss of staining was present in negative controls and in viable myocardium. Immunostains provided new diagnoses in 2 cases, including evidence of reinfarction and a newly diagnosed acute myocardial infarction.

Conclusions.—C4d and C9 have comparable reactivity and specificity for necrotic myocytes. C4d and C9 staining of necrotic myocytes is apparent before the influx of inflammatory cells, demonstrating utility in early myocardial infarction. Patchy loss of Troponin T in some cases of histologically normal myocardium limited its usefulness as a sole marker of infarction.

▶ Like many immunohistochemical stains, following initial discovery and use for a primary indication, which show good sensitivity and specificity, over time other indications are often identified. This article identifies an additional diagnostic use for C4d immunohistochemistry over antibody-mediated rejection. Early histologic features of acute myocardial infarction (AMI), including hypereosinophilia, contraction bands, and focal early inflammatory cell infiltration, may be difficult to identify by routine light microscopy alone, particularly in the time period before inflammatory cell infiltration. Therefore, a more definitive marker for damaged myocytes may be of interest. The authors describe how C4d is readily available in paraffin-embedded tissues and may assist in confirming suspected AMI. One of the limitations of this study was the sole comparison of normal myocardium to myocardial infarction. Additional studies are required to evaluate C4d immunohistochemical characteristics in damaged muscle of other disease processes, such as myocarditis and acute cellular rejection. Should the hypothesis hold true in further studies, C4d may be of use in patients who have recently undergone transplantation when the differential diagnosis is acute cellular rejection versus AMI.

M. L. Smith, MD

Utility of Routine Immunofluorescence Staining for C4d in Cardiac Transplant Recipients

Gupta S, Mitchell JD, Lavingia B, et al (Univ Hosp-St Paul, Dallas, TX; et al)
J Heart Lung Transplant 28:776-780, 2009

Background.—Immunofluorescence staining of endomyocardial biopsy (EMB) specimens to detect the complement fragment C4d is used to diagnose antibody-mediated rejection. However, data are limited regarding the utility of routine staining for C4d in clinical care.

Methods.—This study retrospectively reviewed the clinical course of adult cardiac transplant recipients who underwent $\geq$ 2 EMBs with immunofluorescence C4d staining at the University of Texas Southwestern Medical Center since September 2006. C4d staining was performed by the immunohistochemistry laboratory and interpreted by the members of the surgical pathology department, in conjunction with interpretation of the routine hematoxylin and eosin staining. Donor-specific antibodies (DSA) were routinely assessed at the time of clinical rejection.

Results.—Of 67 patients, specimens were positive for C4d (C4d+) in 14 and negative for C4d (C4d−) in 53. The frequency of acute cellular rejection (ACR) in these 2 groups was 57% (8 of 14, designated C4d+/ACR+) vs 11% (6 of 53, designated C4d−/ACR+; $p < 0.001$). Significantly more patients with a positive C4d specimen had a positive retrospective donor

TABLE 2.—Post-transplant Variables Stratified by the Presence of C4d, Acute Cellular Rejection, or Both

Post-Tx Variables[a]	C4d−/ACR− (n = 47)	C4d+/ACR− (n = 6)	C4d−/ACR+ (n = 6)	C4d+/ACR+ (n = 8)	p-Value
DSA+, %[b]	2	75	0	100	<0.01
LVEF, %[c]	60 (55–64)	38 (17–51)	60 (55–65)	43 (36–58)	<0.01
IVS, cm[c]	1.10 (0.99–1.20)	1.20 (1.20–1.35)	1.20 (1.10–1.40)	1.40 (1.30–1.60)	0.02
LVPW, cm[c]	1.10 (1.00–1.20)	1.20 (1.10–1.35)	1.30 (1.10–1.50)	1.35 (1.20–1.55)	<0.01

ACR, acute cellular rejection; DSA, donor-specific antibody; LVEF, left ventricular ejection fraction; IVSD, interventricular septum thickness; LVPW, left ventricular posterior wall thickness; Tx, transplantation.
[a]Data are presented as percentages and median (interquartile range [25th–75th]).
[b]Data available for 46, 4, 6, 8, respectively, for DSA.
[c]At the time of the first abnormal biopsy specimen or were recorded from the latest echocardiogram done in C4d−/ACR− patients.

specific crossmatch, presence of DSA after transplantation, and depressed graft function ($p < 0.01$ for each).

Conclusions.—Positive C4d immunofluorescence staining on EMB specimens was associated with ACR, reduced allograft function, a positive retrospective crossmatch, and the presence of DSA after transplantation. The latter 2 observations support the contention that C4d deposition is a marker of antibody-mediated rejection. Routine evaluation of C4d staining is feasible in the clinical setting and may identify variable patterns of rejection (Table 2).

▶ Much of the recent controversy and discussion in cardiac transplant pathology is centered on the diagnosis of antibody-mediated rejection (AMR). The current International Society for Heart and Lung Transplantation (ISHLT) recommendations require both histologic findings and evidence of humoral immune system activation within perimyocyte capillaries. Histologic features include endothelial cell swelling, intravascular macrophage accumulation, interstitial hemorrhage and edema, and increased neutrophils. Evidence of humoral immune system activation includes the demonstration of immunoglobulin and compliment components by immunofluorescence or intervascular macrophages and perimyocyte C4d by immunohistochemistry. Isolated staining for C4d, either by immunofluorescence or immunohistochemistry, has become the most common way to assess for compliment activation. The ISHLT suggestion is to workup only the cases that show these histologic features in the presence of unexplained cardiac dysfunction. Unfortunately, the sensitivity of the histologic features as a screening tool has been shown to be unacceptably low. A logical next step may be to perform routine C4d analysis to screen for AMR. This retrospective study of 67 heart transplant recipients (669 biopsy events) evaluated the use of routine C4d immunofluorescence. While the sample size is relatively small for generalizations, the correlation between positive C4d and the presence of donor-specific antibodies (DSA), decreased ejection fraction, and positive retrospective crossmatch supports the importance of C4d status (Table 2). As in the renal transplant population, one must use caution when comparing immunofluorescence to immunohistochemistry, as immunofluorescence may have a slightly higher sensitivity. However, further investigation is required for the subset of patients who are C4d positive but do not have a decreased ejection fraction or presence of DSA. If widespread screening for C4d is undertaken, this is the population that will generate most clinical management questions.

M. L. Smith, MD

8 Female Genital Tract

Differentiated vulvar intraepithelial neoplasia contains *Tp53* mutations and is genetically linked to vulvar squamous cell carcinoma
Pinto AP, Miron A, Yassin Y, et al (Federal Univ of Paraná, Curitiba, Brazil; Dana Farber Cancer Inst, Boston, MA; et al)
Mod Pathol 23:404-412, 2010

Differentiated vulvar intraepithelial neoplasia is a unique precursor to vulvar squamous cell carcinoma that is typically HPV-negative and frequently associated with nuclear p53 staining. These features imply a mode of pathogenesis involving somatic mutations. However, the genetic relationship of differentiated vulvar intraepithelial neoplasm and vulvar squamous cell carcinoma and the role of *Tp53* mutations in this process have not been resolved. We analyzed 11 differentiated vulvar intraepithelial neoplasms and 6 associated vulvar squamous cell carcinomas. Sections were stained for p53 and p63 and DNA from multiple epithelial sites, representing normal control tissues ($n = 10$), differentiated vulvar intraepithelial neoplasias ($n = 18$), and vulvar squamous cell carcinomas ($n = 6$), were obtained by laser capture microdissection, and sequenced for exons 2–11 of *Tp53*. Six of 10 cases contained at least one *Tp53* mutation-positive differentiated vulvar intraepithelial neoplasia focus; 4 strongly p53 immuno-positive and 2 negative. Staining for p53 and p63 co-localized, targeting the immature epithelium, but surface epithelium was *Tp53* mutation-positive. Four of five vulvar squamous cell carcinomas were *Tp53* mutation-positive; two shared identical *Tp53* mutation with adjacent differentiated vulvar intraepithelial neoplasia. Disparate foci of differentiated vulvar intraepithelial neoplasia often showed different mutations consistent with multiple neoplastic clones. Differentiated vulvar intraepithelial neoplasia is, with few exceptions, associated with *Tp53* mutations and will be p53 immunopositive when missense mutations (*versus* some nonsense and all deletion mutations) are present. Multiple *Tp53* mutations in different sites support the presence of multiple independent genetic events, but shared *Tp53* mutations in both differentiated vulvar intraepithelial neoplasia and vulvar squamous cell carcinoma support a genetic relationship between the two. The confinement of p53 staining to immature cell nuclei is consistent with maturation-dependent degradation of mutant p53 protein.

▶ Although human papillomavirus (HPV) is the causative agent in more than 90% of cervical cancers, it is only linked to approximately 40% of vulvar malignancies, which are typically preceded by classic vulvar intraepithelial neoplasms and share a common hematoxylin and eosin (H&E) appearance to their cervical counterparts. In contrast, the 60% of non-HPV-associated vulvar malignancies are often coupled to simplex or differentiated vulvar intraepithelial neoplasia (d-VIN). Although lacking the pronounced cytologic atypia of the HPV-associated lesions, they can usually be identified by their distinctive histology and positivity for p53 by immunohistochemistry. What has not yet been demonstrated and this article attempts to address, is whether d-VIN contains *Tp53* mutations, whether these mutations correlate with p53 positivity and whether d-VIN and vulvar squamous cell carcinomas (SCCs) share identical mutations.

The authors selected 11 cases of d-VIN on which to test their hypothesis, including 6, which also contained SCC. They stained these for p53, p16, and p63, then tested them for HPV DNA, and analyzed them for *Tp53* mutations. They found that *Tp53* mutations are highly associated with d-VIN (6/10 cases) and that multiple mutations occur in some cases, supporting the idea of independent neoplastic clones. Two of 6 cases showed identical *Tp53* mutations to those in the adjacent d-VIN, and 70% of the mutations in either d-VIN or SCCs were located in exons 5 through 9. They did prove that expression of mutated p53 protein is confined to immature epithelium (that which also stained with p63), suggesting degradation of the protein as keratinocytes mature, despite the retained *Tp53* mutation.

The study is primarily limited by the inclusion of a small number of cases. Additionally, the fact that only 2 cases with both d-VIN and SCC share an identical mutation makes it difficult to draw conclusions about the origin of one lesion from the other, although the finding of multiple *Tp53* mutations in different areas of d-VIN within the same case to some extent explains this discrepancy. The authors do point out the salient H&E features of d-VIN and highlight the importance of recognizing this deceptively bland lesion, as it has been linked to non-HPV-associated vulvar SCCs. For additional reading see the reference section.[1,2]

M. D. Post, MD

References

1. McCluggage WG. Recent developments in vulvovaginal pathology. *Histopathology.* 2009;54:156-173.
2. Terlou A, Blok LJ, Helmerhsorst TJ, van Beurden M. Premalignant epithelial disorders of the vulva: squamous vulvar intraepithelial neoplasia, vulvar Paget's disease and melanoma in situ. *Acta Obstet Gynecol Scand.* 2010;89:741-748.

Conjunctive p16[INK4a] Testing Significantly Increases Accuracy in Diagnosing High-Grade Cervical Intraepithelial Neoplasia

Bergeron C, for the European CINtec Histology Study Group (Laboratoire Cerba, Cergy Pontoise, France; et al)
Am J Clin Pathol 133:395-406, 2010

The histopathologic interpretation of cervical intraepithelial neoplasia (CIN) is subject to a high level of interobserver variability and a substantial number of false-positive and false-negative results. We assessed the impact of the conjunctive interpretation of p16[INK4a]-immunostained slides on the accuracy of community-based pathologists in diagnosing high-grade cervical intraepithelial neoplasia (CIN; CIN 2 and CIN 3) in biopsy specimens. Twelve pathologists rendered independent diagnoses on a set of 500 H&E-stained cervical punch and conization specimens. Results were compared with a dichotomized "gold standard" established by consensus of 3 gynecopathology experts. When p16[INK4a]-immunostained slides were added and conjunctively interpreted with the H&E-stained slides, a significant increase in diagnostic accuracy for the detection of high-grade CIN was observed ($P = .0004$). Sensitivity for high-grade CIN was increased by 13%, cutting the rate of false-negative results in half. Agreement of community-based pathologists in diagnosing high-grade CIN was significantly improved (mean κ values advanced from 0.566 to 0.749; $P < .0001$). Reproducibility of p16[INK4a] stain interpretation was excellent (κ = 0.899). Our results show that conjunctive interpretation

TABLE 3.—Cross-Tabulation of Diagnostic Results of Community-Based Pathologists for Interpretation of H&E-Stained Slides and H&E- and p16-Stained Slides Compared With the "Gold Standard" Diagnoses*

Community-Based Pathologists' Diagnoses	Gold Standard Diagnosis			
	Negative	CIN 1	CIN 2	CIN 3
H&E				
Negative	1,742	306	130	114
CIN1	485	555	186	87
CIN2	82	198	340	326
CIN3	18	92	172	926
Invasive carcinoma	1	1	0	23
Total	2,328	1,152	828	1,476
H&E and p16				
Negative	1,732	146	47	13
CIN1	543	630	158	68
CIN2	44	313	447	390
CIN3	9	63	174	1,002
Invasive carcinoma	0	0	2	3
Total	2,328	1,152	828	1,476

CIN, cervical intraepithelial neoplasia.
*Data are given as number of cases. Negative is negative for dysplasia. There was no invasive carcinoma diagnosed according to the gold standard result.

of p16^{INK4a}-stained slides could significantly improve the routine interpretation of cervical histopathology (Table 3).

▶ This article attempts to address the question of whether routine immunostaining for p16^{INK4a} (p16) ought to be undertaken in general practice pathology as a means of improving diagnostic accuracy for high-grade cervical intraepithelial neoplasia (CIN) 2 or 3. Perhaps the most problematic aspect of this study is the gold standard that was chosen, namely, the consensus diagnosis of 3 expert gynecopathologists based solely on a hematoxylin and eosin (H&E) review. The initial review showed complete concordance in only 253 cases (50.6%) and revealed 3 separate opinions in 92 cases (18.4%). This discordance highlights the difficulty facing pathologists trying to diagnose both cervical biopsies and excision specimens on a regular basis.

With that caveat in mind, the authors did demonstrate a significantly improved accuracy (taking the gold standard diagnosis as truth) in dichotomous sorting of cases into high grade (CIN 2 or 3) versus non–high grade (CIN 1 or negative for dysplasia) with the adjunctive use of p16 immunohistochemistry (Table 3). Importantly, the gain in sensitivity for detecting high-grade lesions was not associated with a loss of specificity.

Benefits to this study include the large number of cases examined (n = 500) and the incorporation of community pathologists rather than dedicated specialists. The findings do suggest that routine staining of cervical biopsies and excision specimens may provide diagnostic benefit and more appropriate patient management. Each laboratory, however, needs to assess the feasibility of incorporating an immunohistochemical stain into the evaluation of such a common specimen and perform a cost-benefit analysis based on its particular circumstances. For additional reading, see the reference section.[1,2]

M. D. Post, MD

References

1. Mulvany NJ, Allen DG, Wilson SM. Diagnostic utility of p16INK4a: a reappraisal of its use in cervical biopsies. *Pathology*. 2008;40:335-344.
2. Wentzensen N, von Knebel Doeberitz M. Biomarkers in cervical cancer screening. *Dis Markers*. 2007;23:315-330.

Metastatic Carcinomas in the Cervix Mimicking Primary Cervical Adenocarcinoma and Adenocarcinoma in Situ: Report of a Series of Cases
McCluggage WG, Hurrell DP, Kennedy K (Belfast Health and Social Care Trust, Northern Ireland)
Am J Surg Pathol 34:735-741, 2010

Metastatic tumors within the cervix are uncommon if one excludes endometrial carcinoma, which involves the cervix by direct spread. A variety of other neoplasms rarely metastasize to the cervix and, in most cases, the diagnosis is straightforward because of a combination of clinical and pathologic parameters, common features of metastatic carcinoma within the cervix including predominant involvement of the deep stroma, absence of surface involvement and of an in situ component, and prominent lymphovascular permeation. We describe 6 cases of metastatic adenocarcinoma involving the cervix with superficial "mucosal" involvement mimicking primary cervical adenocarcinoma or adenocarcinoma in situ. In 5 cases, the primary adenocarcinoma was in the ovary or peritoneum and was of serous (4 cases) or clear-cell (1 case) type. In the other case, the primary neoplasm was in the pancreas and this was initially interpreted as a primary cervical adenocarcinoma. In the cases of primary ovarian or peritoneal carcinoma, the mucosal tumor within the cervix, which was discovered at the same time as the ovarian or peritoneal neoplasm, raised the possibility of synchronous independent lesions or metastasis from the cervix to the ovary or peritoneum. Positive staining for WT1, p53, and estrogen receptor in the cases of serous carcinoma and an absence of human papillomavirus by linear array genotyping in all cases was of value in excluding a primary cervical neoplasm, although these ancillary studies are supplementary to microscopic examination. In those cases with an ovarian or peritoneal primary, the likely pathogenesis of the cervical involvement is transtubal and intrauterine spread. It is important for the pathologist to be aware of the possibility of cervical mucosal metastasis to avoid an erroneous diagnosis of a primary cervical adenocarcinoma or adenocarcinoma in situ.

▶ With the exception of endometrial carcinomas, cervical metastases are relatively rare occurrences and typically have features readily suggestive of a metastatic lesion, such as deep stromal involvement, lack of an in situ component, and prominent lymphovascular invasion (LVI). This article relates a series of 6 cases of tumors metastatic to the cervix, which show the opposite pattern, namely, they have predominantly or exclusively surface involvement and no identifiable LVI. These lesions could readily be mistaken for primary endocervical adenocarcinomas, leading to inappropriate treatment and suboptimal postsurgical chemotherapy or radiation.

Of the 6 cases, 5 originated from the ovary or peritoneum and 4 of those showed a serous phenotype, while the other case was a clear cell carcinoma. Although these morphologies would be very unusual as primary lesions in the cervix, they have been reported previously. The predominantly mucosal involvement was morphologically reminiscent of an in situ component, leading to further potential diagnostic confusion. Although all diagnoses were ultimately determined based on routine histologic examination, the authors note that immunohistochemistry may be of some limited value in this setting. Particularly in serous carcinomas, it has been previously demonstrated that those arising from the ovaries or peritoneum strongly and diffusely express WT1, while those of uterine origin are typically WT1-negative. Although no systematic study has been undertaken examining WT1 expression in endocervical serous carcinomas, the authors suppose that they would most likely be negative. In the cases reported here, there was strong and diffuse WT1 reactivity, supporting an interpretation of disease metastatic to the cervix. Interestingly, p16 was positive in these lesions, highlighting the caveat that it cannot be used as a specific marker of endocervical adenocarcinoma. However, all cases tested for human papillomavirus DNA were negative, similar to that seen in most p16-positive carcinomas of the ovary. They assert that spread of tumor from the ovaries/peritoneum to the endocervix (of note, all lesions were proximal to the transition zone [TZ], in contrast to primary endocervical adenocarcinomas, which typically arise at the TZ) was likely one of direct extension via the fallopian tubes and uterine cavity, essentially representing a skip lesion, similar to those frequently found in endometrial carcinomas involving the cervix.

The final case of mucosal cervical disease was metastatic from a primary pancreatic lesion and the means of spread to the cervix were less obvious. Aids to diagnosis here were an overtly mucinous phenotype existing in both the cervix and bilateral ovaries and lack of an in situ component. While typically this sort of metastasis is supposed to spread via lymphovascular spaces, there was no LVI identified, and instead, a mechanism of direct spread from the ovarian metastases is suggested.

While usually cervical involvement by a metastatic tumor would be readily identified as part of a larger staging procedure, there does exist the possibility for detection in a cone biopsy perhaps done for atypical glandular cells in a Papanicolaou test. Additionally, there are reported cases of primary cervical lesions metastasizing to the ovaries, thus involvement of both sites does not confirm either as the definitive origin. The description by the authors of cases of adenocarcinomas metastatic to the surface of the endocervix highlights the needs for pathologists to consider this possibility when confronted with unusual histologic subtypes (such as serous, clear cell, or mucinous) or lack of an identifiable in situ component.[1]

M. D. Post, MD

Reference

1. Mazur MT, Hsueh S, Gersell DJ. Metastases to the female genital tract. Analysis of 325 cases. *Cancer.* 1984;53:1978-1984.

PAX2 Distinguishes Benign Mesonephric and Mullerian Glandular Lesions of the Cervix From Endocervical Adenocarcinoma, Including Minimal Deviation Adenocarcinoma

Rabban JT, McAlhany S, Lerwill MF, et al (Univ of California San Francisco; Massachusetts General Hosp, Boston)
Am J Surg Pathol 34:137-146, 2010

Mesonephric remnants of the cervix are vestiges of the embryonic mesonephric system which typically regresses during female development. Uncommonly, hyperplasia of the mesonephric remnants may occur. The differential diagnosis of exuberant mesonephric hyperplasia includes minimal deviation adenocarcinoma of the cervix, a tumor with deceptively bland morphology for which no reliable diagnostic biomarkers currently exist. PAX2 encodes a transcription factor necessary in the development of the Wolffian duct system, and the protein is expressed in several tumors of mesonephric origin, including renal cell carcinoma, Wilm tumor, and nephrogenic adenoma. We hypothesized that PAX2 may also be expressed in mesonephric lesions of the cervix and may distinguish mesonephric hyperplasia from minimal deviation adenocarcinoma of the cervix. We demonstrated that PAX2 was strongly and diffusely expressed in mesonephric remnants (6 of 6) and in mesonephric hyperplasia (18 of 18); however, no expression was noted in mesonephric adenocarcinoma (0 of 1). PAX2 was expressed in normal endocervical glands (including tunnel clusters and Nabothian cysts) (86 of 86), lobular endocervical glandular hyperplasia (5 of 5), tubal/tuboendometrioid metaplasia (8 of 8), and cervical endometriosis (13 of 14). In contrast, only 2 cases of endocervical adenocarcinoma were positive for PAX2 [invasive adenocarcinoma of the minimal deviation type (0 of 5), usual type (1 of 22), and endometrioid type (1 of 1)]. Adjacent adenocarcinoma in situ, as well as cases of pure adenocarcinoma in situ (0 of 6), were also PAX2 negative. PAX2 expression in the 2 positive endocervical adenocarcinomas was patchy and weak. Most (11 of 15) stage II endometrial endometrioid adenocarcinomas lacked PAX2 expression but 1 of 10 grade 1 tumors and 3 of 5 grade 2 tumors did express PAX2. These results suggest that PAX2 immunoreactivity may be useful to (1) distinguish mesonephric hyperplasia from minimal deviation adenocarcinoma, (2) to distinguish lobular endocervical glandular hyperplasia from minimal deviation adenocarcinoma, and (3) to distinguish endocervical tubal metaplasia or cervical endometriosis from endocervical adenocarcinoma in situ. Overall, a strong, diffuse nuclear PAX2 expression pattern in a cervical glandular proliferation predicts a benign diagnosis (positive predictive value 90%, negative predictive value 98%; $P < 0.001$); however, PAX2 should not be interpreted in isolation from the architectural and cytologic features of the lesion as it may be expressed in some stage II endometrial adenocarcinomas involving the cervix.

▶ Although relatively uncommonly encountered in routine clinical practice, the presence of mesonephric remnants in the cervical wall can prove problematic.[1,2] While routine histomorphology typically distinguishes benign remnants or hyperplasia from malignant processes, there can exist a degree of overlap between these and endocervical adenocarcinoma, particularly the minimal deviation type (adenoma malignum). There is no reliable immunohistochemistry to definitively identify one entity versus another, particularly as adenoma malignum is frequently p16 negative. Further, although there are markers of variable utility to identify cells of mesonephric origin (calretinin, vimentin, inhibin, and androgen receptor), none of these are useful in determining whether a lesion is benign or malignant. This article explores the use of a novel biomarker, PAX2, to differentiate benign endocervical and mesonephric lesions from their malignant counterparts.

The authors studied a number of cases, 86 of which contained at least some normal endocervical glandular tissue, with diagnoses including mesonephric remnants, mesonephric hyperplasia, mesonephric adenocarcinoma, endocervical adenocarcinoma of usual and minimal deviation types, tubal metaplasia, cervical endometriosis, endocervical lobular hyperplasia, and endometrial endometrioid carcinomas involving the cervix. Overall, they found 100% of benign mesonephric lesions to express PAX2, virtually all in a strong diffuse nuclear pattern. Ninety-seven percent of benign endocervical lesions expressed PAX2, while only 6% of malignant endocervical lesions were positive, often weakly or in a patchy distribution. Eleven of 15 endometrioid carcinomas were negative, introducing a potential pitfall in overreliance on the immunostain; however, the authors note that all cases had obviously malignant features on routine histology. They found a 90% positive predictive value of strong diffuse nuclear staining for PAX2 in benign lesions and a 98% negative predictive value (absence of PAX2 favored a malignant diagnosis).

The article briefly touches on the embryologic expression pattern of this member of the *PAX* gene family and raises the question (as yet unanswered) regarding why it is expressed in Müllerian epithelium. Also unknown is the mechanism by which *PAX* alterations affect tumors (initiation of tumorigenesis vs contribution to progression vs other). The major significance is in the strong positive and negative predictive values convincingly demonstrated for PAX2 staining in benign and malignant lesions in the endocervix of mesonephric or endocervical glandular origin. The caveat is repeated that the immunostain cannot be used in isolation, particularly if extension of endometrial carcinoma is a consideration; however, other routine morphologic and cytologic features should be sufficient for that determination.

M. D. Post, MD

References

1. Gilks CB, Young RH, Aguirre P, DeLellis RA, Scully RE. Adenoma malignum (minimal deviation adenocarcinoma) of the uterine cervix. A clinicopathological and immunohistochemical analysis of 26 cases. *Am J Surg Pathol.* 1989;13: 717-729.
2. Dressler GR, Douglass EC. Pax-2 is a DNA-binding protein expressed in embryonic kidney and Wilms tumor. *Proc Natl Acad Sci U S A.* 1992;89:1179-1183.

An Immunohistochemical Study of Cervical Neuroendocrine Carcinomas: Neoplasms That are Commonly TTF1 Positive and Which May Express CK20 and P63
McCluggage WG, Kennedy K, Busam KJ (Belfast Health and Social Care Trust, Northern Ireland; Memorial Sloan-Kettering Cancer Centre, NY)
Am J Surg Pathol 34:525-532, 2010

Cervical small cell neuroendocrine carcinoma (SCNEC) and large cell neuroendocrine carcinoma (LCNEC) are uncommon but highly aggressive neoplasms. From a diagnostic point of view, there may be problems both in distinguishing these from other neoplasms and in confirming a cervical origin. This is important as management is critically dependent on the correct histologic diagnosis. We undertook a detailed immunohistochemical analysis of a relatively large series of primary cervical SCNEC (n = 13) and LCNEC (n = 8). Cases were stained with AE1/3, chromogranin, CD56, synaptophysin, PGP9.5, TTF1, p16, p63, CK7, CK20, neurofilament, and CD99. CK20 and neurofilament staining was undertaken to investigate whether some of these neoplasms might exhibit a Merkel cell immunophenotype and CD99 staining to assess whether there is immunohistochemical overlap with neoplasms in the Ewing family of tumors (EFT). For all markers, staining was classified as negative, 1+ (<10% cells immunoreactive), 2+ (10 to 50% cells immunoreactive), or 3+ (>50% cells immunoreactive). Eleven and 6 SCNEC and LCNEC, respectively were positive with AE1/3. Chromogranin, CD56, synaptophysin, and PGP9.5 were positive in 11, 19, 19, and 9 cases, respectively. Altogether 15 cases (71%) (11 SCNEC, 4 LCNEC) exhibited nuclear positivity, often diffuse, with TTF1. All but 1 case was diffusely positive with p16. p63 was positive in 9 cases, including 5 with diffuse nuclear immunoreactivity. Ten and 4 neoplasms were positive with CK7 and CK20, respectively. Neurofilament was positive in 7 tumors. The 4 neoplasms that were CK20 positive were stained with the monoclonal antibody CM2B4, generated against an antigenic epitope on the Merkel cell polyomavirus T antigen; all were negative. CD99 was positive in 6 cases. In 2 cases, adjacent foci of adenocarcinoma in situ (AIS) contained scattered individual chromogranin positive cells, raising the possibility that some cervical neuroendocrine carcinomas arise from neuroendocrine cells in AIS. Four of 13 cases of pure AIS also contained scattered chromogranin positive cells. Our results illustrate that a proportion of cervical neuroendocrine carcinomas are negative with broad spectrum cytokeratins and some of the commonly used neuroendocrine markers. TTF1 positivity is extremely common and may be a useful marker of a neuroendocrine carcinoma. It is of no value in exclusion of a pulmonary primary. p16 is almost always positive in cervical neuroendocrine carcinomas, possibly owing to an association with oncogenic human papillomavirus, although other mechanisms of expression are also possible. Cervical neuroendocrine carcinomas may be p63 positive, illustrating that this marker is not specific for squamous differentiation. CK20 and neurofilament positivity in some cervical neuroendocrine carcinomas is in keeping with a Merkel cell immunophenotype, similar to that described in SCNECs in other organs. However, the absence of staining with CM2B4 argues against a true Merkel cell tumor. CD99 staining in a cervical neuroendocrine carcinoma should not result in misdiagnosis as a neoplasm in the Ewing family of tumors (Fig 2).

▶ This article examines the immunophenotype of 21 cases of small cell neuroendocrine carcinoma (SCNEC, 13 cases) and large cell neuroendocrine carcinoma (LCNEC, 8 cases) of the cervix—uncommon lesions that pursue an aggressive course and have a predilection for systemic spread. The authors

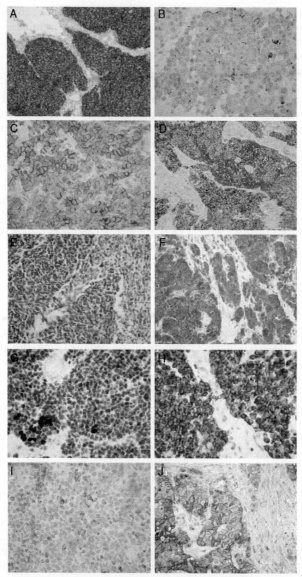

FIGURE 2.—Cervical small cell neuroendocrine carcinoma (SCNEC) exhibiting diffuse immunoreactivity with chromogranin (A). Another SCNEC exhibits focal immunoreactivity with chromogranin with a punctuate pattern (B), diffuse membranous positivity with CD56 (C) and diffuse cytoplasmic staining with synaptophysin (D). Cervical SCNEC exhibiting diffuse nuclear immunoreactivity with TTF1 (E). Cervical large cell neuroendocrine carcinoma (LCNEC) exhibiting diffuse nuclear and cytoplasmic p16 staining (F). Cervical SCNEC exhibiting diffuse nuclear p63 immunoreactivity (G). Cervical SCNEC exhibiting diffuse CK20 immunoreactivity (H). Cervical SCNEC exhibiting focal neurofilament immunoreactivity (I). Cervical SCNEC exhibiting CD99 membranous immunoreactivity (J). (Reprinted from McCluggage WG, Kennedy K, Busam KJ. An immunohistochemical study of cervical neuroendocrine carcinomas: Neoplasms that are commonly TTF1 positive and which may express CK20 and P63. *Am J Surg Pathol.* 2010;34:525-532.)

found results consistent with those of previous studies, namely that most of tumors express cytokeratin AE1/3 (81%), p16 (95%), and at least 1 of the 4 examined neuroendocrine markers (CD56—90%, synaptophysin—90%, chromogranin—52%, PGP9.5—43%, 100% of cases had at least 1 marker positive). Additionally, they found frequent expression of thyroid transcription factor 1 (71%), as has been detected in small cell carcinomas arising in other sites and make the point that this should not be interpreted as evidence of a pulmonary metastasis. Immunohistochemistry for p63 also showed frequent nuclear positivity (43%), which is significant as some SCNEC or LCNEC can resemble squamous cell carcinomas but are treated quite differently. Representative images are shown in Fig 2.

The point is repeatedly made that while immunohistochemistry can be quite valuable in identifying these rare lesions, the diagnosis can be made even in the absence of cytokeratin or neuroendocrine marker staining, provided the typical morphologic features are present, including hyperchromatic nuclei with molding and streaming, scant cytoplasm, and absence of squamous or glandular differentiation for SCNEC and large polygonal cells with low nuclear to cytoplasmic ratio, coarse chromatin with prominent nucleoli, and greater than 10 mitoses per 10 high-powered fields for LCNEC.

The primary importance of this study lies in its focus on the recognition of a rare but highly aggressive neoplasm seen in the cervix and delineation of commonly seen immunophenotypes. The authors explore the possibility of dividing cervical neuroendocrine carcinomas into pulmonary type and Merkel cell type, as has been done in the major salivary glands,[1] although they conclude that further study is needed to determine if this has a similar prognostic significance in the cervix. They also address the differential diagnosis of tumors in the Ewing family of tumors (EFT) and demonstrate that at least 2 of the 4 CD99-positive cases also contained an oncogenic strain of human papillomavirus (HPV), arguing against EFT, as those tumors are not known to be HPV associated.

For further reading on this subject, see also articles by Connor et al[2] and Gilks et al.[3]

M. D. Post, MD

References

1. Nagao T, Gaffey TA, Olsen KD, Serizawa H, Lewis JE. Small cell carcinoma of the major salivary glands: clinicopathologic study with emphasis on cytokeratin 20 immunoreactivity and clinical outcome. *Am J Surg Pathol.* 2004;28:762-770.
2. Conner MG, Richter H, Moran CA, Hameed A, Albores-Saavedra J. Small cell carcinoma of the cervix: a clinicopathologic and immunohistochemical study of 23 cases. *Ann Diagn Pathol.* 2002;6:345-348.
3. Gilks CB, Young RH, Gersell DJ, Clement PB. Large cell neuroendocrine carcinoma of the uterine cervix: a clinicopathologic study of 12 cases. *Am J Surg Pathol.* 1997;21:905-914.

Endometrial carcinoma: controversies in histopathological assessment of grade and tumour cell type

Clarke BA, Gilks CB (Univ of Toronto, Ontario, Canada; Univ of British Columbia, Vancouver, Canada)

J Clin Pathol 63:410-415, 2010

Histopathological assessment of tumour grade and cell type is central to the management of endometrial carcinoma, guiding the extent of surgery and the use of adjuvant radiation therapy and chemotherapy. Endometrioid carcinomas are usually low grade but high grade examples are encountered, and they have a significantly worse prognosis, similar to that of high grade subtypes such as serous and clear cell carcinoma. This article reviews the various grading systems that have been proposed for use with endometrioid endometrial carcinoma, and discusses the recent progress in cell type assignment, including the use of immunohistochemistry as a diagnostic adjunct.

▶ This article first addresses the universal International Federation for Gynecology and Obstetrics (FIGO) grading system for endometrial cancers and attempts to elucidate whether modification or switching to another system would prove beneficial. The most important factors in developing any grading system for cancers are reproducibility and clinical significance. After a brief review of multiple recently proposed modifications, the authors conclude that histopathological assessment can only reproducibly distinguish 2 prognostic groups of endometrioid carcinoma: high grade and low grade. Of the proposed binary systems, they advocate for combining FIGO grades 1 and 2 into a low-grade category based on familiarity, ease of use, and support by available data. They do reiterate that adjunctive molecular tests may ultimately prove much more useful for risk stratification.

The next aspect of tumor analysis they tackle is assignment of cell type in endometrial cancers. This too is of critical importance, as various histological subtypes have dramatically different prognoses and may respond to different chemotherapeutic agents. The primary difficulties lie in distinguishing between endometrioid and serous, clear cell and serous, and undifferentiated and endometrioid cell types. The authors briefly review a variety of immunohistochemical stains that may be used as an adjunct to careful hematoxylin and eosin (H&E) assessment, concluding that a panel consisting of p53, PTEN, estrogen receptor, and p16 is likely to be most helpful.

The strength of this article lies in its bringing forward a key issue in gynecological pathology and in trying to determine whether the currently universal grading system for endometrial cancers is in fact the best one. Although any widespread change in the field will take some time, by highlighting the pitfalls and arbitrary nature of the current system, these authors do a good job of beginning the dialogue to move this field toward a more reproducible and clinically significant goal. Similarly, the importance of accurately classifying tumor cell types cannot be overemphasized, and here is a nice review of commonly available immunohistochemical markers for those rare cases in which H&E

analysis alone is insufficient for definitive determination. For additional reading, see the reference section.[1,2,3]

M. D. Post, MD

References

1. Lax SF, Kurman RJ, Pizer ES, Wu L, Ronnett BM. A binary architectural grading system for uterine endometrial endometrioid carcinoma has superior reproducibility compared with FIGO grading and identifies subsets of advance-stage tumors with favorable and unfavorable prognosis. *Am J Surg Pathol.* 2000;24:1201-1208.
2. Kapucuoglu N, Bulbul D, Tulunay G, Temel MA. Reproducibility of grading systems for endometrial endometrioid carcinoma and their relation with pathologic prognostic parameters. *Int J Gynecol Cancer.* 2008;18:790-796.
3. Alkushi A, Clarke BA, Akbari M, et al. Identification of prognostically relevant and reproducible subsets of endometrial adenocarcinoma based on clustering analysis of immunostaining data. *Mod Pathol.* 2007;20:1156-1165.

Evaluation of vascular space involvement in endometrial adenocarcinomas: laparoscopic *vs* abdominal hysterectomies
Folkins AK, Nevadunsky NS, Saleemuddin A, et al (Brigham and Women's Hosp, Boston, MA)
Mod Pathol 23:1073-1079, 2010

Recent reports have described 'vascular pseudoinvasion' in total laparoscopic hysterectomies with endometrial carcinoma. To better understand this phenomenon, we compared pathologic findings in these laparoscopic and total abdominal hysterectomies performed for uterine endometrioid adenocarcinoma. Reports from 58 robotically assisted laparoscopic and 39 abdominal hysterectomies with grade 1 or 2 endometrioid endometrial adenocarcinomas were reviewed for stage, depth of invasion, vascular space involvement, uterine weight, and lymph node metastases. In addition, attention was given to possible procedural artifacts, including vertical endomyometrial clefts, and inflammatory debris, benign endometrial glands, and disaggregated tumor cells in vascular spaces. All foci with vascular involvement were reviewed by three gynecologic pathologists. Nine of the 58 (16%) laparoscopic and 3 of the 39 (7%) abdominal hysterectomies contained vascular space involvement based on the original pathology reports (P-value = 0.0833). No one histologic feature consistently distinguished laparoscopic from abdominal cases on blind review of the available cases. Disaggregated intravascular tumor cells were significantly associated with *reported* vascular involvement in both procedures (P-values < 0.001 and 0.016), most of which were corroborated on review. Laparoscopic procedures tend to have a higher index of vascular involvement, which is associated with lower stage, fewer lymph node metastases, and less myometrial invasion; however, pathologists cannot consistently determine the procedure on histologic findings alone. Moreover, there is significant interobserver variability in distinguishing true from artifactual vascular space involvement, even among pathologists at the same institution. The clinical

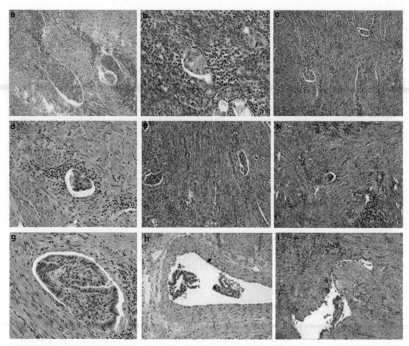

FIGURE 2.—Microscopic fields reflecting a consensus diagnosis of vascular space involvement (a–c), suspicious for vascular space involvement (d–f), and presumed artifact (g–i). (Reprinted from Folkins AK, Nevadunsky NS, Saleemuddin A, et al. Evaluation of vascular space involvement in endometrial adeno-carcinomas: laparoscopic vs abdominal hysterectomies. *Mod Pathol.* 2010;23:1073-1079. Reprinted by permission from Macmillan Publishers Ltd: Modern Pathology, copyright 2010.)

significance of apparent true vascular space involvement seen adjacent to artifacts is unclear, as is the impact of laparoscopic hysterectomy on recurrence risk (Fig 2 and Table 1).

▶ The presence or absence of vascular space involvement in grade 1 and 2 endometrioid carcinomas can have a major impact on posthysterectomy treatment options. This article examines whether a difference exists in artifactual pseudoinvasion depending on the type of procedure (total laparoscopic hysterectomy vs total abdominal hysterectomy) and characterized those features useful to distinguish true from artifactual vascular space involvement. The use of a large number of cases and independent blinded reviewers lends strength to their findings, although these showed that there is the potential for marked disagreement as to what constitutes true vascular space involvement even among pathologists in the same department. In contrast to previous studies, these authors did not find a significant difference in vascular space involvement based on type of hysterectomy performed, although there was a trend toward increased vascular space involvement in laparoscopic procedures, perhaps as an artifactual result of increased intrauterine pressure from the balloon tip manipulator typically used. The authors believe that the most likely reason for

TABLE 1.—Criteria for True and Artifactual Lymphovascular Involvement

True Lymphovascular Space Involvement	Artifactual Lymphovascular Space Involvement
Smooth bordered cohesive clusters of tumor cells	Disaggregated tumor cells, often intermixed with inflammation
Conform to the contours of the lymphovascular space	Floating in the lymphovascular space
Often a change in morphology with more eosinophilic cytoplasm	Similar morphology to intact tumor, sometimes as intact fragments
Lymphatic space adjacent to larger vessels	Spaces are immediately adjacent to invasive tumor with retraction artifact

this is related to varied pathologist interpretation of true vascular space invasion rather than actual procedural differences. The criteria that they felt to be most indicative of true versus artifactual vascular space invasion are depicted in Table 1 and Fig 2.

Here examined are cases of laparoscopic and abdominal hysterectomies performed for grade 1 or 2 endometrioid carcinoma, looking specifically at the phenomenon of artifactual vascular space involvement. They conclude that the determination of real versus artifactual vascular space involvement cannot be reliably sorted out by a single reviewer. This suggests that changes be made where necessary to grossing procedures to minimize the likelihood of artifact arising from that source and potentially having multiple pathologists review cases of suspected vascular space involvement to arrive at a consensus regarding the veracity of this finding. The importance of the article is in highlighting the variability that can exist in interpretation of a pathologic finding with critical clinical implications.

M. D. Post, MD

Expression profiling of 22 genes involved in the PI3K–AKT pathway identifies two subgroups of high-grade endometrial carcinomas with different molecular alterations

Catasus L, D'Angelo E, Pons C, et al (Autonomous Univ of Barcelona, Spain)
Mod Pathol 23:694-702, 2010

Previously, we showed that *PIK3CA* and *p53* alterations in uterine endometrial carcinomas correlate with poor prognosis. However, the contribution of phosphatidylinositol 3-kinase (PI3K) –AKT deregulation to endometrial carcinogenesis is not completely understood. The purpose of this study was to analyze alterations of this pathway in endometrial carcinomas and correlate them with the most common genetic abnormalities. Expression profiling of 22 genes involved in PI3K–AKT signaling pathway was analyzed in 38 endometrial carcinomas using TaqMan low-density array (TLDA) analysis. The gene expression pattern was analyzed by hierarchical clustering analysis. Unsupervised clustering divided the high-grade endometrial carcinomas into two clusters. One cluster identified tumors with alterations in the PI3K–AKT signaling pathway (exon 20 *PIK3CA* mutations and/or *PTEN* mutations 9/15; 60%), and p16 protein overexpression (8/13; 62%). Almost all nonendometrioid adenocarcinomas (serous and clear cell adenocarcinomas) were segregated into this cluster. In contrast, the other cluster identified tumors with *p53* alterations (6/6; 100%), p16 protein overexpression (5/5; 100%), and exon 9 *PIK3CA* mutations (2/6; 33%). Exon 20 *PIK3CA* and *PTEN* mutations were not found in this subgroup. Low-grade endometrial carcinomas clustered in a third subgroup characterized by high frequency of *PTEN* mutations (10/17; 59%) and microsatellite instability (6/17; 35%). Our results show that gene expression profile differences in the PI3K–AKT signaling pathway identify two subgroups of high-grade endometrial carcinomas with different molecular alterations (PI3K–AKT pathway *vs* p53 alterations) that may have distinct roles in endometrial carcinogenesis. Identification of these subgroups can provide insight into the biology of these tumors and may facilitate the development of future treatments.

▶ While it is well recognized that there are 2 major types of endometrial carcinoma with proposed different molecular mechanisms propelling tumorigenesis, the exact mechanisms have yet to be fully elucidated. Using TaqMan low-density array (TLDA) analysis of 22 genes involved in the phosphatidylinositol 3-kinase (PI3K)-AKT signaling pathway, the authors were able to separate 38 endometrial tumors into 3 clusters, which had corresponding clinicopathologic distinctions. The analysis of genes differentially over- or underexpressed in each cluster provides insight into the biology of endometrial carcinomas and offers potential targets for chemotherapeutic agents.

They selected a similar number of high-grade tumors (n = 21) and low-grade tumors (n = 17) for analysis and included endometrioid carcinomas of all 3 grades as well as serous carcinomas, clear cell carcinomas, and mixed-type carcinomas. Following TLDA and hierarchical clustering analysis, the tumors separated into 3 groups. The first contained 15 tumors, 14 (93%) of which were high-grade carcinomas. Many genes were upregulated (arbitrarily designated for this study as twice that seen in the reference sample) in this group, most notably *CCND1* and *E-CADH*, which were both upregulated by more than 8-fold. Cluster 2 contained 17 tumors, including all grade 1 and most grade 2 endometrioid carcinomas (15/17). These tumors showed upregulation of *p21*, *FAK*, *PAK1*, and *CCND1* and downregulation of *CASP3*, *Foxo1A*, *PIK3CA*, *p27*, and *NFKB*. The final cluster contained 6 tumors, 5 (83%) of which were high grade. These showed overexpression of *PTEN* and underexpression of *XIAP*. Statistically significant clinicopathological prognostic parameters, which varied by cluster, included histological subtype and grade. *PTEN* mutations were significantly more frequent in cluster 2 tumors than in cluster 1 tumors (59% vs 27%), while *p53* alterations were present in all cluster 3 tumors compared with 29% (4/14) cluster 1 tumors and no cluster 2 tumors. Expression of p16 protein also varied significantly, as it was strongly positive in all cluster 3 tumors compared with 62% (8/13) cluster 1 tumors and 7% (1/15) cluster 2 tumors. Interestingly, the 2 clusters containing most high-grade carcinomas both had *PIK3CA* mutations but in different axons (exon 20 in cluster 1 and exon 9 in cluster 3). Based in part on this information, the authors advance the idea for the existence of a dualistic model for high-grade endometrial carcinomas.

The primary limitations of this study include the relatively small sample size and the as-yet undetermined significance of finding over- or underexpression of various genes in different subgroups of endometrial carcinomas. However, it had been well established that deregulation of the PI3K-AKT signaling pathway has profound effects on genes that inhibit apoptosis and promote cell proliferation. By coupling gene expression profiling with hierarchical cluster analysis, it becomes possible to evaluate genetic heterogeneity in carcinomas and is useful to develop expression-based classifications that may facilitate development of novel treatments for endometrial cancers. For additional reading, please see the reference section.[1]

M. D. Post, MD

Reference

1. Hayes MP, Ellenson LH. Molecular alterations in uterine serous carcinoma. *Gynecol Oncol.* 2010;116:286-289.

---

p16 Expression in Squamous and Trophoblastic Lesions of the Upper Female Genital Tract

Chew I, Post MD, Carinelli SG, et al (Massachusetts General Hosp, Boston; Univ of Colorado, Denver; Mangiagalli e Regina Elena, Milano, Italy; et al)
Int J Gynecol Pathol 29:513-522, 2010

---

p16, a surrogate marker for human papillomavirus (HPV) infection, is uniformly present in HPV-related carcinomas. This study aims to further characterize p16 expression in trophoblastic lesions and squamous lesions of the upper female genital tract, as little data exists. p16 immunostaining was performed on sections from ichthyosis uteri (1), primary uterine corpus squamous cell carcinoma (UCSCC) (2), primary ovarian SCC (OSCC) (5; 2 associated with a dermoid cyst), endometrial endometrioid adenocarcinoma with extensive squamous differentiation (EC-SD) (5), ovarian endometrioid adenocarcinoma with extensive squamous differentiation (OCSD) (4), placental site nodule (5), and placental site trophoblastic tumor (PSTT) (6). We evaluated the percentage of positive cytoplasmic and nuclear staining (focal = < 10%, multifocal = 10% to 50%, and diffuse = > 50%) and staining intensity (weak, moderate, and strong). HPV-DNA analysis by polymerase chain reaction was performed on 5 OSCC. Ichthyosis uteri, all UCSCC and 1 OSCC (arising in a dermoid) were negative; the other dermoid-associated OSCC showed focal moderate staining, the remaining OSCC displayed strong (100%), diffuse

(2), or multifocal (1) p16 positivity. Three of the 5 ECSD cases showed strong diffuse staining of the squamous component. The glandular component focally showed strong p16 positivity (2), with variably intense focal staining in 3 cases. The squamous component of all OC-SD showed focal moderate staining, with variable staining of the glandular component. Overall, 3 EC-SD had 80% to 90% p16 positivity. Five of the 5 placental site nodules and 4 of the 6 PSTT showed focal weak staining, whereas 2 PSTT were p16 negative. HPV-DNA analysis was negative in 3 of the 5 OSCC, the other 2 cases being technical failures. p16 is expressed in OSCC and in the squamous and glandular components of EC-SD and OC-SD. As p16 is negative in UCSCC, it may help to identify the origin of SCC diffusely involving the corpus and cervix, and suggests different pathogeneses for SCC of the upper female genital tract, likely to be unrelated to HPV infection. In contrast to earlier data, we found weak and focal p16 expression in trophoblastic lesions. Thus, when considering the differential diagnosis of cervical SCC and trophoblastic lesions, only strong diffuse p16 staining should be considered helpful.

▶ It is widely recognized that p16^{INK4a} (p16) is useful as a surrogate marker for human papillomavirus (HPV) infection in carcinomas of cervical origin; however, less is known about the expression pattern in lesions of the upper female genital tract or whether expression in this location is related to HPV infection. Although uncommon, primary squamous cell carcinomas of the uterine corpus and ovary do occur, and distinguishing these from metastatic cervical lesions has important clinical implications. Furthermore, p16 has been reported to be negative in trophoblastic lesions, which occasionally enter the differential diagnosis of squamous carcinomas; however, a relatively small number of cases has been studied.

In this article, the authors explore the immunohistochemical expression pattern of p16 in 28 lesions from the uterine corpus and ovary, including pure squamous cell carcinomas, endometrioid carcinomas with extensive squamous differentiation, and trophoblastic lesions (placental site nodule and placental site trophoblastic tumor). They also examine the connection between p16 positivity in ovarian squamous cell carcinoma (seen in all 3 cases not arising from dermoid cysts) and HPV infection. None of the cases were found to have HPV DNA by polymerase chain reaction, implying that p16 staining does not serve as a useful surrogate of infection in this setting. While most of the findings here support those previously reported, the one area in which the current findings differ is the one showing focal moderate staining of trophoblastic lesions (Fig 7 in the original article).

The importance of these findings is to serve as a caveat to practicing pathologists regarding overreliance on any single immunohistochemical stain. Despite a lack of association with HPV infection, there are multiple lesions described here that show varying levels of p16 expression, potentially leading to serious misdiagnoses if unduly relied upon. Although p16 is a very useful marker in cases of cervical biopsies that are indeterminant for dysplasia, it is increasingly being shown to be positive in a host of other lesions, limiting its more global utility. For additional reading, see reference section.[1,2]

M. D. Post, MD

References

1. O'Neill CJ, McCluggage WG. p16 expression in the female genital tract and its value in diagnosis. *Adv Anat Pathol.* 2006;13:8-15.
2. Pins MR, Young RH, Crum CP, Leach IH, Scully RE. Cervical squamous cell carcinoma in situ with intraepithelial extension to the upper genital tract and invasion of tubes and ovaries: report of a case with human papilloma virus analysis. *Int J Gynecol Pathol.* 1997;16:272-278.

Are All Pelvic (Nonuterine) Serous Carcinomas of Tubal Origin?

Przybycin CG, Kurman RJ, Ronnett BM, et al (The Johns Hopkins Univ School of Medicine, Baltimore, MD)
Am J Surg Pathol 34:1407-1416, 2010

It has been proposed that the presence of tubal intraepithelial carcinoma (TIC), in association with one-third to nearly half of pelvic serous carcinomas, is evidence of fallopian tube origin for high-grade serous carcinomas that would have been otherwise classified as primary ovarian or peritoneal. To address this hypothesis, we evaluated a series of 114 consecutive pelvic (nonuterine) gynecologic carcinomas at our institution (2006 to 2008) to determine the frequency of TIC in 52 cases in which all the resected fallopian tube tissue was examined microscopically. These 52 cases were classified as ovarian (n = 37), peritoneal (n = 8), or fallopian tube (n = 7) in origin as per conventional criteria based on disease distribution. The presence of TIC and its location and relationship to invasive carcinoma in the fallopian tubes and ovaries were assessed. Among the 45 cases of ovarian/peritoneal origin, carcinoma subtypes included 41 high-grade serous, 1 endometrioid, 1 mucinous, 1 high-grade, not otherwise specified, and 1 malignant mesodermal mixed tumor. TIC was identified in 24 cases (59%) of high-grade serous carcinoma but not among any of the other subtypes; therefore, the term serous TIC (STIC) is a more specific appellation. STICs were located in the fimbriated end of the tube in 22 cases (92%) and in the ampulla in 2 (8%); they were unilateral in 21 (88%) and bilateral in 3 (13%). STICs in the absence of an associated invasive carcinoma in the same tube were detected in 7 cases (30%) and with invasive carcinoma in the same tube in 17 (71%). Unilateral STICs were associated with bilateral ovarian involvement in 15 cases and unilateral (ipsilateral) ovarian involvement in 5 (the remaining case with a unilateral STIC had a primary peritoneal tumor with no ovarian involvement); the bilateral STICs were all associated with bilateral ovarian involvement. Six of the 7 primary tubal tumors were high-grade serous carcinomas, and 4 of these 6 (67%) had STICs. Based on conventional criteria, 70%, 17%, and 13% of high-grade serous carcinomas qualified for classification as ovarian, peritoneal, and tubal in origin, respectively; however, using STIC as a supplemental criterion to define a case as tubal in origin, the distribution was modified to 28%, 8%, and 64%, respectively. Features of tumors in the ovary that generally suggest metastatic disease (bilaterality, small size, nodular growth pattern, and surface plaques) were identified with similar frequency in cases with and without STIC and were, therefore, not predictive of tubal origin. The findings, showing that nearly 60% of high-grade pelvic (nonuterine) serous carcinomas are associated with STICs, are consistent with the proposal that the fallopian tube is the source of a majority of these tumors. If these findings can be validated by molecular studies that definitively establish that STIC is the earliest form of carcinoma rather than intraepithelial spread from adjacent invasive serous carcinoma of ovarian or peritoneal origin, they will have important clinical implications for screening, treatment, and prevention.

▶ This article further explores the relationship between tubal intraepithelial carcinoma (TIC) and identification of primary site of origin of pelvic (nonuterine) carcinomas. Although limited by a relatively small number of cases (n = 52), the authors performed a comprehensive examination of these cases and drew some important conclusions, namely that the incidence of pelvic serous carcinomas originating in the fallopian tube (64% in this study) may be much higher than the classically quoted incidence (2%-6%) when TIC is used as a supplemental criterion to define a case as tubal in origin. While currently treatment of pelvic serous cancers does not vary based on site of origin, accurate classification and knowledge about the earliest form of this devastating disease may have significant implications for development of methods of early detection, treatment, and prevention. Furthermore, developing consensus among pathologists is important for future epidemiologic studies using cancer registry databases.

Here the authors examined consecutive cases of pelvic gynecologic carcinomas spanning a 2-year period at their institution in which all visible fallopian tube tissue was resected and processed for microscopic examination (using the sectioning and extensively examining the fimbria (SEE-FIM) protocol, which extensively examines the fimbriated end of the tube[1]). Fifty-two cases fit these criteria, of which 47 were high-grade serous carcinomas, shown to be the only histologic subtype associated with TIC. By conventional criteria, the site of origin was considered ovarian, peritoneal, and tubal in 71%, 15%, and 13% cases, respectively. Of the high-grade serous carcinoma cases classified as ovarian or peritoneal primaries (n = 41), TIC was identified in 24 cases (59%), predominantly in the fimbriated end of the fallopian tube (22 cases). Four of the 6 cases classified as primary tubal serous carcinomas had TIC (67%). In cases with or without TIC, there was not a significant difference (although formal statistics were not performed) between size of ovarian tumor, frequency of bilateral ovarian involvement, or tumor growth pattern in the ovary. By incorporating the presence of TIC into determination of site of origin, the studied cases were reclassified as ovarian, peritoneal, or tubal carcinomas in 28%, 8%, and 64%, respectively (see Fig 8 in the original article).

Because the only histologic subtype associated with TIC was high-grade serous carcinomas, the authors support the previously proposed change in nomenclature to serous TIC (STIC). There are 3 proposed explanations to account for the concurrent presence of STIC and primary ovarian or peritoneal high-grade serous carcinoma. The first is that these are primary fallopian tube carcinomas with secondary involvement of the ovary/peritoneum, the second is that they originate in the ovary or peritoneum with intraepithelial spread to the fallopian tube, or lastly that they are independent primary lesions. Based on this and previous studies, the authors conclude that the weight of evidence supports the first interpretation. They do acknowledge that although there is mounting evidence that ovarian high-grade serous carcinomas in fact originate in the fallopian tube, not every case was associated with STIC. They offer a variety of explanations for this but ultimately conclude that more definitive molecular genetic studies are required to determine if fallopian tube epithelium gives rise to the vast majority of pelvic serous carcinomas. For additional reading see the reference section.[1,2]

M. D. Post, MD

References

1. Medeiros F, Muto MG, Lee Y, et al. The tubal fimbria is a preferred site for early adenocarcinoma in women with familial ovarian cancer syndrome. *Am J Surg Pathol.* 2006;30:230-236.
2. Lee Y, Miron A, Drapkin R, et al. A candidate precursor to serous carcinoma that originates in the distal fallopian tube. *J Pathol.* 2007;211:26-35.

Diagnosis of Ovarian Carcinoma Cell Type is Highly Reproducible: A Transcanadian Study

Köbel M, Kalloger SE, Baker PM, et al (Univ of Calgary, Canada; Vancouver General Hosp and British Columbia Cancer Agency, Canada; Univ of Manitoba, Winnipeg, Canada; et al)
Am J Surg Pathol 34:984-993, 2010

Reproducible diagnosis of ovarian carcinoma cell types is critical for cell type-specific treatment. The purpose of this study was to test the reproducibility of cell type diagnosis across Canada. Analysis of the interobserver reproducibility of histologic tumor type was performed among 6 pathologists after brief training in the use of modified World Health Organization criteria to classify ovarian carcinomas into 1 of 6 categories: high-grade serous, endometrioid, clear cell, mucinous, low-grade serous, and other. These 6 pathologists independently reviewed a test set of 40 ovarian carcinomas. A validation set of 88 consecutive ovarian carcinomas drawn from 5 centers was subject to local review by 1 of the 6 study pathologists, and central review by a single observer. Interobserver agreement was assessed through calculation of concordance and κ values for pair-wise comparison. For the test set, the paired concordance between pathologists in cell type diagnosis ranged from 85.0% to 97.5% (average 92.3%), and the κ values were 0.80 to 0.97 (average 0.89). Inclusion of immunostaining results did not significantly improve reproducibility ($P = 0.69$). For the validation set, the concordance between original diagnosis and local review was 84% and between local review and central review was 94%. The κ values were 0.73 and 0.89, respectively. With a brief training exercise and the use of defined criteria for ovarian carcinoma subtyping, there is excellent interobserver reproducibility in diagnosis of cell type. This has implications for clinical trials of subtype-specific ovarian carcinoma treatments.

▶ One of the most challenging areas of gynecological pathology is the accurate classification of the histologic subtype of some ovarian carcinomas. Multiple studies have historically shown a lack of reproducibility in such diagnoses, despite increasingly commonly recognized features shared by carcinomas of the same cell type (Fig 2 in the original article). Although, to date, the histologic subtype of ovarian carcinomas has not had a major impact on treatment decisions, this is changing, as there is increasing evidence that these are biologically distinct entities with varied responses to different chemotherapeutic or radiation treatments.[1]

For this study, the authors participated in a training session consisting of individual then group review of 40 cases focusing on current criteria for diagnosis of different histologic subtypes. They then assessed the test sample of 40 cases, first by hematoxylin and eosin (H&E) alone, then with immunohistochemical results. Lastly, they evaluated 88 cases from clinical practice at 5 medical centers. Selected immunohistochemical results were provided following H&E review and initial diagnosis. The authors found that a relatively brief orientation was followed by a high level of concordance (average $\kappa = 0.9$) in the test set and only slightly lower agreement (average $\kappa = 0.77$) in the validation set.

The implications of this study are far reaching, as greater accuracy in subclassification of ovarian tumors could have a marked impact on treatment decisions and future studies of tumor pathogenesis. Interestingly, the authors found that the addition of immunohistochemistry only slightly improved their agreement, although they do point out that for pathologists who see relatively few ovarian carcinoma cases, ancillary studies may be of greater benefit, as they are in small biopsy samples. The slides reviewed for the test and training sets in this article are available online at: http://www.gpecimage.ubc.ca/aperio/images/transcanadian/. For additional reading, see references.[2,3]

M. D. Post, MD

References

1. Köbel M, Kalloger SE, Santos JL, Huntsman DG, Gilks CB, Swenerton KD. Tumor type and substage predict survival in stage I and II ovarian carcinoma: insights and implications. *Gynecol Oncol.* 2010;116:50-56.

2. Malpica A, Deavers MT, Tornos C, et al. Interobserver and intraobserver variability of a two-tier system for grading ovarian serous carcinoma. *Am J Surg Pathol.* 2007;31:1168-1174.

3. McCluggage WG. My approach to and thoughts on the typing of ovarian carcinomas. *J Clin Pathol.* 2008;61:152-163.

The clinicopathological characteristics of 'triple-negative' epithelial ovarian cancer

Liu N, Wang X, Sheng X (Shandong Cancer Hosp and Inst, Jinan, PR China)
J Clin Pathol 63:240-243, 2010

Background.—'Triple-negative' is traditionally used to define a specific subtype of breast cancer with negative oestrogen receptor (ER), progesterone receptor (PR) and human epidermal growth factor receptor-type 2 (HER2) expressions. ER/PR and HER2 testing is also widely used in the informative classification of ovarian cancer.

Aim.—To investigate whether a 'triple-negative' subtype also exists in ovarian cancer.

Methods.—ER, PR and HER2 expressions in 116 Chinese women with primary epithelial ovarian cancer were reviewed. Triple-negative epithelial ovarian cancer (TNEOC) was defined based on negative ER, PR and HER2 expression. The clinicopathological characteristics and Ki-67, P53 and epidermal growth factor receptor (EGFR) expression in the TNEOC and non-TNEOC group were compared.

Results.—15.5% of cases (18/116) were identified as TNEOC among 116 ovarian carcinomas. Histological grade 3 was found in a higher percentage of the TNEOC than of the non-TNEOC group (94.4% vs 62.2%). TNEOC also correlated with a high level of Ki-67 and p53 expression. EGFR overexpression and other clinicopathological characteristics were not significantly associated with TNEOC subtype. TNEOC was associated with a shorter progression free survival and overall survival in univariate and multivariate analyses.

Conclusions.—A novel subtype of ovarian carcinoma, which is negative for ER, PR and HER2 expression, has been identified; this specific ovarian subtype tends to have aggressive characteristics and a poor prognosis, which is similar to triple-negative breast cancer in most respects. TNEOC should be considered in future investigations of informative classification of ovarian cancer.

▶ There is a subset of breast carcinomas (approximately 10%-19%) that are negative for estrogen receptor (ER) and progesterone receptor (PR) and lack HER2 overexpression; these are referred to as triple-negative breast cancers (TNBCs). Similarly, there is a newly evolving concept of TN epithelial ovarian cancers (TNEOCs); however, these are not well characterized with regard to associated clinicopathologic parameters or outcome data. This article examines 116 cases of EOC to determine expression patterns of hormone receptors and other markers as well as clinicopathologic characteristics potentially associated with these tumors. All cases were pathologically examined to determine histopathologic subtype, grade, and stage. Immunohistochemistry was performed on all cases to look at ER, PR, p53, epidermal growth factor receptor (EGFR), and Ki-67, while chromogenic in situ hybridization (CISH) was performed to look for HER2 amplification (defined as > 6 copies in > 50% of cancer cell nuclei). Clinical information was collected with respect to optimal cytoreduction (defined as < 1 cm residual disease following surgery) and response to cisplatin-based chemotherapy, which all patients received postoperatively. Follow-up was on average 43 months.

The authors found that 15.5% (18/116) cases were TN; however, there was no statistically significant link to age, histology, stage, cytoreduction, or response to treatment. The only factor significantly linked to TN status was grade (94.4% of TNEOC were grade 3 compared with 62.2% of non-TNEOC). Although p53 and Ki-67 were more frequent in TNEOC, EGFR overexpression was not correlated to TN status, unlike what is seen in breast cancer. This suggests that there are different molecular mechanisms operating in cases of TNEOC compared with TNBC, an area which needs to be explored in more detail in the future. Similar to what is seen in TNBC, the TNEOC cases had a shorter progression-free survival and overall survival, with TN status being an independent prognostic factor. This last point is perhaps the most pertinent conclusion the authors draw, as routine testing for ER, PR, and HER2 is not currently universally used in ovarian cancer cases yet could influence clinical management and counseling. The finding that TNEOC is associated with cancer grade offers a possible way to selectively screen cases for TN status, particularly in situations where global screening is not an option. The authors acknowledge that they have evaluated a relatively small sample size in this study and that further investigation into the area is needed; it will be very interesting to see whether recommendations for changes in either evaluation or management of ovarian cancers are forthcoming as more research is performed.[1,2]

M. D. Post, MD

References

1. Reis-Filho JS, Tutt AN. Triple negative tumors: a critical review. *Histopathology.* 2008;52:108-118.
2. García-Velasco A, Mendiola C, Sánchez-Muñoz A, Ballestín C, Colomer R, Cortés-Funes H. Prognostic value of hormonal receptors, p53, ki67 and HER2/neu expression in epithelial ovarian carcinoma. *Clin Transl Oncol.* 2008; 10:367-371.

Tumor associated endothelial expression of B7-H3 predicts survival in ovarian carcinomas

Zang X, Sullivan PS, Soslow RA, et al (Howard Hughes Med Inst, NY; David Geffen School of Medicine at UCLA; Memorial Sloan-Kettering Cancer Ctr, NY)
Mod Pathol 23:1104-1112, 2010

B7-H3 and B7x are members of the B7 family of immune regulatory ligands that are thought to attenuate peripheral immune responses through co-inhibition. Previous studies have correlated their overexpression with poor prognosis and decreased tumor-infiltrating lymphocytes in various carcinomas including uterine endometrioid carcinomas, and mounting evidence supports an immuno-inhibitory role in ovarian cancer prognosis. We sought to examine the expression of B7-H3 and B7x in 103 ovarian borderline tumors and carcinomas and study associations with clinical outcome. Using immunohistochemical tissue microarray analysis on tumor specimens, we found that 93 and 100% of these ovarian tumors express B7-H3 and B7x, respectively, with expression found predominantly on cell membranes and in cytoplasm. In contrast, only scattered B7-H3-and B7x-positive cells were detected in non-neoplastic ovarian tissues. B7-H3 was also expressed in the endothelium of tumor-associated vasculature in 44% of patients, including 78% of patients with high-stage tumors (FIGO stages III and IV), nearly all of which were high-grade serous carcinomas, and 26% of patients with low-stage tumors (FIGO stages I and II; $P < 0.001$), including borderline tumors. Analysis of cumulative survival time and recurrence incidence revealed that carcinomas with B7-H3-positive tumor vasculature were associated with a significantly shorter survival time ($P = 0.02$) and a higher incidence of recurrence ($P = 0.03$). The association between B7-H3-positive tumor vasculature and poor clinical outcome remained significant even when the analysis was limited to the high-stage subgroup. These results show that ovarian borderline tumors and carcinomas aberrantly express B7-H3 and B7x, and that B7-H3-positive tumor vasculature is associated with high-grade serous histological subtype, increased recurrence and reduced survival. B7-H3 expression in tumor vasculature may be a reflection of tumor aggressiveness and has diagnostic and immunotherapeutic implications in ovarian carcinomas.

▶ Recent research into multiple cancers have shown that overall survival and recurrence rates are associated with the state of the local adaptive immune response, specifically the presence and activity of T-cells. T-cell costimulation and coinhibition are primarily generated by interactions between members of the B7 family of immuno regulatory ligands, which has been divided into 3 groups. The most recently identified group consists of B7-H3 and B7x, which are believed to attenuate peripheral immune responses through coinhibition. Their expression has been studied in other carcinomas and associated with aggressive behavior; however, the same investigation had not previously been conducted in ovarian carcinoma vasculature.

The authors selected 63 low-stage ovarian tumors (37 carcinomas and 26 borderline tumors) and 68 high-stage (International Federation of Gynecology and Obstetrics stage III or IV) tumors, then performed immunohistochemical analysis of B7-H3 and B7x expression in tumor cells and tumor-associated endothelial cells. Both were expressed in the vast majority (93%-100%) of tumors but not in nonneoplastic ovary. No difference in expression was noticed based on histologic subtype, although with the borderline tumors excluded, there was a significant correlation between expression and tumor stage. Although B7x was not expressed in tumor-associated endothelium, there was a statistically significant association between B7-H3 expression in these cells and histologic subtype, stage, shorter survival times, and cumulative recurrence incidence. These findings show that B7-H3 expression in tumor-associated vasculature predicts poorer survival, particularly in high-stage ovarian cancer patients. The authors postulate that ovarian tumor development and progression may be associated with downregulation of T cell-mediated antitumor immunity. It is not currently known what triggers B7-H3 expression in tumor vasculature; however, other studies have suggested that it may be involved in tumor angiogenesis. The significance of this study lies in its identification of a protein whose expression has the potential to be used as a diagnostic and prognostic aid for ovarian tumors. For additional reading see the reference section.[1,2]

M. D. Post, MD

References

1. Sato E, Olson SH, Ahn J, et al. Intraepithelial CD8+ tumor-infiltrating lymphocytes and a high CD8+/regulatory T cell ratio are associated with a favorable prognosis in ovarian cancer. *Proc Natl Acad Sci U S A.* 2005;102:18538-18543.
2. Miyatake T, Tringler B, Liu W, et al. B7-H4 (DD-O110) is overexpressed in high risk uterine endometrioid adenocarcinomas and inversely correlated with tumor T-cell infiltration. *Gynecol Oncol.* 2007;106:119-127.

Characterization of the molecular differences between ovarian endometrioid carcinoma and ovarian serous carcinoma
Madore J, Ren F, Filali-Mouhim A, et al (Centre de Recherche du Centre Hospitalier de l'Université de Montréal (CHUM)/Institut du Cancer de Montréal, Canada; et al)
J Pathol 220:392-400, 2010

The histopathological diagnosis of high-grade endometrioid and serous carcinoma of the ovary is poorly reproducible under the current morphology based classification system, especially for anaplastic, high-grade tumours. The transcription factor Wilms' tumour-1 (*WT1*) is differentially expressed among the gynaecological epithelia from which epithelial ovarian cancers (EOCs) are believed to originate. In EOCs,

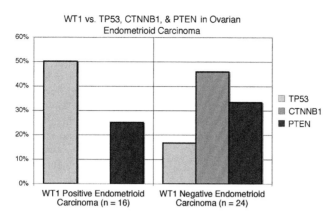

FIGURE 4.—Detection of aberrant β-catenin signalling, aberrant TP53 signalling and loss of PTEN protein expression, in WT1 determined subgroups of ovarian endometrioid carcinoma by IHC-TMA. CHUM-ND cohort ($n = 40$). (Reprinted from Madore J, Ren F, Filali-Mouhim A, et al. Characterization of the molecular differences between ovarian endometrioid carcinoma and ovarian serous carcinoma. *J Pathol.* 2010;220:392-400.)

WT1 protein is observed in the majority of serous carcinomas and in up to 30% of endometrioid carcinomas. It is unclear whether the latter is a reflection of the actual incidence of WT1 protein expression in endometrioid carcinomas, or whether a significant number of high-grade serous carcinomas have been misclassified as endometrioid carcinoma. Several genetic aberrations are reported to occur in EOCs. These include mutation of the *TP53* gene, aberrant activation of β-catenin signalling and loss of PTEN protein expression, among others. It is unclear whether these aberrations are histotype-specific. The aim of this study was to better define the molecular characteristics of serous and endometrioid carcinomas in an attempt to address the problems with the current histopathological classification methods. Gene expression profiles were analysed to identify reproducible gene expression phenotypes for endometrioid and serous carcinomas. Tissue microarrays (TMA) were used to assess the incidence of TP53, β-catenin and PTEN aberrations in order to correlate their occurrence with WT1 as an immunohistochemistry based biomarker of serous histotype. It was found that nuclear WT1 protein expression can identify misclassified high-grade endometrioid carcinomas and these tumours should be reassigned to serous histotype. Although low-grade endometrioid carcinomas rarely progress to high-grade carcinomas, a combined WT1-negative, TP53-positive immunophenotype may identify an uncommon high-grade subtype of ovarian endometrioid carcinoma. GEO database: array data accession number *GSE6008* (Fig 4).

▶ This article examines a number of endometrioid and serous ovarian carcinomas via molecular and immunohistochemical methods to explore whether current classification systems are sufficiently accurate. Using both previously published data and a cohort of their own cases, the authors reviewed Wilms tumor type-1 (WT1), p35, PTEN, and β-catenin expression in a relatively large number of ovarian tumors. Two groups of endometrioid ovarian cancers were revealed (Fig 4). The first tended to be of higher nuclear grade, had an overall poorer prognosis and showed p53 and WT1 immunoexpression. In contrast, the other group had mutations in the PI3K-PTEN pathway or β-catenin activation. They ultimately concluded that there may be a rationale presented here to reclassify high-grade endometrioid adenocarcinomas that are WT1 positive as serous carcinomas. As the authors point out, currently, virtually all ovarian carcinomas are treated with approximately the same chemotherapeutic regimens; however, as more data are accrued relating to the biologic potential and progression of different subtypes, more directed therapies may be used. For this reason, it is crucial to continue searching for similarities and differences that exist between tumors as they are currently classified. For additional reading, see the reference section.[1,2]

M. D. Post, MD

References

1. Willner J, Wurz K, Allison KH, et al. Alternate molecular genetic pathways in ovarian carcinomas of common histological types. *Hum Pathol*. 2007;38:607-613.
2. Köbel M, Kalloger SE, Boyd N, et al. Ovarian carcinoma subtypes are different diseases: implications for biomarker studies. *PLoS Med*. 2008;5:e232.

Alternate mucoid and hyalinized stroma in clear cell carcinoma of the ovary: manifestation of serial stromal remodeling
Kato N, Takeda J, Fukase M, et al (Yamagata Univ School of Medicine, Japan; Shonai Hosp, Tsuruoka, Japan)
Mod Pathol 23:881-888, 2010

The stroma in ovarian clear cell carcinoma often shows alternate mucoid and hyalinized change. The hyalinized stroma is recognized to be an aberrant deposition of basement membrane material produced by tumor cells. The mucoid stroma, however, has drawn far less attention, and its significance remains unclear. We examined 60 ovarian clear cell carcinomas for the distribution and nature of the mucoid stroma. For comparison, 125 other surface epithelial ovarian tumors were examined. Twenty-nine of 60 (48%) clear cell carcinomas showed a mucoid stroma, either focally (21 cases) or diffusely (8 cases). The mucoid stroma in clear cell carcinomas was distinct from that in other surface epithelial tumors as follows: it showed a compact spherule-like appearance, commonly occupying the cores of small papillae. It also exhibited a cribriform pattern, resembling that of adenoid cystic carcinoma. It was rarely associated with stromal cells, despite the presence of abundant glycosaminoglycan including hyaluronan. Alternatively, it was strongly associated with hyalinized stroma. Among 40 clear cell carcinomas that had at least one type of stroma, 26 (65%) had both, either concomitantly or separately. The mucoid stroma tended to attenuate if the hyalinized stroma developed. *In vitro*, a clear cell carcinoma cell line, HAC-2, formed a spherule-like structure containing hyaluronan in the center, and a significant amount of hyaluronan was detected by latex agglutination immunoturbidimetry, indicating that HAC-2 itself has the potential to produce hyaluronan. All of these facts indicate that the spherule-like mucoid stroma and hyalinized stroma represent different phases of the stromal remodeling process, which is promoted by the deposition of different extracellular matrices produced by clear cell carcinoma cells. The spherule-like mucoid stroma and hyalinized stroma are considered complementary diagnostic signatures of ovarian clear cell carcinoma.

▶ Accurate recognition of clear cell carcinoma (CCC) of the ovary is essential— as it has a relatively poor prognosis—and should not to be confused with other epithelial subtypes. This article is a morphologic comparison of stromal features of ovarian CCCs with those of other subtypes and an investigation into the cells responsible for 2 distinct stromal morphologies. One of the hallmarks of CCC is densely hyalinized stroma, formerly shown to be produced by tumor cells. Less well described and characterized, however, is the compact spherule-like mucoid stroma. The authors found that 29 of 60 cases (48%) of CCC did have basophilic mucoid stroma of compact spherule-like appearance and that this was most commonly found in papillary areas. Furthermore, they observed an inverse relationship between the amount of hyalinized stroma and mucoid stroma. The mucoid stroma was found in areas with a paucity of stromal cells, and by using a CCC cell line (HAC-2), the authors demonstrated that the malignant cells are capable of producing glycosaminoglycan (including hyaluronan). In contrast, relatively few of the other epithelial subtypes studied had any mucoid stroma, and those that did tended to show a looser architecture and to have this stromal type only in areas of abundant stromal cells, suggesting production by stromal rather than malignant epithelial cells. Conclusions drawn based on this study were that ovarian CCC frequently displays 1 or both characteristic stromal types (hyalinized and basophilic mucoid spherule-like), both of which appear to be produced by the malignant epithelial cells. Based on attenuation of the mucoid stroma in areas of extensive hyalinized stroma, the authors posit that these are 2 phases of stromal remodeling, similar to that seen in adenoid cystic carcinoma. The significance of the study is to provide additional morphologic clues to the diagnosis of ovarian CCC and to avoid misdiagnosis of another epithelial carcinoma subtype.[1,2]

M. D. Post, MD

References

1. Scully RE, Young RH, Clement PB. Atlas of Tumor Pathology. Tumors of the Ovary, Maldeveloped Gonads, Fallopian Tube, and Broad Ligament, Washington, DC. *Armed Forces Institute of Pathology.* 1998:141-151.
2. Sangoi AR, Soslow RA, Teng NN, Longacre TA. Ovarian clear cell carcinoma with papillary features: a potential mimic of serous tumor of low malignant potential. *Am J Surg Pathol.* 2008;32:269-274.

Comparison of Fluorescence In Situ Hybridization, p57 Immunostaining, Flow Cytometry, and Digital Image Analysis for Diagnosing Molar and Nonmolar Products of Conception

Kipp BR, Ketterling RP, Oberg TN, et al (Mayo Clinic, Rochester, MN)
Am J Clin Pathol 133:196-204, 2010

Pathologic examination of products of conception (POC) is used to differentiate hydropic abortus (HA), partial hydatidiform mole (PM), and complete hydatidiform mole (CM). Histologic classification of POC specimens can be difficult, and ancillary testing is often required for a definitive diagnosis. This study evaluated 66 POC specimens by flow cytometry, digital image analysis, p57 immunohistochemical analysis, and fluorescence in situ hybridization (FISH). The final diagnosis, based on the combined analysis of all test results, included 33 HAs, 24 PMs, and 9 CMs. The p57 immunostain identified 9 CMs that were evaluated as nontriploid by all other techniques. FISH seems to have the best accuracy (100%) for determining whether a specimen contains a triploid chromosome complement. These data suggest that the combination of p57 and FISH seems to be the best ancillary testing strategy to aid pathologists in the appropriate identification of CM, PM, and HA in POC specimens (Table 1).

▶ Products of conception are among the most common specimens encountered in pathology practices. In most cases, the clinically relevant question pertaining to this specimen is whether there exists a molar pregnancy and/or chromosomally abnormal conceptus. Although there are characteristic histologic features used to distinguish hydropic abortus from partial hydatidiform mole from complete hydatidiform mole, these can be difficult to apply definitively, particularly early in gestation. Because of the significant clinical implications of the diagnosis of a molar pregnancy (need for additional maternal serum, β-human chorionic gonadotropin monitoring, latency before next pregnancy, and risk of progression), there has been increased emphasis recently on providing the most accurate diagnosis possible with the aid of ancillary

TABLE 1.—Microscopic and Genetic Distinctions in Hydropic Abortuses, Partial Moles, and Complete Moles

	Hydropic Abortus	Partial Mole	Complete Mole
Pathology			
Villous trophoblasts	Attenuated	Focally hyperplastic	Diffusely hyperplastic
Villous population	Spectrum of sizes	2 populations	Spectrum of sizes
Trophoblast atypia	None	Rarely present	Prominent
Digital image analysis	Diploid	Triploid	Diploid
Flow cytometry	Diploid	Triploid	Diploid
Fluorescence in situ hybridization	Disomy or single trisomy/monosomy	Trisomy of all autosomes	Disomy
p57 Staining	Diffuse	Diffuse	Absent

techniques. The most commonly used include flow cytometry, digital image analysis and fluorescence in situ hybridization (FISH) (all to evaluate for the presence of triploidy, considered diagnostic for a partial mole), and p57 immunohistochemistry to identify complete moles (Table 1).

This study took a subset of histologically challenging cases and performed all 4 ancillary techniques on them to evaluate the ideal method or combination of methods for accurate diagnosis. They show that while each method has advantages and disadvantages, the use of some ancillary technique can improve upon histologic examination alone. They acknowledge that there is absolutely no single algorithm that fits every laboratory, but rather, they try to highlight strengths and weaknesses in each method (eg, barriers to interpretation, need for fresh vs formalin-fixed tissue, and overall cost) to highlight some available tests. They do not include molecular genotyping in this study but briefly discuss its possible contribution as well. In our clinical practice, we have found results similar to those published, namely that the combination of p57 immunohistochemistry and FISH analysis provide the most efficient and accurate means for diagnosing molar pregnancies. For additional reading, please see the reference section.[1,2,3]

M. D. Post, MD

References

1. Wells M. The pathology of gestational trophoblastic disease: recent advances. *Pathology.* 2007;39:88-96.
2. Berkowitz RS, Goldstein DP. Current management of gestational trophoblastic diseases. *Gynecol Oncol.* 2009;112:654-662.
3. Bifulco C, Johnson C, Hao L, Kermalli H, Bell S, Hui P. Genotypic analysis of hydatidiform mole: an accurate and practical method of diagnosis. *Am J Surg Pathol.* 2008;32:445-451.

Placental pathology in egg donor pregnancies

Gundogan F, Bianchi DW, Scherjon SA, et al (Women and Infants Hosp, Providence, RI; Tufts Med Ctr, Boston, MA; Leiden Univ Med Ctr, The Netherlands; et al)
Fertil Steril 93:397-404, 2010

Objective.—To determine placental pathology and immune response at the maternal-fetal interface in pregnancies conceived by IVF via egg donation compared with nondonor IVF pregnancies.

Design.—Retrospective case-control study.

Setting.—Academic medical center.

Patient(s).—The study population included 20 egg donor and 33 nondonor IVF pregnancies of >24 weeks' gestation.

Intervention(s).—None.

Main Outcome Measure(s).—Perinatal complications (gestational hypertension, abruption, preterm delivery, cesarean section), microscopic features indicating an immune response and trophoblast damage, and characterization of inflammatory cells using immunohistochemistry.

Result(s).—There was an increase in gestational hypertension and preterm delivery in egg donor pregnancies. Dense fibrinoid deposition in the basal plate with severe chronic deciduitis containing significantly increased numbers of T helper and natural killer cells were demonstrated in egg donor placentas. Trophoblast damage was also increased in the preterm egg donor group.

Conclusion(s).—There are significant histological and immunohistochemical differences between the placentas of egg donor and nondonor IVF pregnancies. The increased immune activity and fibrinoid deposition at the maternal-fetal interface of egg donor pregnancies could represent a host versus graft rejection-like phenomenon.

▶ With the advent of new technologies, it is now possible for women otherwise unable to conceive to bear children from donor eggs fertilized by in vitro fertilization (IVF). As this becomes more common, researchers have begun to examine whether there are differences in the pregnancies or placentas resulting from egg donor IVF and whether these provide any insight into pathophysiologic mechanisms of common diseases of pregnancy, such as preeclampsia. It is believed that preeclampsia results from defective implantation/invasion of fetal trophoblast into maternal decidua and myometrium, potentially related to immunologic interactions between mother and fetus. It has been previously shown that egg donor pregnancies have a higher incidence of preeclampsia,[1,2] although interestingly without significant difference in fetal weight, suggesting a possibly different mechanism for preeclampsia in this population. Other immune-mediated pathologies that can be detected on placental examination include: villitis of unknown etiology, chronic deciduitis (CD), massive chronic intervillositis, and maternal floor infarct. This study examined a group of placentas from women who underwent IVF from either donor or nondonor eggs, looking at a variety of placental lesions with particular focus on the maternal inflammatory response with respect to egg donor status.

Placentas from 53 IVF-conceived pregnancies at 1 institution (20 following egg donation) delivered at gestational age 24 weeks or greater were characterized by a variety of clinical factors, examined by routine staining for placental lesions, immunohistochemically stained for various inflammatory cell markers, and then analyzed by image analysis. Significant differences in clinical characteristics included maternal age, presence of gestational hypertension, and preterm delivery. There was significantly higher incidence of syncytial knots (upregulated in preeclampsia) in egg donor pregnancies and the presence of CD (with or without plasma cells). Further, the deciduitis diffusely involved the basal plate and was uniformly associated with markedly increased fibrinoid in the basal plate of egg donor placentas but was focal and without fibrinoid in nonegg donor cases. By image analysis, it was demonstrated that placentas from egg donor IVF pregnancies had a significant increase in basal plate cellularity secondary to increased numbers of CD45-positive inflammatory cells. The numbers of CD4-positive T helper cells and CD56-positive natural killer cells were also significantly increased in egg donor placentas.

Despite the small study size, these findings convincingly demonstrate differences in placental lesions present in pregnancies derived from egg donors. The most striking of these was the presence of diffuse CD, and the authors hypothesize that diffuse CD with fibrinoid deposition may be a characteristic lesion of egg donor pregnancies. The clinical significance behind these findings relates to the increased incidence of preeclampsia in egg donor pregnancies, as this can pose abundant risks to the mother and fetus. Further investigation is needed to determine whether the preeclampsia found in these pregnancies differs from that seen in pregnancies where there is shared genetic material between mother and fetus. The study highlights the need for a detailed placental examination to elucidate factors that might contribute to successful pregnancy outcomes.

M. D. Post, MD

References

1. Huppertz B. The feto-maternal interface: setting the stage for potential immune interactions. *Semin Immunopathol.* 2007;29:83-94.
2. Perni SC, Predanic M, Cho JE, Baergen RN. Placental pathology and pregnancy outcomes in donor and non-donor oocyte in vitro fertilization pregnancies. *J Perinat Med.* 2005;33:27-32.

9 Urinary Bladder and Male Genital Tract

A Multiplexed, Particle-Based Flow Cytometric Assay Identified Plasma Matrix Metalloproteinase-7 to Be Associated With Cancer-Related Death Among Patients With Bladder Cancer

Svatek RS, Shah JB, Xing J, et al (The Univ of Texas M. D. Anderson Cancer Ctr, Houston)

Cancer 116:4513-4519, 2010

Background.—The current study was conducted to demonstrate the utility of a multiplexed, particle-based flow cytometric assay for the simultaneous analysis of a panel of matrix metalloproteinases (MMPs) using small volumes of plasma samples from patients with bladder cancer. In addition, the authors attempted to test the hypothesis that plasma levels of MMPs are associated with time to cancer-related death.

Methods.—Plasma MMP concentrations (MMP-1, -2, -3, -7, -8, -9, and -12) in 135 patients presenting with high-grade $\geq$T1 bladder cancer were measured. Data regarding clinical and pathologic features was ascertained in a retrospective fashion.

Results.—The median duration of follow-up was 30.4 months. At the time of analysis, 61 patients had died, including 45 (33.3%) who died of bladder cancer. Plasma MMP-12 was not measurable. For all other MMPs, the intra-assay coefficient of variation varied from 6.12% to 9.82%. MMP-1, -2, -3, -8, and -9 were not found to be significantly associated with time to cancer-related death. Plasma MMP-7 levels were significantly associated with time to cancer-related death after adjustment for competing clinical and pathologic features (hazard ratio [HR], 2.2; 95% confidence interval [95% CI], 1.1-4.5 [$P = .022$]). The 5-year median cancer-specific survival rates for those patients with MMP-7 levels above and below the median value (300 pg/mL) were 73.6% (95% CI, 60.0-83.2%) and 48.0% (95% CI, 32.5-61.9%), respectively ($P = .01$).

Conclusions.—Multiplexed, particle-based flow cytometric assay allows for the high throughput measurement of multiple plasma or serum proteins simultaneously. By using this new technology in a cohort of

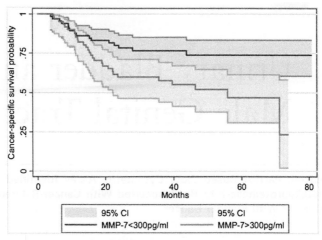

FIGURE 1.—Kaplan-Meier cancer-specific survival probability curves are shown for patients with plasma matrix metalloproteinase-7 (MMP-7) levels above and below the median. 95% CI indicates 95% confidence interval. (Reprinted from Svatek RS, Shah JB, Xing J, et al. A multiplexed, particle-based flow cytometric assay identified plasma matrix metalloproteinase-7 to be associated with cancer-related death among patients with bladder cancer. *Cancer.* 2010;116:4513-4519, copyright 2010 American Cancer Society. This material is reproduced with permission of Wiley-Liss, Inc., a subsidiary of John Wiley & Sons, Inc.)

patients with bladder cancer, plasma levels of MMP-7 were identified as being significantly associated with time to cancer-related death (Fig 1).

▶ Recent advances in biomarker development combined with newer technologies have provided clinicians and researchers with additional tools for both diagnosis and prognosis of human cancers.[1] In this study, the authors describe a novel technology of multiplexed particle-based flow cytometric assay that allows for the high-throughput measurement of multiple plasma or serum proteins simultaneously. The investigators have used this new and novel technology in a group of patients with high-stage bladder cancer for the simultaneous analysis of a panel of matrix metalloproteinases (MMPs) using small volumes of plasma samples from the group of patients diagnosed with bladder cancer. The second goal of this study was to test the hypothesis that plasma levels of MMPs are associated with time to death from bladder cancer.

The results were striking and demonstrated that the multiplexed, particle-based flow cytometric assay worked well and a panel of MMPs (MMP-1, -2, -3, -7, -8, -9, and -12) could be reliably measured in a small volume of plasma sample. Interestingly, only the plasma MMP-7 levels were significantly associated with time to cancer-related death after adjustment for competing clinical and pathologic features ($P = .022$). This correlated well when the death rates were compared and it was found that the 5-year median cancer-specific survival rates for those patients with MMP-7 levels above and below the median value (300 pg/mL) were 73.6% (95% CI, 60.0%-83.2%) and 48.0% (95% CI, 32.5%-61.9%), respectively ($P = .01$) (Fig 1).

The results presented in this study are very convincing and will allow for improved and rapid noninvasive tests for risk stratification of bladder cancer patients. A biomarker such as MMP7 may be a useful marker to provide for prognostic information about patients with bladder cancer. Additional studies are needed to further strengthen the evidence presented here. In addition, because there were no age-matched controls included in this study, addition of control cases would be of immense value, particularly to measure the baseline levels of MMP7 in control populations.

A. V. Parwani, MD, PhD

Reference

1. Thrailkill KM, Moreau CS, Cockrell G, et al. Physiological matrix metalloproteinase concentrations in serum during childhood and adolescence, using Luminex Multiplex technology. *Clin Chem Lab Med*. 2005;43:1392-1399.

Comparative Analysis of Whole Mount Processing and Systematic Sampling of Radical Prostatectomy Specimens: Pathological Outcomes and Risk of Biochemical Recurrence
Salem S, Chang SS, Clark PE, et al (Vanderbilt Univ Med Ctr, Nashville, TN; et al)
J Urol 184:1334-1340, 2010

Purpose.—Whole mount processing is more resource intensive than routine systematic sampling of radical retropubic prostatectomy specimens. We compared whole mount and systematic sampling for detecting pathological outcomes, and compared the prognostic value of pathological findings across pathological methods.

Materials and Methods.—We included men (608 whole mount and 525 systematic sampling samples) with no prior treatment who underwent radical retropubic prostatectomy at Vanderbilt University Medical Center between January 2000 and June 2008. We used univariate and multivariate analysis to compare the pathological outcome detection rate between pathological methods. Kaplan-Meier curves and the log rank test were used to compare the prognostic value of pathological findings across pathological methods.

Results.—There were no significant differences between the whole mount and the systematic sampling groups in detecting extraprostatic extension (25% vs 30%), positive surgical margins (31% vs 31%), pathological Gleason score less than 7 (49% vs 43%), 7 (39% vs 43%) or greater than 7 (12% vs 13%), seminal vesicle invasion (8% vs10%) or lymph node involvement (3% vs 5%). Tumor volume was higher in the systematic sampling group and whole mount detected more multiple surgical margins (each p <0.01). There were no significant differences in the likelihood of biochemical recurrence between the pathological methods when patients were stratified by pathological outcome.

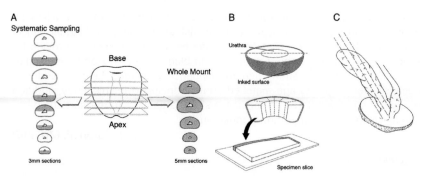

FIGURE 1.—Gross dissection techniques for prostate SS and WM processing. *A*, difference between 2 techniques in slice thickness and amount of tissue submitted (gray areas). *B*, apex and base are sectioned identically in 2 methods and designed to highlight surgical margins (gray areas) for evaluation. *C*, seminal vesicle is sectioned longitudinally in each method through its junction with prostate (dashed lines) to identify seminal vesicle invasion. (Reprinted from Salem S, Chang SS, Clark PE, et al. Comparative analysis of whole mount processing and systematic sampling of radical prostatectomy specimens: pathological outcomes and risk of biochemical recurrence. *J Urol*. 2010;184:1334-1340, with permission from American Urological Association.)

Conclusions.—Except for estimated tumor volume and multiple margins whole mount and systematic sampling yield similar pathological information. Each method stratifies patients into comparable risk groups for biochemical recurrence. Thus, while whole mount is more resource intensive, it does not appear to result in improved detection of clinically important pathological outcomes or prognostication (Fig 1).

▶ Prostate cancer is the most common solid (noncutaneous) tumor in men in the United States, and many men with localized cancer choose to have a radical prostatectomy performed. There have been attempts to standardize the protocols for the pathological evaluation of radical prostatectomy specimens, including recommendations from the Association of Directors of Anatomic and Surgical Pathology and the College of American Pathologists for the required and optional elements for the reporting of radical prostatectomy specimens.

In this study, the investigators have compared 2 methods of evaluation of radical prostatectomy specimens including whole mount processing and systematic sampling. The whole mount method provides a better evaluation of the whole organ and tumor involvement in relation to the capsule and surgical margin but is more resource intensive. The whole mount processing system is not widely used and requires more clinical resources for handling and processing because of the nonstandard larger blocks and slides. Using the whole mount processing method, the prostate is completely embedded in paraffin and the pathologist evaluates full colonal sections perpendicular to the rectal surface on oversized glass slides cut on specialized microtomes. On the other hand, the systematic sampling method is more widely used, does not involve the use of specialized microtomes or slides, and is not as resource intensive (Fig 1).

The investigators in this study have compared the pathological outcomes and the risk of biochemical recurrence between the 2 methods of evaluation. The study included a large number of patients for each group (608 whole mount and 525 systematic sampling samples), and the various pathological parameters such as extraprostatic extension, seminal vesicle involvement, and Gleason score were compared.

The results showed that there were no significant differences between the whole mount and systematic sampling groups in the detection of surgical margins, extraprostatic extension, pathological Gleason score, seminal vesicle invasion, and lymph node involvement. In addition, there were no significant differences in the likelihood of biochemical recurrence between whole mount and systematic sampling methods when patients were stratified by pathological outcome.

These results are useful for practicing surgical pathologists as they make decisions about which method to use for the evaluation of radical prostatectomy specimens, particularly if they do not want to continue to use whole mount because of the additional resources and specialized equipment needed. This study highlights the similarity of results obtained when either method is used.

A. V. Parwani, MD, PhD

Detection of *TMPRSS2-ETS* Fusions by a Multiprobe Fluorescence *in Situ* Hybridization Assay for the Early Diagnosis of Prostate Cancer: A Pilot Study
Sun Q-P, Li L-Y, Chen Z, et al (Sun Yat-Sen Univ, Guangzhou, China; Univ of Utah School of Medicine, Salt Lake City)
J Mol Diagn 12:718-724, 2010

Fusion of the prostate-specific and androgen-regulated transmembrane-serine protease gene (*TMPRSS2*) with the erythroblast transformation-specific (*ETS*) family members is the most common genetic alteration in prostate cancer. However, the biological and clinical role of *TMPRSS2-ETS* fusions in prostate cancer, especially in problematic prostate needle core biopsies, has not been rigorously evaluated. We randomly collected 85 specimens including 50 archival prostate cancer tissue blocks, 15 normal prostate specimens, and 20 benign prostatic hyperplasia specimens for *TMPRSS2-ETS* fusion analyses. Moreover, the fusion status in an additional 20 patients with initial negative biopsies who progressed to biopsy-positive prostate cancer at subsequent follow-ups was also characterized. Fluorescently labeled probes specific for *ERG*-related rearrangements involving the *TMPRSS2-ERG* fusion as well as *TMPRSS2-ETV1* and *TMPRSS2-ETV4* were used to assess samples for gene rearrangements indicative of malignancy under a design of sequential trial. Rearrangements involving *TMPRSS2-ETS* fusions were detected in 90.0% of the 50 postoperative prostate cancer samples. The positive rate for the rearrangements in the initial prostate cancer-negative biopsies of 20 patients who eventually progressed to prostate cancer was 60.0% (12/20). Our preliminary study demonstrates that the clinical utility of *TMPRSS2-ETS* fusion detection as a biomarker and ancillary diagnostic tool for the early diagnosis of prostate cancer is promising, given this approach shows significant high sensitivity and specificity in detection.

▶ *TMPRSS2* is highly expressed in prostate carcinoma and contains androgen-responsive elements in its promoter. *ERG* is an erythroblast transformation-specific family transcription factor, involved in Ewing tumor translocations. Fusion protein results in androgen-stimulated overexpression of *ERG*. Multiple studies have shown the diagnostic utility in the evaluation of small foci of atypical glands. *TMPRSS2-ERG* gene rearrangement is seen in about half of clinically localized prostate cancers, yet controversy exists with regard to its prognostic implications.

This study has evaluated 50 cases of prostate cancers from formalin-fixed paraffin-embedded tissue for the detection of *ERG*-related rearrangements, *TMPRSS2-ETV1* and *TMPRSS2-ETV4* fusion genes. The authors have used a multiprobe fluorescence in situ hybridization (FISH) assay. An additional 20 cases were included in which the patients had an initial negative prostate biopsy and then subsequently progressed to biopsy-positive cancer.

The results in this study showed that *ERG* rearrangements were present in 78% of cases (39/50). The latter is consistent with some previous studies by other investigators who have reported such rearrangements in the range of 40% to 80% of cases.

There is a need for rapid and reliable molecular diagnostic assays for the early detection of prostate cancer, and the detection of *TMPRSS2-ETS* fusion genes in prostate cancer holds much promise as shown in this study and multiple recent studies. Although the study number is small, this is a useful study, and the authors have demonstrated the usefulness of a multiprobe FISH assay on paraffin-embedded samples instead of frozen tissue, making the test easier to use for the clinical laboratories. The results are promising, and the authors have showed that there is high sensitivity and specificity in the detection of the rearrangements.

A. V. Parwani, MD, PhD

External Validation of Urinary *PCA3*-Based Nomograms to Individually Predict Prostate Biopsy Outcome
Auprich M, Haese A, Walz J, et al (Med Univ Graz, Austria; Univ Clinic Eppendorf, Hamburg, Germany; Institut Paoli-Calmettes Cancer Center, Marseille, France; et al)
Eur Urol 58:727-732, 2010

Background.—Prior to safely adopting risk stratification tools, their performance must be tested in an external patient cohort.

Objective.—To assess accuracy and generalizability of previously reported, internally validated, prebiopsy prostate cancer antigen 3 (*PCA3*) gene-based nomograms when applied to a large, external, European cohort of men at risk of prostate cancer (PCa).

Design, Setting, and Participants.—Biopsy data, including urinary *PCA3* score, were available for 621 men at risk of PCa who were participating in a European multi-institutional study.

Intervention.—All patients underwent a $\geq$10-core prostate biopsy. Biopsy indication was based on suspicious digital rectal examination, persistently elevated prostate-specific antigen level (2.5–10 ng/ml) and/or suspicious histology (atypical small acinar proliferation of the prostate, $>/=$ two cores affected by high-grade prostatic intraepithelial neoplasia in first set of biopsies).

Measurements.—PCA3 scores were assessed using the Progensa assay (Gen-Probe Inc, San Diego, CA, USA). According to the previously reported nomograms, different *PCA3* score codings were used. The probability of a positive biopsy was calculated using previously published logistic regression coefficients. Predicted outcomes were compared to the actual biopsy results. Accuracy was calculated using the area under the curve as a measure of discrimination; calibration was explored graphically.

Results and Limitations.—Biopsy-confirmed PCa was detected in 255 (41.1%) men. Median *PCA3* score of biopsy-negative versus biopsy-positive men was 20 versus 48 in the total cohort, 17 versus 47 at initial biopsy, and 37 versus 53 at repeat biopsy (all $p \leq 0.002$). External validation of all four previously reported *PCA3*-based nomograms demonstrated equally high accuracy (0.73–0.75) and excellent calibration. The main limitations of the study reside in its early detection setting, referral scenario, and participation of only tertiary-care centers.

Conclusions.—In accordance with the original publication, previously developed *PCA3*-based nomograms achieved high accuracy and sufficient calibration. These novel nomograms represent robust tools and are thus generalizable to European men at risk of harboring PCa. Consequently, in presence of a *PCA3* score, these nomograms may be safely used to assist clinicians when prostate biopsy is contemplated.

▶ This is an important study that attempts to externally validate urinary prostate cancer antigen 3 (*PCA3*) gene-based nomograms to individually predict prostate biopsy outcomes. Recent studies have shown that *PCA3* is a noncoding RNA and is the most specific clinically available prostate malignancy marker described so far. *PCA3* has a high level of expression in prostate tumors (median 66-fold increase) with low expression in benign prostate tissue but undetectable levels of expression in normal tissues from all major organs. *PCA3* and prostate-specific antigen (PSA) messenger RNA (mRNA) in urine samples are collected after a digital rectal examination. PSA mRNA is required to normalize for the total mRNA present in a sample. PSA mRNA levels in prostate cells released into urine are completely unrelated to PSA protein levels in blood and are essentially unchanged in prostate cancer. Results are represented as a ratio of *PCA3* mRNA/PSA mRNA, referred to as the *PCA3* score. *PCA3* scores were assessed using the Progensa assay (Gen-Probe Inc, San Diego,

CA). Previous studies have established that a high *PCA3* score correlates with an increased probability of a positive prostate biopsy.[1]

This study evaluated the biopsy results as well as the *PCA3* score for a European cohort of 621 patients. The results were good and showed that the median *PCA3* score of biopsy-negative versus biopsy-positive men was 20 versus 48 in the total cohort, 17 versus 47 at initial biopsy, and 37 versus 53 at repeat biopsy (all *P* < .002). These results confirmed the previously described internal validation studies. This is the first external validation study of *PCA3*-based nomograms showing the validity and utility of the *PCA3* score in a large European multi-institutional patient cohort. Overall, the current and previous studies have established that a high *PCA3* score correlates with an increased probability of a positive prostate biopsy.

A. V. Parwani, MD, PhD

Reference

1. Deras IL, Aubin SM, Blase A, et al. *PCA3*: a molecular urine assay for predicting prostate biopsy outcome. *J Urol.* 2008;179:1587-1592.

Extraprostatic extension of prostatic adenocarcinoma on needle core biopsy: report of 72 cases with clinical follow-up
Miller JS, Chen Y, Ye H, et al (Johns Hopkins School of Medicine, Baltimore, MD)
BJU Int 106:330-333, 2010

Objective.—To describe the histological findings and prognosis that are associated with extraprostatic extension (EPE) on needle core biopsy of prostatic adenocarcinoma.

Patients and Methods.—We retrieved 99 cases of prostatic adenocarcinoma with EPE at initial diagnosis on biopsy from the consultation files of one of the authors between 1997 and 2009. The 72 cases that had available clinical follow-up data formed the basis of this study.

Results.—The mean (range) age of the patients was 64 (48–87) years, the median (mean, range) serum prostatic specific antigen level was 7.8 (64.8, 0.3–1505) ng/mL, and 60 of the patients (83%) had abnormalities on a digital rectal examination. The mean (range) number of malignant cores was 7.7 (1–23); the mean percentage of carcinoma in each core was 69.6%, and that in the core(s) with EPE was 76.8%. The mean Gleason score in the core(s) with EPE was 8, with a mean highest Gleason score per case of 8.4. Perineural invasion was detected in 54 cases (75%). Ten of 11 patients treated surgically had EPE on the radical prostatectomy (RP) specimen; also six had positive resection margins, five showed invasion into the seminal vesicles and one had lymph node metastasis. The Gleason scores in nine of the RP specimens did not differ from the highest grade found in the associated biopsies (score 9 in three, 8 in two, 7 in four); in one case it increased (from score 6 to 8) and in one it decreased (from score 9 to 8). Patients were followed for a mean (median, range) of 2.9 (2, 0.1–9) years, with metastases identified in 29 (40%); 10 (14%) died from the disease.

Conclusion.—EPE on needle core biopsy of the prostate is strongly associated with extensive, high-grade prostatic adenocarcinoma, such that its usefulness as an isolated prognostic factor is relatively limited.

▶ This study is very interesting because the authors have evaluated the outcome of a relatively rare finding on prostate needle biopsy, namely the presence or absence of extraprostatic extension (EPE) assessed on needle biopsies. The finding of EPE on radical and clinical outcomes has been very well characterized in a number of studies. However, the significance of EPE discovery on needle biopsies has not been well characterized.

The authors obtained follow-up information on 71 of 99 cases where EPE was recorded on the needle biopsy. The results are very interesting and showed that the mean Gleason score in the core(s) with EPE was 8, with a mean highest Gleason score per case of 8.4. Perineural invasion was detected in 54 cases (75%). Additional findings included the presence of EPE in 10 of 11 patients treated with radical prostatectomy (RP). Of these, 6 patients had positive resection margins, 5 showed invasion into the seminal vesicles and one had lymph node metastasis. Interestingly, the Gleason scores in 9 of the RP specimens did not differ from the highest grade found in the associated biopsies.

Overall, these findings suggest that EPE on needle core biopsy correlated with extensive high-grade prostatic adenocarcinoma. Therefore, by itself, the presence of EPE in needle biopsies has a very limited role as a prognostic marker.

A. V. Parwani, MD, PhD

Histologic Changes Associated With Neoadjuvant Chemotherapy Are Predictive of Nodal Metastases in Patients With High-Risk Prostate Cancer
O'Brien C, True LD, Higano CS, et al (Oregon Health & Science Univ, Portland; Univ of Washington, Seattle)
Am J Clin Pathol 133:654-661, 2010

Clinical trials are evaluating the effect of neoadjuvant chemotherapy on men with high-risk prostate cancer. Little is known about the clinical significance of postchemotherapy tumor histopathologic features. We assessed the prognostic and predictive value of histologic features (intraductal carcinoma, vacuolated cell morphologic features, inconspicuous glands, cribriform architecture, and inconspicuous cancer cells) observed in 50 high-risk prostate cancers treated with preprostatectomy docetaxel and mitoxantrone. At a median follow-up of 65 months, the overall relapse-free survival (RFS) rates at 2 and 5 years were 65% and 49%, respectively. In univariate analyses (using the Kaplan-Meier method and log-rank tests), intraductal ($P = .001$) and cribriform ($P = .014$) histologic features were associated with shorter RFS. In multivariate analyses, using the Cox proportional hazards regression, baseline prostate-specific antigen ($P = .004$), lymph node metastases ($P < .001$), and cribriform histologic features ($P = .007$) were associated with shorter RFS. In multivariable logistic regression analysis, only intraductal pattern ($P = .007$) predicted lymph node metastases. Intraductal and cribriform histologic features apparently predict postchemotherapy outcome.

▶ There is a paucity of information in the literature about the histologic patterns observed in radical prostatectomy specimens obtained from patients at high risk for prostate cancer progression who were treated with neoadjuvant docetaxel and mitoxantrone. This is a timely and pivotal article that evaluates the spectrum of the histological findings and, in addition, highlights the prognostic and predictive value of some of the histologic features such as intraductal carcinoma, vacuolated cell morphologic features, inconspicuous glands, cribriform architecture, and inconspicuous cancer cells.

Two important findings emerge from this study including the[1] histological patterns seen in this group of patients and[2] two of these histological features; intraductal carcinoma and cribriform architecture have power in predicting outcome after neoadjuvant chemotherapy. Histological patterns most commonly seen in this group of patients included inconspicuous, collapsed glands, small inconspicuous tumor, prominently vacuolated tumor cell cytoplasm, cribiform architecture, and an intraductal growth pattern (Fig 1 in the original article). Based on statistical analysis done in this study, it was determined that the intraductal ($P = .001$) and cribriform ($P = .014$) histologic features were associated with shorter relapse-free survival rates. In multivariable logistic regression analysis, only intraductal pattern ($P = .007$) predicted lymph node metastases.

These are important findings, particularly the association of intraductal carcinoma with shorter relapse-free survival, as this is a relatively controversial area of prostate pathology, and many authors have argued if intraductal carcinoma is a variant of prostatic intraepithelial neoplasia or if it represents a variant of prostatic adenocarcinoma that invades into prostate ducts and glands. The description of the histological findings in radical prostatectomy specimens seen in association with a treatment of neoadjuvant docetaxel and mitoxantrone will be of value to pathologists as they encounter similar or related cases in their practice.

A. V. Parwani, MD, PhD

References

1. Dawkins HJ, Sellner LN, Turbett GR, et al. Distinction between intraductal carcinoma of the prostate (IDC-P), high-grade dysplasia (PIN), and invasive prostatic adenocarcinoma, using molecular markers of cancer progression. *Prostate.* 2000;44:265-270.
2. Magi-Galluzzi C, Zhou M, Reuther AM, Dreicer R, Klein EA. Neoadjuvant docetaxel treatment for locally advanced prostate cancer: a clinicopathologic study. *Cancer.* 2007;110:1248-1254.

Improved Resolution of Diagnostic Problems in Selected Prostate Needle Biopsy Specimens by Using the ASAP Workup: A Prospective Study of Interval Sections vs New Recut Sections

Strand CL, Aponte SL, Chatterjee M, et al (PLUS Diagnostics Laboratory, Union, NJ)
Am J Clin Pathol 134:293-298, 2010

This study assessed the value of an atypical small acinar proliferation (ASAP) workup consisting of preparing new recut sections from the paraffin block and performing H&E-stained sections and immunostains (using the antibody cocktail for p63, cytokeratins 5 and 14, and α-methylacyl coenzyme A racemase) on the slides. We compared the ASAP workup with the interval workup, the common practice of performing the same immunostains on the saved interval sections, in 105 cases because of focal glandular atypia on the original H&E-stained sections. There were no specimens in which only the interval workup showed a changed diagnosis, but there were 23 specimens (21.9%) in which the preliminary diagnosis was changed to a definitive diagnosis of carcinoma (10 specimens) or a specific benign diagnosis (13 specimens) based solely on the findings of the ASAP workup. The ASAP workup is recommended as a very useful histologic tool for resolving diagnostic problems in prostate needle biopsy specimens (Fig 2).

▶ This is an interesting article that evaluates the usefulness of an atypical small acinar proliferation (ASAP) workup. The latter is a difficult diagnostic area when prostate needle biopsies with small foci of atypical glands are reviewed by the pathologist, both general and subspeciality-based. The ASAP workup

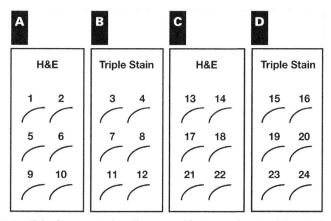

FIGURE 2.—Slides for an atypical small acinar proliferation workup. **A**, Slide stained with H&E. **B**, Interval section slide stained with triple stain. **C**, Recut section slide stained with H&E. **D**, Recut slide with triple stain. (Reprinted from Strand CL, Aponte SL, Chatterjee M, et al. Improved resolution of diagnostic problems in selected prostate needle biopsy specimens by using the ASAP workup: a prospective study of interval sections vs new recut sections. *Am J Clin Pathol.* 2010;134:293-298, with permission from © American Society for Clinical Pathology.)

comprises of preparing new recut sections from the paraffin block and performing hematoxylin and eosin (H&E)-stained sections and immunostains (using the antibody cocktail for p63, cytokeratins 5 and 14, and alpha-methylacyl coenzyme A racemase) on the slides (Fig 2). As a baseline for comparison, the authors compared the ASAP workup to an interval workup in which immunostains are performed on the saved interval sections. An interval type of work is more commonly used by surgical pathologists with the rationale being that if there is a minute focus of atypical glands present in the H&E-stained slides, the intervening slides will most likely have the atypical focus in question. If additional levels are taken, there is a possibility that the focus will not be represented.

The results from this study, although only based on 105 cases, demonstrate that there were no specimens in which only an interval workup showed a changed diagnosis. Using the interval workup, the most interesting and convincing finding was that there were 23 cases in which the preliminary diagnosis was changed. Of these 23 ASAP cases, in 10 cases a definite diagnosis of carcinoma was rendered, while a definite diagnosis of benign was rendered on the remaining 13 cases.

Based on the results of this study, it seems that the ASAP workup presents a useful protocol for the evaluation of minute foci of atypical glands in the prostate. Additional number of cases and a more broader testing by additional laboratories will be of value and may lead to a wide-scale adoption of the ASAP workup.

A. V. Parwani, MD, PhD

Initial Atypical Diagnosis With Carcinoma on Subsequent Prostate Needle Biopsy: Findings at Radical Prostatectomy
Chen Y-B, Pierorazio PM, Epstein JI (The Johns Hopkins Hosp, Baltimore, MD)
J Urol 184:1953-1957, 2010

Purpose.—Limited data exist on radical prostatectomy findings performed for cancer on repeat biopsy following an initial atypical biopsy (atypical glands suspicious but not diagnostic for carcinoma).

Materials and Methods.—We compared 169 such men to 15,810 without an initial diagnosis of atypical glands suspicious for carcinoma who underwent radical prostatectomy from 1993 to 2008.

Results.—Median time between atypical biopsy and repeat biopsy showing cancer was 6.1 months (range 0.7 to 94.8). An initial diagnosis of atypical glands suspicious but not diagnostic for carcinoma correlated significantly with nonpalpable disease, biopsy Gleason score 6 and lower tumor volume on needle cores. Compared to radical prostatectomy without prior atypical findings, radical prostatectomy cases with an initial atypical biopsy had a significantly lower Gleason score (p <0.0001) and pathological stage (p = 0.001), with 126 (74.5%) Gleason score 6 and 140 (83.0%) organ confined. Only 2 (1.2%) cases showed seminal vesicle

TABLE 3.—Radical Prostatectomy Findings

	With Initial ATYP	Without Initial ATYP	p Value
No. Gleason score (%):			
5–6	126 (74.5)	9,660 (61.1)	—
7	42 (24.9)	5,240 (33.2)	—
8	1 (0.6)	541 (3.4)	—
9–10	0 (0)	369 (2.3)	—
Mean	6.20	6.45	<0.0001
No. pathological stage (%):			
Organ confined	140 (83.0)	10,934 (69.2)	0.001
EPE	28 (16.6)	4,028 (25.5)	—
Margin pos	22 (13.0)	2,121 (13.4)	0.8
Seminal vesicle pos	2 (1.2)	835 (5.3)	—
Lymph node pos	0 (0.0)	266 (1.7)	—

involvement and none had lymph node metastases. In addition to known preoperative parameters (clinical stage and biopsy Gleason score), the presence of initial atypical biopsy was an independent predictor of organ confined disease at radical prostatectomy. However, when tumor volume on needle biopsy was included in the multivariate analysis a diagnosis of atypical glands suspicious but not diagnostic for carcinoma lost its independent predictive value.

Conclusions.—Prostate cancer diagnosed on needle biopsy following a diagnosis of atypical glands suspicious but not diagnostic of carcinoma demonstrates a significantly lower tumor grade and pathological stage at radical prostatectomy than cancer without such a diagnosis. Correlating with lower tumor volume on biopsy, the presence of initial atypical biopsy predicts organ confined disease at radical prostatectomy. However, a few cases with high Gleason score and advanced pathological stage in this group emphasize the importance of re-biopsy within 3 to 6 months following such a diagnosis (Table 3).

▶ The presence of small foci of atypical glands in prostate needle biopsies often presents the pathologist with diagnostic difficulty because the foci often lack sufficient architectural and cytological atypia, making this finding suspicious but not diagnostic for carcinoma. Immunostains for basal cell markers (p63 and CK903) or racemase are often used by the pathologist to make a more definite diagnosis, but in spite of all the ancillary testing and initial review, up to 5% of all needle biopsies get an "atypical" or "atypical small acinar proliferation" diagnosis. In up to 40% of the cases with an atypical diagnosis, the repeat biopsy will show cancer, and interestingly, this risk of cancer is much higher than the risk of a cancer diagnosis followed by a diagnosis of benign or prostatic intraepithelial neoplasia.

There are only limited data available of the histopathological findings including Gleason scores (GSs) at radical prostatectomy in patients with an initial atypical diagnosis, followed by a diagnosis of carcinoma. This is a very important study because the authors have studied the histopathological findings in a large series (n = 169) of radical prostatectomy specimens from patients with an initial atypical diagnosis followed by a second biopsy with established carcinoma diagnosis.

The results from this study are interesting and showed that an initial atypical diagnosis on biopsy was a significant independent predictor of organ-confined disease at radical prostatectomy. Of the 169 cases in this study, 126 (74.5%) were GS 6 or less and 140 (83.0%) were organ confined. Only 2 of 169 (1.2%) cases showed seminal vesicle involvement and none of the cases had pelvic lymph node metastases. Compared with radical prostatectomy cases without a previous atypical diagnosis, radical prostatectomy specimens from patients with an initial atypical diagnosis showed a significantly lower GS and pathological stage (Table 3).

The findings from this study are important because they emphasize that patients with an initial atypical diagnosis have a significantly lower GS and pathological stage, but there is a minor subset of patients with an initial atypical diagnosis who may have a higher GS and extraprostatic extension. The pathology report should document the atypical findings, and the pathologist should convey to the urologist the significance of an atypical diagnosis. Based on the findings of higher GS and cases of extraprostatic extension in the study population, the urologist should be informed of the importance of a follow-up biopsy within 3 to 6 months of an atypical diagnosis on prostate needle biopsy.

A. V. Parwani, MD, PhD

Invasive micropapillary urothelial carcinoma of the bladder
Lopez-Beltran A, Montironi R, Blanca A, et al (Univ of Cordoba Faculty of Medicine, Spain; Polytechnic Univ of the Marche Region School of Medicine, Ancona, Italy; Univ Hosp, Cordoba, Spain; et al)
Hum Pathol 41:1159-1164, 2010

In this report, we present the clinicopathologic features of 13 cases of the invasive micropapillary variant of urothelial carcinoma. This is a rare and aggressive variant of bladder cancer recognized by the current World Health Organization classification of urologic tumors. The micropapillary component varied from 50% to 100% of the tumor specimen; in 10 cases, the micropapillary component composed greater than 70% of the tumor, with 5 cases showing pure micropapillary carcinoma. The architectural pattern of the tumor varied from solid expansile nests with slender papillae within tissue retraction spaces to pseudoglandular growth with prominent ring-like structures (2 cases, 15%) and invasive micropapillary carcinoma with squamous differentiation (2 cases, 15%); a streaking solid architectural pattern of micropapillary carcinoma was additionally present in 2 cases (15%). At histology, the individual tumor cells had abundant eosinophilic cytoplasm and nuclei with prominent nucleoli and irregular distribution of chromatin, and frequent mitotic figures. Most neoplastic cells had nuclei of low to intermediate nuclear grade with occasional nuclear pleomorphism. Eight mixed cases had concurrent conventional high-grade urothelial carcinoma with squamous or glandular differentiation in 3 and 1 case(s), respectively. All patients had advanced-stage cancer (>pT2), and 8 (62%) had lymph node metastasis. Immunohistochemical staining demonstrated that both micropapillary and associated conventional urothelial carcinomas were positive for MUC1 and 2, cytokeratin 7, PTEN, p53, and Ki-67. Her2Neu, uroplakin, cytokeratin 20, 34βE12, CA125, and p16 were positive in 4, 10, 8, 7, 3, and 3 cases, respectively. MUC5A, MUC6, and CDX2 were negative in all micropapillary cases. Follow-up information was available in all cases (range, 2-21 months; mean, 10 months). Eleven of patients died of disease from 2 to 14 months, and 2 patients were alive with disease at 14 and 21 months. Univariate statistical analysis showed survival differences between invasive micropapillary and conventional urothelial carcinomas ($P < .0001$). In summary, invasive micropapillary variant of urothelial carcinoma is an aggressive variant associated with poor prognosis that presents at an advanced clinical stage. The immunophenotype of invasive micropapillary carcinoma supports urothelial origin; the immunoreactivity to Her2Neu and PTEN might be relevant in terms of future targeting therapy. The morphologic diversity of micropapillary carcinoma may represent a diagnostic pitfall in limited samples, where

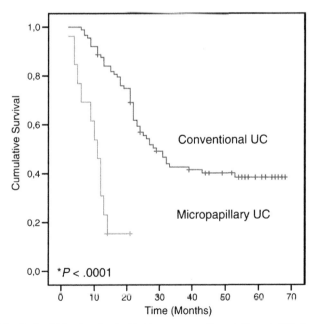

FIGURE 2.—Kaplan-Meier plots showing bladder cancer–specific mortality probability for conventional urothelial carcinoma compared with invasive micropapillary carcinoma. *P value based on log-rank test. (Reprinted from Lopez-Beltran A, Montironi R, Blanca A, et al. Invasive micropapillary urothelial carcinoma of the bladder. *Hum Pathol.* 2010;41:1159-1164, with permission from Elsevier Inc.)

TABLE 2.—Summary of the Immunostains Results[a]

Case	MUC1	MUC2	Uroplakin	CK7	CK20	34βE12	CA125	Her2Neu[b]	P16	PTEN	P53	Ki-67
1	+	+	+	+	Neg	+	Neg	+	+	+	+	+
2	+	+	+	+	+	Neg	Neg	Neg	Neg	+	+	+
3	+	+	+	+	Neg	Neg	Neg	+	+	+	+	+
4	+	+	+	+	+	+	+	Neg	+	+	+	+
5	+	+	Neg	+	Neg	+	Neg	Neg	Neg	+	+	+
6	+	+	+	+	+	Neg	Neg	Neg	+	+	+	+
7	+	+	+	+	+	+	+	+	+	+	+	+
8	+	+	+	+	+	+	Neg	Neg	+	+	+	+
9	+	+	Neg	+	Neg	Neg	Neg	Neg	Neg	+	+	+
10	+	+	+	+	+	Neg	Neg	Neg	+	+	+	+
11	+	+	+	+	Neg	Neg	Neg	+	Neg	+	+	+
12	+	+	Neg	+	+	+	+	Neg	+	+	+	+
13	+	+	+	+	+	+	Neg	Neg	+	+	+	+
Range (%)	80-100	80-100	10-30	90-100	30-60	30-60	10-20	80-100	30-60	80-90	5-30	30-50

Abbreviation: Neg, negative immunostaining.

[a]Other immunohistochemical markers performed in the differential diagnosis context include MUC5A, MUC6, and CDX2; and all were negative.

[b]Using 3+ membranous reactivity for Her2Neu as positive based on the 2007 College of American Pathologists/American Society of Clinical Oncology guidelines for invasive breast carcinoma (defined as uniform intense membrane staining of >30% of tumor cells).

its distinction from conventional urothelial carcinoma is critical for its clinical management (Fig 2 and Table 2).

▶ Invasive micropapillary urothelial carcinoma (IMUC) is a rare variant of urothelial carcinoma and shares its histological appearance to micropapillary carcinomas arising in the ovary, breast, or lung as well as some other anatomical locations. IMUC has been recognized in the World Health Organization.

This entity may present with diagnostic dilemma for the practicing pathologist because of the unusual histological appearance and wide spectrum of morphological diversity leading to a broad differential diagnosis. Recently, there have been some published case series on this entity, but the information on immunostaining profile and long-term follow-up is limited or controversial.[1,2] This publication is important as the authors not only describe their clinicopathological and follow-up experience with 13 consecutive cases of IMUC but also provide the results of an extensive immunohistochemistry evaluation of this entity in an attempt to confirm or establish the staining profile of known immunomarkers with IMUC.

The study is well illustrated, and the authors have provided good images to illustrate the morphological spectrum of this rare variant of urothelial carcinomas. The immunostaining profile further confirms the consistent positive immunostaining with MUC1 in 100% of the cases in the current series (Table 2). The clinicopathological review of the cases in this series revealed that all had a poor outcome and presented at an advanced stage with poor outcome (Fig 2).

This study is an important one because even though IMUC represents a rare variant of urothelial carcinoma and may present the pathologist with a diagnostic challenge. The recognition and accurate classification of IMUC by the pathologist is critical for the appropriate clinical management of the patient.

A. V. Parwani, MD, PhD

References

1. Kamat AM, Dinney CP, Gee JR, et al. Micropapillary bladder cancer: a review of the University of Texas M.D. Anderson Cancer Center experience with 100 consecutive patients. *Cancer.* 2007;110:62-67.
2. Amin MB, Ro JY, el-Sharkawy T, et al. Micropapillary variant of transitional cell carcinoma of the urinary bladder. Histologic pattern resembling ovarian papillary serous carcinoma. *Am J Surg Pathol.* 1994;18:1224-1232.

MicroRNA profiling of clear cell renal cell carcinoma by whole-genome small RNA deep sequencing of paired frozen and formalin-fixed, paraffin-embedded tissue specimens
Weng L, Wu X, Gao H, et al (City of Hope Natl Med Ctr and Beckman Res Inst, Duarte, CA)
J Pathol 222:41-51, 2010

Renal cell carcinoma (RCC) is one of the leading causes of cancer mortality. Characterization of microRNA (miRNA) expression of RCC

TABLE 2.—Top 20 Dysregulated miRNAs in ccRCC Detected by Frozen and FFPE Sample Deep-Sequencing Analysis

	miRNAs	Frozen Log2 Ratio	p	Alteration	miRNAs	FFPE Log2 Ratio	p	Alteration
1	*hsa-miR-122*	7.43	0.0003	Up	*hsa-miR-184*	9.15	0.0012	Down
2	*hsa-miR-184*	7.02	0.0336	Down	*hsa-miR-122*	7.05	0.0162	Up
3	*hsa-miR-200c*	6.43	0.0004	Down	*hsa-miR-138*	6.28	0.0045	Down
4	*hsa-miR-141*	6.05	0.0003	Down	hsa-miR-509-3p	5.54	0.0165	Down
5	*hsa-miR-875-5p*	5.43	0.0023	Up	*hsa-miR-200c*	5.45	0.0002	Down
6	hsa-miR-9	4.69	0.0007	Down	hsa-miR-508-3p	5.38	0.0064	Down
7	hsa-miR-934	4.43	0.0397	Down	hsa-miR-514	5.37	0.0100	Down
8	*hsa-miR-138*	4.30	0.0007	Down	hsa-miR-891a	5.04	0.0000	Down
9	*hsa-miR-599*	4.06	0.0153	Up	hsa-miR-509-5p	4.74	0.0055	Down
10	hsa-miR-135b	3.52	0.0113	Down	*hsa-miR-210*	4.67	0.0001	Up
11	hsa-miR-335	3.45	0.0261	Down	hsa-miR-224	4.65	0.0036	Up
12	*hsa-miR-210*	3.38	0.0072	Up	*hsa-miR-875-5p*	4.50	0.0387	Up
13	hsa-miR-199b-5p	3.36	0.0242	Up	*hsa-miR-885-5p*	4.42	0.0121	Up
14	*hsa-miR-375*	3.32	0.0208	Down	*hsa-miR-155*	4.21	0.0123	Up
15	*hsa-miR-885-5p*	3.20	0.0038	Up	hsa-miR-506	4.08	0.0370	Down
16	hsa-miR-1270	3.15	0.0031	Up	hsa-miR-206	3.98	0.0006	Down
17	hsa-miR-592	2.94	0.0004	Up	*hsa-miR-375*	3.91	0.0231	Down
18	hsa-miR-129-5p	2.90	0.0127	Down	*hsa-miR-599*	3.80	0.0356	Up
19	*hsa-miR-155*	2.84	0.0173	Up	hsa-miR-486-3p	3.76	0.0145	Up
20	hsa-miR-483-3p	2.78	0.0183	Down	*hsa-miR-141*	3.73	0.0043	Down

ccRCC, clear cell renal cell carcinoma; Frozen, frozen sample set; FFPE, formalin-fixed paraffin-embedded tissue set. Bold italic indicates dysregulated miRNAs in both lists. (minor forms of miRNA excluded).

will help disclose new pathogenic pathways in tumourigenesis and progression and may lead to the development of molecular biomarkers and target-specific therapies for diagnosis, prognostication and treatment. With limitations in test specificity and the ability to detect novel miRNA and other small non-coding RNAs (smRNAs), microarray and RT–PCR techniques are being replaced by the evolving deep-sequencing technologies, at least in the discovery phase. Until now, cancer miRNA profiling of human benign and tumour specimen sets, using smRNA deep-sequencing (smRNA-seq), has not been reported. Specifically, due to concern over possible poor RNA quality/integrity, formalin-fixed paraffin-embedded (FFPE) samples have not been used for such studies. Here, we performed whole-genome smRNA-seq analysis using a benign and RCC specimen set and have successfully profiled the miRNA expression. Studies performed on paired frozen and FFPE specimens showed very similar results. Moreover, a comparison study of microarray, deep-sequencing and RT–PCR methodologies also showed a high correlation among the three technologies. To our knowledge, this is the first study to demonstrate that FFPE specimens can be used reliably for miRNA deep-sequencing analysis, making future large-scale clinical cohort/trial-based studies possible (Table 2).

▶ MicroRNA (miRNA) is a group of small single-stranded noncoding RNAs of 19 to 22 nucleotides in size and regulates gene expression, as do other noncoding small RNAs (smRNAs). In recent years, several hundred miRNAs have been discovered and investigations have revealed alterations in miRNA expression in multiple malignancy types.

This is a timely study in which the investigators have performed whole-genome smRNA sequencing in paired, frozen, and formalin-fixed paraffin-embedded (FFPE) specimens of benign kidney and clear cell renal cell carcinomas (RCCs). Another strength of the study is that the investigators have performed these assays on FFPE samples and evaluated their performance for next-generation sequencing technology.

The authors have successfully profiled miRNA expression associated with its renal neoplasia. The data were based on the benign and the RCC cases and the measured miRNA expression levels. The investigators used the unsupervised clustering method, and using this method, the investigators were successfully able to subclassify the benign and tumor samples. One of the limitations of the study was that the specimen set was small, and therefore, the statistical power of the profiling was limited. Although there was a high correlation between the identified lists of differentially expressed miRNAs between the frozen and FFPE samples, they were not identical.

The results showed that there were 133 types of mature miRNAs, which were differentially expressed between cancer and benign samples ($P < .05$). Of these, 66 types of miRNA were upregulated, while 57 were downregulated in the tumor cases. When the authors classified the top 20 dysregulated miRNAs by rank, interestingly, 11 of these were found in both the frozen and FFPE sample sets (Table 2). These data support the use of FFPE specimens for molecular testing and the feasibility of using deep sequencing for tumor types such as RCC for the analysis of noncoding smRNAs.

A. V. Parwani, MD, PhD

10 Kidney

A Novel Tumor Grading Scheme for Chromophobe Renal Cell Carcinoma: Prognostic Utility and Comparison With Fuhrman Nuclear Grade

Paner GP, Amin MB, Alvarado-Cabrero I, et al (Cedars-Sinai Med Ctr, Los Angeles, CA; Emory Univ School of Medicine, Atlanta, GA; et al)
Am J Surg Pathol 34:1233-1240, 2010

Chromophobe renal cell carcinoma (RCC) is a histologic subtype of RCC that portends a favorable prognosis. It is controversial whether the Fuhrman nuclear grade of chromophobe RCC has prognostic utility. Irregular nuclei, prominent nucleoli, and nuclear pleomorphism are inherently present in chromophobe RCC. Hence, the Fuhrman nuclear grade is higher even though the majority of these tumors have a favorable outcome. In this study, the prognostic utility of a novel 3-tiered tumor grading system in which the innate nuclear atypia of chromophobe RCC was discounted, herein referred to as chromophobe tumor grade from a series of 124 chromophobe RCC, was compared with Fuhrman nuclear grade. Chromophobe tumor grade is based on the assessment of geographic nuclear crowding and anaplasia. The Fuhrman nuclear grade distribution between the tumors was grade 1 (1%), grade 2 (19%), grade 3 (74%), and grade 4 (6%), whereas the chromophobe tumor grade distribution was grade 1 (74%), grade 2 (16%), and grade 3 (10%). Neither Fuhrman nuclear grade nor chromophobe tumor grade was significantly associated with patient's age or sex and chromophobe RCC cell types, but both showed a significant association with tumor size. Both Fuhrman nuclear grade and chromophobe tumor grade showed statistically significant positive associations with broad alveolar growth, necrosis, vascular invasion, and with pathologic stage; however, all these associations tended to be dictated by tumors with sarcomatoid change. When tumors with sarcomatoid change were excluded, a strong positive association persisted between chromophobe tumor grade and pathologic stage. In contrast, there was no such association between Fuhrman nuclear grade and stage in nonsarcomatoid chromophobe RCCs. Characterizing aggressive chromophobe RCC with aggressive behavior with the time from surgery to first occurrence of metastasis, local recurrence, or death owing to disease, we found that both Fuhrman nuclear grade and chromophobe tumor grade were highly associated with adverse outcome. However, as with the pathologic stage, only a significant association between chromophobe tumor grade and outcome was retained among nonsarcomatoid chromophobe RCCs. Multivariable Cox regression analysis also tended to support chromophobe tumor grade rather than Fuhrman nuclear grade as an independent predictor of adverse outcome, controlling for other univariably significant risk factors [estimated relative hazard $= 3.68$ $(P = 0.026)$ vs. 1.86 $(P = 0.42)$]. In conclusion, the novel chromophobe tumor grading system proposed herewith provides superior prognostic value to that of the Fuhrman nuclear grade in chromophobe RCC and will potentially help stratify patients of chromophobe RCC who are at a greater risk of disease progression.

▶ Fuhrman nuclear grading is currently the most widely used grading system for renal cell carcinoma (RCC) in the United States. The Fuhrman nuclear grade encompasses the nuclear size, shape, and the prominence of nucleoli and stratifies the RCC cases into a 4-tiered grading system. Chromophobe RCC is a subtype of RCC, which has a favorable prognosis. Interestingly, some of the characteristic histological findings in chromophobe RCCs include the presence of irregular nuclei, prominent nucleoli, and nuclear pleomorphism. There is much controversy in the literature[1] as to the applicability of the Fuhrman nuclear grade in stratification of chromophobe RCCs because of the presence of the above high-grade histological features and yet a better clinical outcome.

The authors in this study have addressed this discordance between the current grading system and clinical outcome in cases of chromophobe RCCs by proposing and evaluating a new and novel 3-tiered grading system. A total of 124 cases were evaluated using Fuhrman grading system and the chromophobe grading system. The latter grading system as defined in this study is as follows: (1) Grade 1: chromophobe RCC with (usual) wide constitutive nuclear range but without nuclear crowding and anaplasia (Figs 1A and B in the original article); (2) Grade 2: geographic nuclear crowding (defined as cellular clustering characterized by high geographic nuclear/cytoplasmic density detectable using 10× objective and some nuclei in direct contact with each other when assessed with the 40× objective) and the presence of nuclear pleomorphism (size variation of greater than 3-fold and distinct nuclear chromatin irregularities (Figs 1C and D in the original article); and (3) Grade 3: presence of frank anaplasia (nuclear polylobation and tumor giant cells) (Figs 1E and F in the original article) or sarcomatoid change.

The results showed that on the basis of Fuhrman grading system, most of the cases were graded as Fuhrman grade 3 and very few as grade 1. On the other hand, using the chromophobe grading system, most chromophobe RCCs that are low grade show a declining distribution with increasing tumor grade. There was a more consistent trend toward an increasing proportion of chromophobe RCC with an adverse outcome with increasing nuclear grade using the chromophobe tumor grading system (Fig 5 in the original). The results of the study are also important because the authors have provided a side-by-side comparison with their grading system and the original Fuhrman grading system for chromophobe RCCs (Fig 6 in the original article).

The authors have demonstrated that the novel chromophobe tumor grading system proposed in this article is a more superior grading system than the Fuhrman nuclear grade in stratifying chromophobe RCCs and their correlation with prognosis. Additional larger studies by independent investigators and long-term follow-up of the patients in the future are needed to confirm the risk stratification power of the proposed grading system for chromophobe RCCs.

A. V. Parwani, MD, PhD

Reference

1. Patard JJ, Leray E, Rioux-Leclercq N, et al. Prognostic value of histologic subtypes in renal cell carcinoma: a multicenter experience. *J Clin Oncol*. 2005;23: 2763-2771.

A Novel Tumor Grading Scheme for Chromophobe Renal Cell Carcinoma: Prognostic Utility and Comparison With Fuhrman Nuclear Grade
Paner GP, Amin MB, Alvarado-Cabrero I, et al (Cedars-Sinai Med Ctr, Los Angeles, CA; Emory Univ School of Medicine, Atlanta, GA; et al)
Am J Surg Pathol 34:1233-1240, 2010

Chromophobe renal cell carcinoma (RCC) is a histologic subtype of RCC that portends a favorable prognosis. It is controversial whether the Fuhrman nuclear grade of chromophobe RCC has prognostic utility. Irregular nuclei, prominent nucleoli, and nuclear pleomorphism are inherently present in chromophobe RCC. Hence, the Fuhrman nuclear grade is higher even though the majority of these tumors have a favorable outcome. In this study, the prognostic utility of a novel 3-tiered tumor grading system in which the innate nuclear atypia of chromophobe RCC was discounted, herein referred to as chromophobe tumor grade from a series of 124 chromophobe RCC, was compared with Fuhrman nuclear grade. Chromophobe tumor grade is based on the assessment of geographic nuclear crowding and anaplasia. The Fuhrman nuclear grade distribution between the tumors was grade 1 (1%), grade 2 (19%), grade 3 (74%), and grade 4 (6%), whereas the chromophobe tumor grade distribution was grade 1 (74%), grade 2 (16%), and grade 3 (10%). Neither Fuhrman nuclear grade nor chromophobe tumor grade was significantly associated with patient's age or sex and chromophobe RCC cell types, but both showed a significant association with tumor size. Both Fuhrman nuclear grade and chromophobe tumor grade showed statistically significant positive associations with broad alveolar growth, necrosis, vascular invasion, and with pathologic stage; however, all these associations tended to be dictated by tumors with sarcomatoid change. When tumors with sarcomatoid change were excluded, a strong positive association persisted between chromophobe tumor grade and pathologic stage. In contrast, there was no such association between Fuhrman nuclear grade and stage in nonsarcomatoid chromophobe RCCs. Characterizing aggressive chromophobe RCC with aggressive

TABLE 3.—Multivariable Cox Regression: Independent Predictors of Chromophobe Renal Cell Carcinoma With Adverse Outcome Using Chromophobe Tumor Grade*

Predictor	Estimated Relative Hazard (P Value)	95% Confidence Interval
Chromophobe nuclear grade (2, 3 vs. 1)	3.68 (0.026)	(1.17-11.59)
Necrosis (1, 2 vs. 0)	4.37 (0.004)	(1.61-11.89)
pT stage (3,4 vs. 1,2)	1.75 (0.36)	(0.53-5.77)
Tumor size (cm)	1.02 (0.67)	(0.94-1.09)

See Ref. 3 for details of distribution of parameters.
*Excluding 12 chromophobe renal cell carcinoma with sarcomatoid change; 102 patients contributed to analysis.

TABLE 4.—Multivariable Cox Regression: Independent Predictors of Chromophobe Renal Cell Carcinoma With Adverse Outcome Using Fuhrman Nuclear Grade*

Predictor	Estimated Relative Hazard (P Value)	95% Confidence Interval
Fuhrman nuclear grade (3, 4 vs. 2)	1.86 (0.42)	(0.41-8.40)
Necrosis (1, 2 vs. 0)	3.67 (0.012)	(1.34-10.07)
pT stage (3, 4 vs. 1,2)	4.15 (0.006)	(1.51-11.40)
Tumor size (cm)	1.01 (0.78)	(0.94-1.09)

*Excluding 12 chromophobe renal cell carcinoma with sarcomatoid change; 116 patients contributed to analysis.

behavior with the time from surgery to first occurrence of metastasis, local recurrence, or death owing to disease, we found that both Fuhrman nuclear grade and chromophobe tumor grade were highly associated with adverse outcome. However, as with the pathologic stage, only a significant association between chromophobe tumor grade and outcome was retained among nonsarcomatoid chromophobe RCCs. Multivariable Cox regression analysis also tended to support chromophobe tumor grade rather than Fuhrman nuclear grade as an independent predictor of adverse outcome, controlling for other univariably significant risk factors [estimated relative hazard = 3.68 ($P = 0.026$) vs. 1.86 ($P = 0.42$)]. In conclusion, the novel chromophobe tumor grading system proposed herewith provides superior prognostic value to that of the Fuhrman nuclear grade in chromophobe RCC and will potentially help stratify patients of chromophobe RCC who are at a greater risk of disease progression (Tables 3 and 4).

▶ As a surgical pathologist, it always feels inadequate to assign a Fuhrman nuclear grade to chromophobe renal cell carcinoma (CRCC). One of the main goals of reporting kidney tumor resection specimens is to provide clinically useful prognostic information. Unfortunately, it seems we overcall the nuclear grade on chromophobe tumors with an otherwise good prognosis. This article proposes a new grading scheme specific for CRCC and compares it with Fuhrman grading and prognosis. The proposed scheme has 3 tiers; Grade 1 tumors show a wide range of nuclear size/shape without nuclear crowding and anaplasia; Grade 2 tumors show geographic nuclear crowding, at least a 3-fold variation in nuclear size, and nuclear chromatin irregularities; Grade 3 tumors show frank anaplasia or sarcomatoid changes. Indeed, while 74% of cases were initially classified as Fuhrman grade 3, application of the chromophobe nuclear grade resulted in 74% of cases being classified as grade 1. Tables 3 and 4 show the multivariate analysis for independent predictors between the chromophobe and Fuhrman nuclear grades, respectively. The average follow-up time with 48 months and 20 adverse events were identified out of 123 patients with follow-up. Although studies with a longer follow-up are needed to validate the chromophobe nuclear grade, this classification seems to add additional value over Fuhrman grading. Perhaps the more difficult challenge will be introducing a new grading system to our clinical colleagues.

M. L. Smith, MD

Fluorescence In Situ Hybridisation in the Diagnosis of Upper Urinary Tract Tumours

Mian C, Mazzoleni G, Vikoler S, et al (Central Hosp of Bolzano, Italy; et al)
Eur Urol 58:288-292, 2010

Background.—Upper urinary tract (UUT) tumours are often a diagnostic challenge. Because of delayed diagnosis at an advanced stage, prognosis is less qualitative when compared to bladder tumours. There is, therefore, a need for reliable markers to improve diagnosis.

Objective.—Because of the difficulty in interpreting washing cytologies of the UUT, we evaluated the reliability of fluorescence in situ hybridisation (FISH) in the detection of upper tract urothelial cancer.

Design, Setting, and Participants.—A prospective, multicentre cohort study was carried out on 55 consecutive patients with a suspected UUT tumour.

Measurements.—Between May 2007 and May 2009, 55 consecutive patients (mean age 71.7 yr; range: 52–93) with a suspected urinary tract tumour were studied with intravenous pyelography, cytology, washing cytology, ureterorenoscopy, and endoscopic biopsies. The patients were followed for a mean observation time of 12.21 mo (range: 0.5–20; standard deviation: 6.12). A multicolour-FISH approach was performed on a liquid-based washing urinary cytology in all cases.

Results and Limitations.—Twenty-one out of 55 patients had a histologically proven urothelial carcinoma, of which 10 had stage pTa disease, 6 had pT1 disease, 2 had pT2 disease, 2 had pTis disease, and 1 had pTx disease (6 G1, 6 G2, and 9 G3). Three patients had a papilloma, 2 had renal cell carcinoma, 27 had a negative histologic report, and 2 had a non-diagnostic histology. In total, 68 analyses were performed. The cytology was negative or doubtful in 60 out of a total 68 specimens (88.2%) and was suspicious or positive for malignancy in 7 (10.3%) specimens. One specimen was not diagnostic. FISH was negative in 37 of 68 analyses

TABLE 2.—Sensitivity, Specificity, and the Predictive Values of Fluorescence In Situ Hybridisation

	Cytology, %	FISH, %
Sensitivity	20.8	100
Specificity	97.4	89.5
PPV	83.3	84.6
NPV	68.5	100

FISH = fluorescence in situ hybridisation; PPV = positive predictive value; NPV = negative predictive value.

(54.4%) and positive in the other 30 analyses (44.1%). One FISH analysis was not diagnostic as a result of insufficient cellular material. The overall sensitivity of the cytology was 20.8% and of FISH 100%. The specificity was 97.4% for cytology and 89.5% for FISH. Even though this is the largest UUT cohort studied with FISH, the sample size is relatively small.

Conclusions.—The UroVysion FISH test is a reliable method in the diagnosis of UUT tumours in cases with clinical suspicion but negative or doubtful cytology and no diagnostic histology (Table 2).

▶ Upper urinary tract urothelial tumors often present with a diagnostic challenge for the surgical pathologist because of the scant material usually available for diagnosis because of the inherent difficulty in sampling the neoplasm. Additionally, there is significant interobserver and intraobserver variability in the diagnosis. Also, there is very limited use for immunohistochemical markers to aid in the diagnostic process. The type of material obtained may also have an impact on the diagnostic process.

This article is important because it targets this difficult area of upper urinary tract and presents the author's experience with using fluorescence in situ hybridization (FISH) in the detection of upper tract urothelial cancer (UroVysion FISH test).

Although only 55 cases were included in this study, the results from this study were very interesting. The studies indicated that there was a highly significant difference between the cytology and FISH data as compared with the histologic diagnosis ($P < .001$). In addition, there was also a highly significant correlation ($P < .001$) between the chromosomal pattern and the tumor grade (Table 2).

Based on these results, it can be concluded that the UroVysion FISH test is reliable for the diagnosis of upper urinary tract tumors, particularly in cases where there is a negative or indeterminate cytology or if the surgical pathology results are nondiagnostic. These results need to be verified in larger number of cases but point to the use of a promising diagnostic test when we encounter a diagnostically challenging urothelial tumor in the renal pelvis or upper urinary tract.

A. V. Parwani, MD, PhD

Clinicopathological characteristics of patients with IgG4-related tubulointerstitial nephritis

Saeki T, Nishi S, Imai N, et al (Nagaoka Red Cross Hosp, Niigata, Japan; Niigata Univ Graduate School of Med and Dental Sciences, Japan; et al)
Kidney Int 2010 [Epub ahead of print]

IgG4-related disease is a recently recognized multi-organ disorder characterized by high levels of serum IgG4 and dense infiltration of IgG4-positive cells into several organs. Although the pancreas was the first organ recognized to be affected by IgG4-related disorder in the syndrome of autoimmune pancreatitis, we present here clinicopathological features of 23 patients diagnosed as having renal parenchymal lesions. These injuries were associated with a high level of serum IgG4 and abundant IgG4-positive plasma cell infiltration into the renal interstitium with fibrosis. In all patients, tubulointerstitial nephritis was the major finding. Although 14 of the 23 patients did not have any pancreatic lesions, their clinicopathological features were quite uniform and similar to those shown in autoimmune pancreatitis. These included predominance in middle-aged to elderly men, frequent association with IgG4-related conditions in other organs, high levels of serum IgG and IgG4, a high frequency of hypocomplementemia, a high serum IgE level, a patchy and diffuse lesion distribution, a swirling fibrosis in the renal pathology, and a good response to corticosteroids. Thus, we suggest that renal parenchymal lesions actually develop in association with IgG4-related disease, for which we propose the term 'IgG4-related tubulointerstitial nephritis.'

▶ Tubulointerstitial nephritis (TIN) is defined by an inflammatory cell infiltrate involving the interstitium and tubules often with tubular injury, edema, fibrosis, and tubular atrophy. TIN is often classified into infectious and noninfectious causes. Noninfectious causes often show prominent mixed inflammation including neutrophils, plasma cells, macrophages, and eosinophils. Occasionally, one of these cell types predominates, which may help suggest a particular diagnosis; however, a definitive diagnosis is often not possible. Saeki et al present a thorough clinicopathologic review of patients with IgG4-related TIN that should be included in the differential diagnosis of TIN. IgG4-related TIN may be suggested histologically by a robust plasma cell infiltrate involving a swirling pattern of interstitial fibrosis, a pathologic finding similar to that seen in the pancreas of patients with autoimmune pancreatitis. Immunohistochemical staining for IgG4-positive plasma cells resulted in greater than 10 positive cells per high-power field. A wide range of renal dysfunction was seen at the time of biopsy with serum creatinine ranging from 0.67 to 6.87. Recognition of this disease process is important as prompt administration of steroids usually results in a good response.

M. L. Smith, MD

Quantitative Real-Time Polymerase Chain Reaction Detection of BK Virus Using Labeled Primers

Gu Z, Pan J, Bankowski MJ, et al (St Jude Children's Res Hosp, Memphis, TN; Univ of Hawaii, Honolulu)
Arch Pathol Lab Med 134:444-448, 2010

Context.—BK virus infections among immunocompromised patients are associated with disease of the kidney or urinary bladder. High viral loads, determined by quantitative polymerase chain reaction (PCR), have been correlated with clinical disease.

Objective.—To develop and evaluate a novel method for real-time PCR detection and quantification of BK virus using labeled primers.

Design.—Patient specimens (n = 54) included 17 plasma, 12 whole blood, and 25 urine samples. DNA was extracted using the MagNA Pure LC Total Nucleic Acid Isolation Kit (Roche Applied Science, Indianapolis, Indiana); sample eluate was PCR-amplified using the labeled primer PCR method. Results were compared with those of a userdeveloped quantitative real-time PCR method (fluorescence resonance energy transfer probe hybridization).

Results.—Labeled primer PCR detected less than 10 copies per reaction and showed quantitative linearity from 10^1 to 10^7 copies per reaction. Analytical specificity of labeled primer PCR was 100%. With clinical samples, labeled primer PCR demonstrated a trend toward improved sensitivity compared with the reference method. Quantitative assay comparison showed an R^2 value of 0.96 between the 2 assays.

Conclusions.—Real-time PCR using labeled primers is highly sensitive and specific for the quantitative detection of BK virus from a variety of clinical specimens. These data demonstrate the applicability of labeled primer PCR for quantitative viral detection and offer a simplified method that removes the need for separate oligonucleotide probes.

▶ Many studies have shown that the polyomavirus-associated nephropathy in renal transplant recipients and hemorrhagic cystitis in hematopoietic stem cell transplant recipients are associated with BK virus infection. Pathology laboratories are increasingly receiving specimens to accurately evaluate BK virus load to assess for the presence and severity of BK virus-associated disease. Additionally, such viral load testing is being also used to monitor therapeutic response in transplant patients.

In recent years, polymerase chain reaction (PCR) technology has had a significant impact in the clinical molecular diagnosis of infectious agents. This is an important article that describes the development and use of a new method for real-time PCR detection and quantification of BK viral load using labeled primers. The assay was designed based on the MultiCode-RTx system (EraGen Biosciences, Inc, Madison, Wisconsin). The system uses a real-time PCR based on the use of fluorescence resonance energy transfer (FRET). There is a specific interaction between 2 modified nucleotides (iso-deoxyguanosine triphosphate and iso-deoxycytidine triphosphate). This system is advantageous because there is no need for separate oligonucleotide probes and differs from many other FRET chemistries in that labeled primers are used. Although the number of samples tested is small (n = 54), it encompasses a wide range of clinical specimens, such as urine, plasma, and whole blood.

The results were good and showed that all clinical specimen types were successfully evaluated. The labeled primer PCR assay was able to detect less than 10 copies per reaction with an analytical specificity of 100%. The methods described in this study is valuable for the molecular laboratory because it can reduce the number of reagents required for testing. This also reduces test variability. Similar method can be used for detection of other infectious agents. It is important for the anatomical and clinical pathologist to continuously get involved in the testing of new technology and promising assays such as described in this study to improve their practice and ultimately patient care.

A. V. Parwani, MD, PhD

De novo Thrombotic Microangiopathy in Renal Allograft Biopsies — Role of Antibody-Mediated Rejection

Satoskar AA, Pelletier R, Adams P, et al (Ohio State Univ, Columbus)
Am J Transplant 10:1804-1811, 2010

The most common cause of thrombotic microangiopathy (TMA) in renal allografts is thought to be calcineurin inhibitor toxicity. Antibody-mediated rejection (AMR) can also cause TMA, but its true impact on *de novo* TMA is unknown. In a retrospective review of renal allograft biopsies from January 2003 to December 2008 at our institution, we determined the prevalence of TMA in patients with C4d positive (n = 243) and C4d negative (n = 715) biopsies. Over 90% of patients received cyclosporine in both groups. *De novo* TMA was seen in 59 (6.1%) patients; most of them (55%) with C4d positive biopsy. Among patients with C4d positive biopsies, 13.6% had TMA, as compared to only 3.6% patients with C4d negative biopsies (p < 0.0001). Incidence of graft loss between C4d positive and C4d negative TMA groups was not significantly different, but 70% of patients with C4d positive TMA who received plasmapheresis had slightly lower graft loss rate. In biopsies with AMR-associated TMA, glomerulitis and peritubular capillaritis were significantly more prominent. AMR is the most common cause of TMA in renal allografts in our patient population. It is important to recognize AMR-related TMA because plasmapheresis treatment may be beneficial (Tables 1 and 5).

▶ In the past, most cases of thrombotic microangiopathy (TMA) arising in renal allografts have been attributed to calcineurin inhibitor effect. As the recognition of antibody-mediated rejection (AMR) has become more common and different histopathologic presentations are described, AMR-associated TMA is becoming increasingly recognized. This article seeks to evaluate the prevalence

TABLE 1.—Proportion of Patients with TMA, High PRA and Graft Loss in the C4d Positive and C4d Negative Groups

	PTC C4d Positive (n = 243)	PTC C4d Negative (n = 715)	p-Value[1]
TMA present	33 (13.6%)	26 (3.6%)	<0.0001
High PRA with TMA	26/31 (84%)	3/24 (12.5%)	<0.0001
Graft loss at 2 years	13/33 (40%)	11/26 (42%)	1

TMA = thrombotic microangiopathy; PRA = panel-reactive antibodies; PTC = peritubular capillary.
[1]Fisher's exact p value.

TABLE 5.—Histopathologic Features

Histologic Features	C4d Positive (n = 33)	C4d Negative (n = 26)	p-Value
Interstitial inflammation (i)	1.03 ± 0.95	1 ± 0.98	0.846
Tubulitis (t)	0.13 ± 0.55	0.27 ± 0.72	0.356
Glomerulitis (g)	1 ± 1	0.36 ± 0.81	0.003
Intimal arteritis (i)	0.09 ± 0.39	0.12 ± 0.6	1.000
Peritubular capillary margination	1.45 ± 0.9	0.85 ± 0.97	0.017
Acute tubular necrosis (ATN)	1.58 ± 1.15	1.62 ± 1.3	0.844
Tubular isometric vacuolization	0.24 ± 0.66	0.42 ± 0.86	0.392
Transplant glomerulopathy (cg)	0.76 ± 1.12	0.52 ± 1.16	0.239
Mucoid intimal thickening	0.61 ± 0.83	1.08 ± 1.2	0.136
Tubular atrophy (ct)	0.94 ± 1	1.27 ± 1.25	0.307
Interstitial fibrosis (ci)	0.94 ± 1	1.27 ± 1.25	0.307
Arteriolar hyaline (ah)	0.45 ± 0.79	1.2 ± 1.29	0.025
Arterial intimal fibrosis (cv)	0.64 ± 0.74	0.35 ± 0.49	0.164
Glomerular sclerosis	0.3 ± 0.64	0.32 ± 0.48	0.543
Chronic allograft damage index (CADI)	4.21 ± 4.19	4.62 ± 3.77	0.557
TMA changes in glomeruli alone[1]	17 (51%)	8 (30%)	0.122
TMA changes in glomeruli and arteries/ arterioles[1]	16 (48%)	18 (69%)	

All the histopathologic features were graded semiquantitatively from 0 to 3+. Average of the scores was used for comparison. Nonparametric Wilcoxon rank sum test was used for statistical comparison.
[1]TMA changes in glomeruli and/or arteries were scored as present/absent. The numbers indicate the number of patients. Fisher's exact p-value was calculated.

of TMA changes in 2 groups of patients: those who are C4d positive and those who are C4d negative. One must use caution when using only C4d immunofluorescence as a surrogate marker for AMR. Clinically, in addition to C4d deposition within peritubular capillaries, AMR requires histologic evidence of allograft injury and the presence of donor-specific antibodies. Nevertheless, in this series of patients, most of the C4d-positive patients did show a high panel-reactive antibody level, supporting the use of C4d as a surrogate marker for AMR. The histologic data suggest that peritubular capillaritis and glomerulitis favor AMR-associated TMA, while there was a trend toward increased arteriolar hyaline in C4d-negative TMA cases (Table 5). Overall, regardless of the etiology, the graft loss rate at 2 years in cases of TMA is approximately 41% (Table 1). For centers that do not routinely perform C4d stains on all allograft biopsies, this article provides support for C4d analysis in cases that histologically show TMA.

M. L. Smith, MD

The Association Between Age and Nephrosclerosis on Renal Biopsy Among Healthy Adults

Rule AD, Amer H, Cornell LD, et al (Mayo Clinic, Rochester, MN)
Ann Intern Med 152:561-567, 2010

Background.—Chronic kidney disease is common with older age and is characterized on renal biopsy by global glomerulosclerosis, tubular atrophy, interstitial fibrosis, and arteriosclerosis.

Objective.—To see whether the prevalence of these histologic abnormalities in the kidney increases with age in healthy adults and whether histologic findings are explained by age-related differences in kidney function or chronic kidney disease risk factors.

Design.—Cross-sectional study.

Setting.—Mayo Clinic, Rochester, Minnesota, from 1999 to 2009.

Patients.—1203 adult living kidney donors.

Measurements.—Core-needle biopsy of the renal cortex obtained during surgical implantation of the kidney, and medical record data of kidney function and risk factors obtained before donation.

Results.—The prevalence of nephrosclerosis (≥ 2 chronic histologic abnormalities) was 2.7% (95% CI, 1.1% to 6.7%) for patients aged 18 to 29 years, 16% (CI, 12% to 20%) for patients aged 30 to 39 years, 28% (CI, 24% to 32%) for patients aged 40 to 49 years, 44% (CI, 38% to 50%) for patients aged 50 to 59 years, 58% (CI, 47% to 67%) for patients aged 60 to 69 years, and 73% (CI, 43% to 90%) for patients aged 70 to 77 years. Adjustment for kidney function and risk factor covariates did not explain the age-related increase in the prevalence of nephrosclerosis.

Limitation.—Kidney donors are selected for health and lack the spectrum or severity of renal pathologic findings in the general population.

Conclusion.—Kidney function and chronic kidney disease risk factors do not explain the strong association between age and nephrosclerosis in healthy adults (Table 2).

▶ Chronic kidney disease (CKD) is more common in older patients. The characteristic histological findings on renal biopsy include global glomerulosclerosis, tubular atrophy, interstitial fibrosis, and arteriosclerosis. Clinically, the patient has a reduced estimated glomerular filtration rate (GFR) or elevated urinary albumin excretion. There is limited information on age-related changes in CKD.[1]

This is a comprehensive study on the association between age and nephrosclerosis on renal biopsy among healthy adults. The study population comprised of 1203 adult living kidney donors. Selecting living kidney donors

TABLE 2.—Prevalence of Nephrosclerosis, by Age Group*

Age Group	Crude Prevalence (95% CI), %	Crude Prevalence After Exclusion of Persons Who Received Therapy for Hypertension (95% CI), %
18–29 y	2.7 (1.1–6.7)	2.7 (1.1–6.7)
30–39 y	16 (12–20)	15 (12–20)
40–49 y	28 (24–32)	26 (22–31)
50–59 y	44 (38–50)	42 (36–49)
60–69 y	58 (47–67)	55 (44–66)
70–77 y	73 (43–90)	75 (41–93)
Overall	28 (25–30)	26 (24–29)

*Among 1203 living kidney donors at Mayo Clinic.

as the study population offers an advantage: usually these individuals are healthy donors so the investigators can study the clinical attributes and the histopathologic findings without other variables such as preexisting health conditions. Therefore, the investigators in this study were able to study the prevalence and spectrum of histologic changes in the kidneys of the living donor and were able to assess if they were age-related or not or if there were any associations with risk factors for CKD.

The results from this study were striking and showed that nephrosclerosis increased with age with an overall prevalence of 28% (confidence interval [CI], 25% to 30%). Interestingly, the youngest age group showed a prevalence of only 2.7% (95% CI, 1.1% to 6.7%), and there were no significant differences in the prevalence of nephrosclerosis between men and women (Table 2).

Some of the conclusions from this study are that there is an association between age and nephrosclerosis in healthy adults. The latter association is not attributable to age differences in chronic kidney risk factors, urinary albumin excretion, or GFR. Because this study population was composed of living kidney donors, some of the age-related associations are not valid for the general population. Additional studies are needed to include general population subjects to further characterize the age-related association with CKD, to design and implement prevention and treatment strategies.

A. V. Parwani, MD, PhD

Reference

1. Silva FG. The aging kidney: a review–part I. *Int Urol Nephrol*. 2005;37:185-205.

Expression of Galectin-3 in Renal Neoplasms: A Diagnostic, Possible Prognostic Marker

Dancer JY, Truong LD, Zhai Q, et al (The Methodist Hosp and Res Inst and Weill Med College of Cornell Univ, Houston, TX; M D Anderson Cancer Ctr, Houston, TX)
Arch Pathol Lab Med 134:90-94, 2010

Context.—Galectin-3, a member of the lectin family, was shown to be expressed in normal distal tubular cells and in renal cell carcinomas (RCC). However, its diagnostic and prognostic significance in RCC is as yet undefined.

Objectives.—To describe the expression of Galectin-3 among different histologic subtypes of renal neoplasms and to determine their diagnostic and prognostic significances.

Design.—The expression of Galectin-3 was evaluated in 217 renal neoplasms by tissue microarray and immunohistochemistry with semi-quantitative analysis.

Results.—Strong expression of Galectin-3 was observed in 92 of 217 of renal neoplasms (42.4%). Although 22 of 23 oncocytomas (95.7%) and 19 of 21 chromophobe RCCs (90.5%) express Galectin-3, only 4 of 32 papillary RCCs (12.5%) and 47 of 137 clear cell RCCs (34.3%) express Galectin-3, suggesting that it may be used as a potential diagnostic marker. Galectin-3 expression was seen in 55% of high-grade (Fuhrman nuclear grades 3 and 4) versus 21% low-grade (grades 1 and 2) clear cell RCCs ($P < .001$).

Conclusions.—This study confirms that Galactin-3 is strongly overex-pressed in renal cell neoplasms of distal tubular differentiation, that is, oncocytoma and chromophobe RCCs, suggesting it might be used as a possible differential diagnostic tool for renal cell neoplasm with onco-cytic or granular cells. Furthermore, we observed a strong association of overexpression of Galectin-3 and high nuclear grade in clear cell RCC. These results also suggest a possible pivotal role for Galectin-3 in the differentiation and prognosis of clear cell RCC (Fig 3, Table 1).

▶ Needle core biopsies for smaller renal lesions identified by imaging are increasingly being performed prior to definitive therapy. While the diagnosis is often straightforward, lesions that are difficult to classify are not uncommon. Of particular difficulty are limited samples of lesions comprised of eosinophilic granular or oncocytic cells. The differential diagnosis often includes the eosinophilic variant of clear cell renal cell carcinoma (RCC), oncocytoma, and chromophobe RCC. This retrospective immunohistochemical study confirms that Galectin-3 is more commonly overexpressed in oncocytomas and chromophobe RCCs and may be a useful immunohistochemical marker to add to the panel of stains for renal cell neoplasms, which may include CK7, RCC, CD10, vimentin, and CD117. Table 1 shows the Galectin-3 expres-sion for different renal lesions. Galectin-3 is proposed to be involved in cell proliferation, cell-cell interaction, apoptosis, and characteristics important in

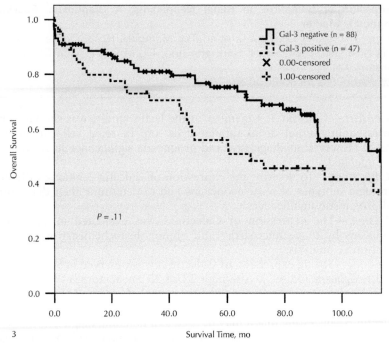

3   Survival Time, mo

FIGURE 3.—Survival of clear cell renal cell carcinoma and expression of Galectin-3 (Gal-3). (Reprinted from Dancer JY, Truong LD, Zhai Q, et al. Expression of Galectin-3 in renal neoplasms: a diagnostic, possible prognostic marker. *Arch Pathol Lab Med.* 2010;134:90-94, with permission from Archives of Pathology & Laboratory Medicine. Copyright 2010. College of American Pathologists.)

TABLE 1.—Expression of Galectin-3 by Different Histologic Types

Histologic Type (No.)	Galectin-3[+] Cases, No. (%)
Clear Cell RCC (137)	47 (34.3)
Papillary RCC (32)	4 (12.5)
Chromophobe RCC (21)	19 (90.5)
Oncocytoma (23)	22 (95.7)
Unclassified RCC (3)	0 (0)
Collecting duct carcinoma (1)	0 (0)
Total (217)	92 (42.4)

Abbreviation: RCC, renal cell carcinoma.

tumor progression and spread. Indeed, Galectin-3 has been associated with increased tumor aggressiveness in gastric, breast, and urothelial malignancies.[1-3] In the subset of clear cell RCCs, the authors demonstrate a trend toward worse prognosis with increased Galectin-3 staining (Fig 3).

M. L. Smith, MD

References

1. Miyazaki J, Hokari R, Kato S, et al. Increased expression of galectin-3 in primary gastric cancer and the metastatic lymph nodes. *Oncol Rep.* 2002;9:1307-1312.
2. Shekhar MP, Nangia-Makker P, Tait L, et al. Alterations in galectin-3 expression and distribution correlate with breast cancer progression: functional analysis of galectin-3 in breast epithelial-endothelial interactions. *Am J Pathol.* 2004;165: 1931-1941.
3. Canesin G, Gonzalez-Peramato P, Palou J, et al. Galectin-3 expression is associated with bladder cancer progression and clinical outcome. *Tumour Biol.* 2010;31: 277-285.

What Is the Role of Percutaneous Needle Core Biopsy in Diagnosis of Renal Masses?
Sofikerim M, Tatlisen A, Canoz O, et al (Erciyes Univ, Kayseri, Turkey)
Urology 76:614-619, 2010

Objective.—To define the accuracy and acceptability of ultrasonography-guided percutaneous needle core biopsy in diagnosis of renal masses.

Methods.—The data of 42 consecutive patients on whom needle biopsies were performed and were surgically treated for suspicious renal masses in our clinic between January 2001 and April 2008 were evaluated. In all patients, needle biopsies were done percutaneously with an 18-gauge needle under local anesthesia in prone position with ultrasonography guidance. Two cores were taken from each tumor. The pathology results of biopsy and surgical specimens were compared.

Results.—The mean age was 56.1 years (range, 21-77 years). The mean follow-up period was calculated as 44.8 months (range, 10-85 months). The abdominal computed tomography imaging showed that the mean mass size was 63.9 mm (range, 25-140 mm). Of 42 patients, 39 were diagnosed (92.8%) after the first biopsy. The accuracy of percutaneous needle biopsy in differentiating between malignant and benign masses was calculated as 90% (36/40). The accuracy of histopathological diagnostic typing as against the postsurgical pathologic examination results was 77.5% (31/40) and the accuracy in the Fuhrman grade was 51.5% (17/33). The sensitivity was calculated as 91.4% and specificity as 60%. Its negative predictive value was 50% and positive predictive value was 94.1%.

Conclusions.—In conclusion, percutaneous renal needle core biopsy has an acceptable sensitivity and specificity in the diagnosis of renal masses. The major limitation of percutaneous core biopsy is the technical failure that leads to insufficient material for accurate diagnosis.

▶ This is an interesting article that describes the experience of the authors with the use of ultrasonography-guided percutaneous needle core biopsy for the diagnosis of renal masses. The latter is a controversial area in cytopathology and surgical pathology because studies have claimed that percutaneous aspiration cytology has low sensitivity and frequently results in a nondiagnostic report. On the other hand, some authors have claimed that percutaneous needle biopsies offer the urologists with a test that has high specificity and sensitivity. Because many small renal masses are often benign, it may be advantageous to use a percutaneous needle biopsy to evaluate them.

Even though the number of cases that were evaluated was only 42, the results are very convincing. For each case, needle core biopsy without aspiration was obtained and 2 cores were taken from each mass. The authors compared the results of biopsy and surgical specimens and found out that accuracy of percutaneous needle biopsy in differentiating between malignant and benign masses was calculated as 90% (36/40). When the histopathological typing accuracy was evaluated, it was found to be 77.5% (31/40) as compared with the resection specimen. Fuhrman grade scoring was only 51.5% (17/33), most likely because of sampling and tumor heterogeneity.

The conclusions from this study were that percutaneous renal needle core biopsy has an acceptable sensitivity and specificity in the diagnosis of renal masses. However, the histopathological typing and grading may present with some difficulties. In the diagnosis of more challenging histological subtypes, ancillary testing such as immunohistochemistry or molecular diagnostics, including fluorescence in situ hybridization assays, may be of additional value in more accurate characterization of the lesions.

Thus, offering this procedure to elderly patients with comorbidity and to patients who are at higher risk for postoperative morbidity and mortality is of immense importance. Such patients may be treated with cryotherapy, radiofrequency ablation, or thermoablation. The role of the pathologist in the accurate diagnosis of tumor histology is pivotal, guiding the appropriate treatment and at the same time decreasing the need for unnecessary surgeries.

A. V. Parwani, MD, PhD

Functional Genomic Analysis of Peripheral Blood During Early Acute Renal Allograft Rejection
Günther OP, for the Biomarkers in Transplantation Team (Univ of British Columbia, Vancouver, Canada; et al)
Transplantation 88:942-951, 2009

Background.—Acute graft rejection is an important clinical problem in renal transplantation and an adverse predictor for long-term graft survival. Peripheral blood biomarkers that provide evidence of early graft rejection may offer an important option for posttransplant monitoring, optimize the utility of graft biopsy, and permit timely and effective therapeutic intervention to minimize the graft damage.

Methods.—In this feasibility study (n = 58), we have used gene expression profiling in a case-control design to compare whole blood samples between normal subjects (n = 20) and patients with (n = 11) or without (n = 22) biopsy-confirmed acute rejection (BCAR) or borderline changes (n = 5).

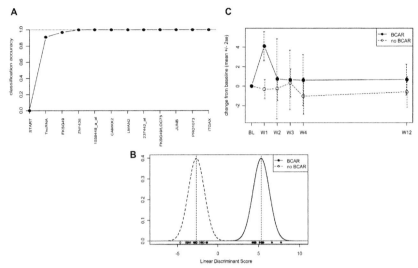

FIGURE 4.—Performance of classifier. (A) Incremental classification accuracy demonstrating step-wise inclusion of 11 common most highly predictive probe sets. (B) Linear discriminant analysis showing performance of 11 probe set classifiers in distinguishing cases with (●) and without (○) biopsy-confirmed acute rejection. (C) Change in classifier score posttransplant relative to individual pretransplant (baseline) value. The difference between cohorts is significant only at the time of rejection (week 1) (P=0.0001). (Reprinted from Günther OP, for the Biomarkers in Transplantation Team. Functional genomic analysis of peripheral blood during early acute renal allograft rejection. *Transplantation.* 2009;88:942-951, with permission from Lippincott Williams & Wilkins.)

Results.—A total of 183 probe sets representing 160 genes were differentially expressed (false discovery rate [FDR] <0.01) between subjects with or without BCAR, from which linear discriminant analysis and cross-validation identified an initial gene signature of 24 probe sets, and a more refined set of 11 probe sets found to classify subject samples correctly. Cross-validation suggested an out-of-sample sensitivity of 73% and specificity of 91% for identification of samples with or without BCAR. An increase in classifier gene expression correlated closely with acute rejection during the first 3 months posttransplant. Biological evaluation indicated that the differentially expressed genes encompassed processes related to immune response, signal transduction, and cytoskeletal reorganization.

Conclusion.—Preliminary evidence indicates that gene expression in the peripheral blood may yield a relevant measure for the occurrence of BCAR and offer a potential tool for immunologic monitoring. These results now require confirmation in a larger cohort (Fig 4).

▶ The holy grail in allograft monitoring is a noninvasive means to detect early allograft rejection prior to substantial graft injury and decreased function. Currently, transplant physicians are required to wait for evidence of graft dysfunction (increasing creatinine, increased liver function testing, and decreased ejection fraction) prior to performing an invasive biopsy of the allograft organ to confirm or exclude rejection. Recently, many groups have turned to peripheral blood-based gene expression profiling to find a pattern of increased or decreased expression that may be used for rejection screening. This article describes the identification of a subset of 11 probes that may be used to classify patients into rejection and nonrejection categories (Fig 4B). It is not surprising that the probes identified are involved in immune response, signal transduction, and cytoskeletal reorganization. The probe with the strongest association was trophoblast noncoding *RNA*, which has been identified as a possible target for p53 indicating a possible role in cell-cycle control or apoptosis (Fig 4A). The probes seem to be accurate in identifying ACR early in the course. After treatment, the change from baseline returns to just slightly increased over baseline levels (Fig 4C). As expected, cases deemed borderline by histologic analysis distributed heterogeneously between cases with and without rejection. While the data are impressive, one must keep in mind the large number of exclusion criteria used in the study design resulting in a highly selected study population. Most notably, participants were required to have had no evidence of infection, recurrence, or other major comorbid events. Obviously, additional studies on more complex subject populations are required.

M. L. Smith, MD

Histopathologic Classification of ANCA-Associated Glomerulonephritis
Berden AE, Ferrario F, Hagen EC, et al (Leiden Univ Med Ctr, Netherlands; San Gerardo Hosp, Monza, Italy; Meander Med Ctr, Amersfoort, Netherlands; et al)
J Am Soc Nephrol 21:2010 [Epub ahead of print]

Anti-neutrophil cytoplasmic antibody (ANCA)-associated vasculitis is the most common cause of rapidly progressive glomerulonephritis worldwide, and the renal biopsy is the gold standard for establishing the diagnosis. Although the prognostic value of the renal biopsy in ANCA-associated glomerulonephritis is widely recognized, there is no consensus regarding its pathologic classification. We present here such a pathologic classification developed by an international working group of renal pathologists. Our classification proposes four general categories of lesions: Focal, crescentic, mixed, and sclerotic. To determine whether these lesions have predictive value for renal outcome, we performed a validation study on 100 biopsies from patients with clinically and histologically confirmed ANCA-associated glomerulonephritis. Two independent pathologists, blinded to patient data, scored all biopsies according to a standardized protocol. Results show that the proposed classification system is of prognostic value for 1- and 5-year renal outcomes. We believe this pathologic classification will aid in the prognostication of patients at the time of diagnosis and facilitate uniform reporting between centers. This classification at some point might also provide means to guide therapy (Table 2).

▶ This article seeks to provide a foundation for international pathologic consensus by proposing a classification scheme for antineutrophil cytoplasmic

TABLE 2.—Classification Schema for ANCA-Associated Glomerulonephritis

Class	Inclusion Criteria[a]
Focal	≥50% normal glomeruli
Crescentic	≥50% glomeruli with cellular crescents
Mixed	<50% normal, <50% crescentic, <50% globally sclerotic glomeruli
Sclerotic	≥50% globally sclerotic glomeruli

[a]Pauci-immune staining pattern on immunofluorescence microscopy (IM) and ≥1 glomerulus with necrotizing or crescentic glomerulonephritis on light microscopy (LM) are required for inclusion in all four classes. See Fig 1 in the original article for hierarchical structure.

antibody-associated glomerulonephritis (Table 2). One of the strengths of this article is the recognition that interobserver agreement in the identification of critical glomerular lesions required for classification within the schema may occur. Thus, the authors provide detailed photomicrographs and microscopic descriptions with detailed inclusion and exclusion criteria. This extra effort should help to standardize reporting in the proposed classification. A second strength is the use of a validation step following consensus expert opinion. One may question the use of a classification scheme without a prognostic implication. Using a flowchart (Fig 1 in the original article) and the detailed microscopic descriptions, all biopsies were able to be classified accordingly and significant prognostic differences were identified. The categories sorted out as expected, from best to worse prognosis: focal, crescentic, mixed, and sclerotic (Fig 4 in the original article). Although tubulointerstitial disease was evaluated, it did not contribute significantly to prognosis and only added complexity to the classification system.

M. L. Smith, MD

Pathologic Classification of Diabetic Nephropathy
Cohen Tervaert TW, on behalf of the Renal Pathology Society (Leiden Univ Med Ctr, The Netherlands; et al)
J Am Soc Nephrol 21:556-563, 2010

Although pathologic classifications exist for several renal diseases, including IgA nephropathy, focal segmental glomerulosclerosis, and lupus nephritis, a uniform classification for diabetic nephropathy is lacking. Our aim, commissioned by the Research Committee of the Renal Pathology Society, was to develop a consensus classification combining type1 and type 2 diabetic nephropathies. Such a classification should discriminate lesions by various degrees of severity that would be easy to use internationally in clinical practice. We divide diabetic nephropathy into four hierarchical glomerular lesions with a separate evaluation for degrees of interstitial and vascular involvement. Biopsies diagnosed as diabetic nephropathy are classified as follows: Class I, glomerular basement

TABLE 1.—Glomerular Classification of DN

Class	Description	Inclusion Criteria
I	Mild or nonspecific LM changes and EM-proven GBM thickening	Biopsy does not meet any of the criteria mentioned below for class II, III, or IV GBM > 395 nm in female and >430 nm in male individuals 9 years of age and older[a]
IIa	Mild mesangial expansion	Biopsy does not meet criteria for class III or IV Mild mesangial expansion in >25% of the observed mesangium
IIb	Severe mesangial expansion	Biopsy does not meet criteria for class III or IV Severe mesangial expansion in >25% of the observed mesangium
III	Nodular sclerosis (Kimmelstiel–Wilson lesion)	Biopsy does not meet criteria for class IV At least one convincing Kimmelstiel–Wilson lesion
IV	Advanced diabetic glomerulosclerosis	Global glomerular sclerosis in >50% of glomeruli Lesions from classes I through III

LM, light microscopy.
[a]On the basis of direct measurement of GBM width by EM, these individual cutoff levels may be considered indicative when other GBM measurements are used.

membrane thickening: isolated glomerular basement membrane thickening and only mild, nonspecific changes by light microscopy that do not meet the criteria of classes II through IV. Class II, mesangial expansion, mild (IIa) or severe (IIb): glomeruli classified as mild or severe mesangial expansion but without nodular sclerosis (Kimmelstiel–Wilson lesions) or global glomerulosclerosis in more than 50% of glomeruli. Class III, nodular sclerosis (Kimmelstiel–Wilson lesions): at least one glomerulus with nodular increase in mesangial matrix (Kimmelstiel–Wilson) without changes described in class IV. Class IV, advanced diabetic glomerulosclerosis: more than 50% global glomerulosclerosis with other clinical or pathologic evidence that sclerosis is attributable to diabetic nephropathy. A good interobserver reproducibility for the four classes of DN was shown (intraclass correlation coefficient = 0.84) in a test of this classification (Table 1).

▶ Diagnostic classification systems can be helpful to standardize terminology and reporting. Adoption and widespread use of any classification system depends on the ease of use, completeness of category descriptions, reproducibility, and clinical significance. This article describes a universal classification system for diabetic nephrology that meets many of these needs. The general classification system is based primarily on glomerular lesions and is relatively straightforward with specific details for inclusion (Table 1). Much of the text of the article is dedicated to explanation and justification of these criteria. As an example, mesangial expansion is defined strictly in the text as increases in extracellular material such that the width of the interspace exceeds 2 mesangial cell nuclei in at least 2 glomerular lobules. A flow chart is included to assist in classification (Fig 2 in the original article). The interclass correlation coefficient of 0.84 demonstrates fairly good reproducibility. However, this was performed by pathologists involved in the formulation of the classification system, and it is likely that in general use, the reproducibility will not be as high. Further studies are required not only to demonstrate reproducibility in the hands of nonstudy pathologists but also to show clinical significance.

M. L. Smith, MD

Primary Leiomyosarcoma of the Kidney: A Clinicopathologic Study of 27 Cases
Miller JS, Zhou M, Brimo F, et al (The Johns Hopkins Hosp, Baltimore, MD; The Cleveland Clinic, OH; et al)
Am J Surg Pathol 34:238-242, 2010

Primary leiomyosarcoma of the kidney is a rare entity that has not been well characterized. We retrieved 27 cases of primary renal leiomyosarcomas diagnosed at 3 institutions between 1986 and 2009. Mean patient age at diagnosis was 58.5 years (range 22 to 85), and 59% were female. Mean tumor size was 13.4 cm (range 4 to 26), and 59% of the tumors were identified in the right kidney. Detailed histologic examination was possible for 24 of the cases. Average mitotic count per 10 high-power fields was 11.1 (range 0 to 50), and the average extent of necrosis was 21% (range 0 to 60). Cellular pleomorphism was classified as either focal (n = 13) or extensive (n = 11) and graded as mild (n = 3), moderate (n = 7) or severe (n = 14). Tumors were either grade 2 (n = 12) or grade 3 (n = 12) using the French Federation of Cancer Centers System. Direct extension beyond the kidney capsule was identified in 55% of the cases, and lymphovascular invasion was identified in 26%. Clinical follow-up information was available for 20 of the cases, and patients were followed for an average of 2.8 years (range 0.25 to 9). Distant metastases were identified in 90% of the patients, and 75% eventually died from their tumor's burden. In conclusion, primary renal leiomyosarcomas have a grim prognosis regardless of the underlying histology.

▶ This retrospective article details the pathologic and clinical features of primary leiomyosarcoma of the kidney. These are rare primary renal tumors, which are often considered when faced with high-grade spindle cell lesions of the kidney. The differential diagnosis is extensive and includes sarcomatoid carcinoma (from either a renal cell carcinoma or urothelial carcinoma), primary leiomyosarcoma of the retroperitoneum, and angiomyolipoma. Differentiating primary renal leiomyoma from leiomyosarcoma may also be difficult and is based on the criteria of smooth muscle lesions at other sites, including the presence of necrosis, mitotic figures, and cellular pleomorphism. Definitive classification often requires thorough sampling and imaging studies. In fact, nearly 50% of the cases initially diagnosed as renal leiomyosarcoma were reclassified following expert review, thus highlighting the difficulty of the diagnosis. The article includes an excellent discussion of the differential diagnosis and how to arrive at the diagnosis. When strictly defined, these malignancies are rare and have a very poor prognosis.

M. L. Smith, MD

The Association Between Age and Nephrosclerosis on Renal Biopsy Among Healthy Adults
Rule AD, Amer H, Cornell LD, et al (Mayo Clinic, Rochester, MN)
Ann Intern Med 152:561-567, 2010

Background.—Chronic kidney disease is common with older age and is characterized on renal biopsy by global glomerulosclerosis, tubular atrophy, interstitial fibrosis, and arteriosclerosis.

Objective.—To see whether the prevalence of these histologic abnormalities in the kidney increases with age in healthy adults and whether histologic findings are explained by age-related differences in kidney function or chronic kidney disease risk factors.

Design.—Cross-sectional study.

Setting.—Mayo Clinic, Rochester, Minnesota, from 1999 to 2009.

Patients.—1203 adult living kidney donors.

Measurements.—Core-needle biopsy of the renal cortex obtained during surgical implantation of the kidney, and medical record data of kidney function and risk factors obtained before donation.

Results.—The prevalence of nephrosclerosis (≥ 2 chronic histologic abnormalities) was 2.7% (95% CI, 1.1% to 6.7%) for patients aged 18 to 29 years, 16% (CI, 12% to 20%) for patients aged 30 to 39 years, 28% (CI, 24% to 32%) for patients aged 40 to 49 years, 44% (CI, 38% to 50%) for patients aged 50 to 59 years, 58% (CI, 47% to 67%) for patients aged 60 to 69 years, and 73% (CI, 43% to 90%) for patients aged 70 to 77 years. Adjustment for kidney function and risk factor covariates did not explain the age-related increase in the prevalence of nephrosclerosis.

Limitation.—Kidney donors are selected for health and lack the spectrum or severity of renal pathologic findings in the general population.

Conclusion.—Kidney function and chronic kidney disease risk factors do not explain the strong association between age and nephrosclerosis in healthy adults (Table 2).

▶ Although one may logically assume that there may be an association between age and the presence of nephrosclerosis, it has yet to be documented as thoroughly as in this article. Using live kidney donors, the authors study the histologic changes related to nephrosclerosis in a healthy patient population, including global glomerulosclerosis, tubular atrophy, interstitial fibrosis, and vascular luminal narrowing. They found a strong linear relationship between age and prevalence of nephrosclerosis (Table 2). Nephrosclerosis was defined as the presence of 2 or more of the histologic abnormalities. Following adjustment for age and sex, the only characteristics associated with nephrosclerosis

TABLE 2.—Prevalence of Nephrosclerosis, by Age Group*

Age Group	Crude Prevalence (95% CI), %	Crude Prevalence After Exclusion of Persons Who Received Therapy for Hypertension (95% CI), %
18–29 y	2.7 (1.1–6.7)	2.7 (1.1–6.7)
30–39 y	16 (12–20)	15 (12–20)
40–49 y	28 (24–32)	26 (22–31)
50–59 y	44 (38–50)	42 (36–49)
60–69 y	58 (47–67)	55 (44–66)
70–77 y	73 (43–90)	75 (41–93)
Overall	28 (25–30)	26 (24–29)

*Among 1203 living kidney donors at Mayo Clinic.

were 24-hour urinary albumin, nocturnal blood pressure, and hypertension. Although glomerular filtration rate declines with age, this decline is not explained by the increased nephrolosclerosis alone (Fig 1 in the original article). In other words, both patients with and without nephrosclerosis show an equal decline in glomerular filtration rate over time. This questions the clinical significance of finding evidence of nephrolosclerosis by renal biopsy.

M. L. Smith, MD

The significance of renal C4d staining in patients with BK viruria, viremla, and nephropathy

Batal I, Zainah H, Stockhausen S, et al (Univ of Pittsburgh Med Ctr, PA)
Mod Pathol 22:1468-1476, 2009

Peritubular capillary C4d staining in allograft kidney is an important criterion for antibody-mediated rejection. Whether BK virus infection can result in complement activation is not known. We studied 113 renal allograft biopsies from 52 recipients with a history of BK virus activation. The samples were classified into four groups according to the concurrent detection of BK virus DNA in urine, plasma, and/or biopsy: BK-negative ($n = 37$), viruria ($n = 53$), viremia ($n = 7$), and nephropathy ($n = 16$) groups. The histological semiquantitative peritubular capillary C4d scores in the viremia (0.3 ± 0.8) and BK nephropathy (0.6 ± 0.9) groups were lower than those in the BK-negative group (1.2 ± 1.1, $P = 0.05$ and $P = 0.06$, respectively) and the viruria group (1.2 ± 1.1, $P = 0.04$ and $P = 0.06$, respectively). Diffuse or focal peritubular capillary C4d staining was present in 9/76 (12%) and 14/76 (19%) of all samples with concurrent BK virus reactivation (viruria, viremia, and nephropathy). The diagnosis of antibody-mediated rejection could be established in 7/9 (78%) and 5/14 (36%) of these samples, respectively. Diffuse tubular basement membrane C4d staining was restricted to BK nephropathy cases (4/16, 25%). Semiquantitative tubular basement membrane C4d scores were higher in BK nephropathy (1.2 ± 1.3) compared with BK-negative

TABLE 4.—Association of Peritubular C4d Staining Patterns with the Presence of Circulating Donor-Specific Antibodies in Different Stages of BK Virus Reactivation

Peritubular Capillary C4d Staining	DSA Present ($n = 42$)	DSA Absent ($n = 55$)
BK virus negative ($n = 37$)		
Diffuse	3/4 (75%)	1/4 (25%)
Focal	7/13 (54%)	6/13 (46%)
Minimal	1/6 (17%)	5/6 (83%)
Negative	2/14 (14%)	12/14 (86%)
Viruria ($n = 48$)		
Diffuse	7/8 (88%)	1/8 (12%)
Focal	4/8 (50%)	4/8 (50%)
Minimal	7/14 (50%)	7/14 (50%)
Negative	7/18 (39%)	11/18 (61%)
Viremia ($n = 7$)		
Diffuse	NA	NA
Focal	1/1	0/1
Minimal	NA	NA
Negative	2/6 (33%)	4/6 (67%)
BK nephropathy ($n = 5$)		
Diffuse	NA	NA
Focal	0/1	1/1
Minimal	NA	NA
Negative	1/4 (25%)	3/4 (75%)
All BK virus reactivation ($n = 60$)		
Diffuse	7/8 (88%)	1/8 (12%)
Focal	5/10 (50%)	5/10 (50%)
Minimal	7/14 (50%)	7/14 (50%)
Negative	10/28 (36%)	18/28 (64%)

DSA, circulating donor specific antibodies.
Only samples with available information concerning DSA are presented in this table (all BK negative, 48 viruria, all viremia, and 5 in-house BK nephropathy).

(0.05 ± 0.3, $P = 0.017$) and viruria (0.0 ± 0.0, $P = 0.008$) groups. Bowman's capsule C4d staining was more frequent in BK nephropathy (5/16) compared with the aforementioned groups (2/36 ($P = 0.023$) and 4/51 ($P = 0.03$), respectively). Within the BK nephropathy group, samples with tubular basement membrane stain had more infected tubular epithelial cells ($12.1 \pm 7.6\%$ vs $4.4 \pm 5.0\%$, $P = 0.03$) and a trend toward higher interstitial inflammation scores. In conclusion, peritubular capillary C4d staining remains a valid marker for the diagnosis of antibody-mediated rejection in the presence of concurrent BK virus infection. A subset of biopsies with BK nephropathy shows tubular basement membrane C4d staining, which correlates with marked viral cytopathic effect (Table 4).

▶ C4d immunoreactivity is part of the diagnostic triad for antibody-mediated rejection (AMR), which includes histologic evidence of renal injury, presence of donor-specific antibodies (DSA), and immunologic evidence of compliment activation in the peritubular capillaries (PTC). While the clinical services typically simplify the evaluation to either positive or negative, localization of the C4d immunoreactivity in the PTC is required for a diagnosis of AMR. Primary polyoma virus infection or reactivation is a common cause of morbidity in patients with renal transplant. Comprehensive analysis of C4d immunoreactivity in patients with polyoma virus infection has yet to be done until this publication. This excellent article comprehensively analyzes C4d immunoreactivity in various stages of polyoma virus infection, including in cases of concurrent acute cellular rejection and AMR. Two main questions are addressed: (1) does PTC C4d expression still correlate with AMR in patients with polyoma virus reactivation and (2) what is the significance of tubular basement membrane staining for C4d? Even in the setting of polyoma virus infection, the presence of diffuse PTC reactivity for C4d was strongly associated with a diagnosis of AMR and the presence of DSA (Table 4). Finally, one can expect cases of polyoma virus nephropathy to show prominent tubular basement membrane reactivity in the setting of prominent viral effect and interstitial inflammation.

M. L. Smith, MD

The width of the basement membrane does not influence clinical presentation or outcome of thin glomerular basement membrane disease with persistent hematuria

Szeto C-C, Mac-Moune Lai F, Kwan BC-H, et al (The Chinese Univ of Hong Kong, Shatin, China)

Kidney Int 2010 [Epub ahead of print]

Thin basement membrane disease (TBMD) typically presents with persistent microscopic hematuria, and is usually defined as a glomerular basement membrane (GBM) thickness <250 nm. Previous studies showed that neither the degree of thinning nor the extent of the abnormality correlate with the patient's clinical presentation or prognosis. To further define this, we enrolled a study group of 41 patients with isolated microscopic hematuria and a normal renal biopsy, except those with a GBM thickness of 250–320 nm, and compared them with 33 patients with traditional TBMD. We found no difference in baseline demographic or clinical parameter between the groups. After follow-up averaging 110 months, there was no significant difference in the risk of detectable or overt proteinuria, hypertension, or impaired renal function between the groups. By the end of the study, only five patients from the study group and four from the TBMD group had no outcome event. By Cox regression analysis, independent predictors of overt proteinuria were male gender, age at biopsy, baseline renal function, proteinuria, and hypertension. Age at biopsy was the only independent predictor for hypertension, and baseline proteinuria was the only independent predictor for impaired renal function. GBM thickness did not predict any outcome event. Hence, lifelong follow-up is advised, as the clinical features and prognosis of these patients with persistent microscopic hematuria and marginally thin GBM are similar to traditional TBMD (Fig 1).

▶ The diagnosis of thin basement membrane disease (TBMD) has been arbitrarily set at approximately 2 standard deviations below the mean of normal

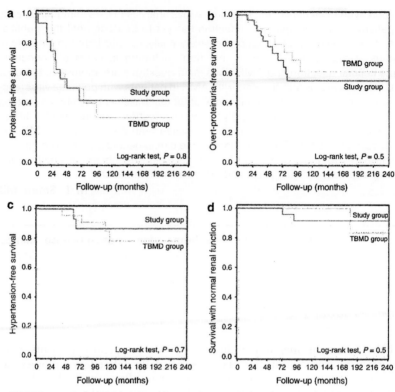

FIGURE 1.—Kaplan-Meier plot of event-free survival. (a) Any detectable proteinuria; (b) proteinuria ≥ 1 g/day; (c) hypertension; and (d) impaired renal function. Data were compared using the log-rank test. TBMD, thin basement membrane disease. (Reprinted with permission from Macmillan Publishers Ltd: Kidney International, Szeto C-C, Mac-Moune Lai F, Kwan BC-H, et al. The width of the basement membrane does not influence clinical presentation or outcome of thin glomerular basement membrane disease with persistent hematuria. *Kidney Int.* 2010 [Epub ahead of print], Copyright 2010.)

adult BM thickness (BM thickness of < 250 nm). In this retrospective case-control study, the authors compare patients with marginally thin glomerular BMs (GBMs) (250-320 nm) with patients who meet criteria for TBMD. The first surprising finding is that most of the patients in both groups eventually had an outcome event. The most common outcome event was low-grade proteinuria and proteinuria greater than or equal to 1 g/d (Fig 1). These findings alone call into question our arbitrary cutoff of 250 nm for a diagnosis of TBMD. In addition, GBM thickness, ranging from 172 to 325 nm, did not correlate with any outcome events. There was no statistical difference between the 2 groups. Study limitations include the possible selection bias for patients undergoing renal biopsy and smaller sample size. Although the authors indicate that failure to screen for glucose intolerance and/or insulin resistance may have resulted in confounding, one would expect increasing thickness of GBM in prediabetic states. Perhaps additional studies comparing even thicker GBM with TBMD are indicated to identify a more data-driven cutoff. Regardless, the data from this article suggest that patients with thin and low normal GBM thickness should be followed for the development of adverse outcomes.

M. L. Smith, MD

Utility of percutaneous renal biopsy in chronic kidney disease
Joseph AJ, Compton SP, Holmes LH, et al (Med Univ of South Carolina, Charleston)
Nephrology 15:544-548, 2010

Background.—We tested the hypothesis that patterns of serum creatinine concentrations (S-cr) prior to percutaneous renal biopsy (PRB) predict the utility of PRB in safely making renal diagnoses, revealing treatable disease, and altering therapy in chronic kidney disease patients.

Methods.—PRB specimens (170 patients) were assigned to 1 of 5 groups: S-cr never greater than 0.11 mM for at least 6 months prior to PRB (Group 1); S-cr greater than 0.11 mM but less than 0.18 mM during the 6 months prior to PRB (Groups 2); S-cr less than 0.18 mM during the 6 months prior to PRB but greater than 0.18 mM prior to these 6 months (Group 3); S-cr greater than 0.18 mM for less than 6 months prior to PRB (Group 4); S-cr greater than 0.18 mM for more than 6 months prior to PRB (Group 5).

Results.—Histopathology chronicity score (0–9) increased with increasing group number: 2.1 (Group 1); 4.4 (Group 2); 4.5 (Group 3); 5.4 (Group 4); 7.0 (Group 5). Post-PRB bleeding was more common with increasing group number. New therapy was instituted after PRB most frequently in Group 4 (62%) and least frequently in Group 5 (24%).

Conclusion.—After more prolonged elevations of S-cr, PRB may be less safe and less likely to reveal treatable disease and opportunities for therapy (Fig 1).

▶ In chronic kidney disease patients, at what point does the likelihood of finding clinically useful information on renal biopsy not justify the risks and are there preprocedural indicators that may help in the decision-making process? These are questions addressed in this article by Joseph et al. The primary preprocedural data used was serum creatinine. Although estimated glomerular filtration rate may have been more optimal, these data were not available in the entire data set. Fig 1 shows how the histologic chronicity score increased with increasing group number, which is expected. Nondiagnostic renal biopsies (normal tissue or end-stage kidney) were most common in groups 2 and 5, occurring 40% and 55% of the time, respectively. Group 2 represents mild disease without significant chronicity, and group 5 represents severe disease with evidence of marked chronicity. Although the risk of complication was less in group 2, the lack of definitive diagnosis suggests renal biopsy may not be as useful. In group 2, the rate of nondiagnostic tissue was approximately equal to the rate of changes in therapy (46%). Group 4 (severe disease without significant chronicity) showed the most frequent changes in therapy

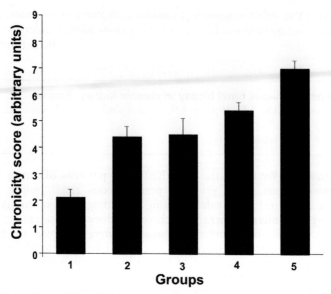

FIGURE 1.—Histopathological chronicity scores in serum creatinine concentration (S-cr) groups. Scores were higher in more highly numbered groups ($P < 0.001$). The number of biopsies in each group can be found in Table 1 in the original article. (Reprinted from Joseph AJ, Compton SP, Holmes LH, et al. Utility of percutaneous renal biopsy in chronic kidney disease. *Nephrology*. 2010;15:544-548.)

(62%). Put in the context of more subacute severe disease, increased changes in therapy and only a low (5%) nondiagnostic rate may be expected. Despite the trends toward more nondiagnostic biopsies and increasing complication rates, renal biopsy remained an important clinical tool confirming diagnoses and altering therapy, even in the most severe and chronic cases. Nevertheless, the decision to perform a percutaneous renal biopsy remains complex and must factor in several different clinical parameters and risks.

M. L. Smith, MD

11 Head and Neck

A survey of methylated candidate tumor suppressor genes in nasopharyngeal carcinoma
Loyo M, Brait M, Kim MS, et al (Greater Baltimore Med Ctr, MD; et al)
Int J Cancer 2010 [Epub ahead of print]

Nasopharyngeal carcinoma (NPC) is a rare malignancy with unique genetic, viral and environmental characteristic that distinguishes it from other head and neck carcinomas. The clinical management of NPC remains challenging largely due to the lack of early detection strategies for this tumor. In our study, we have sought to identify novel genes involved in the pathogenesis of NPC that might provide insight into this tumor's biology and could potentially be used as biomarkers. To identify these genes, we studied the epigenetics of NPC by characterizing a panel of methylation markers. Eighteen genes were evaluated by quantitative methylation-specific polymerase chain reaction (PCR) in cell lines as well as in tissue samples including 50 NPC tumors and 28 benign nasopharyngeal biopsies. Significance was evaluated using Fisher's exact test and quantitative values were optimized using cut off values derived from receiver–operator characteristic curves. The methylation status of *AIM1*, *APC*, *CALCA*, deleted in colorectal carcinomas *(DCC)*, *DLEC*, deleted in liver cancer 1 *(DLC1)*, estrogen receptor alpha *(ESR)*, *FHIT*, *KIF1A* and *PGP9.5* was significantly associated with NPC compared to controls. The sensitivity of the individual genes ranged from 26 to 66% and the specificity was above 92% for all genes except FHIT. The combination of *PGP9.5*, *KIF1A* and *DLEC* had a sensitivity of 84% and a specificity of 92%. Ectopic expression of *DCC* and *DLC1* lead to decrease in colony formation and invasion properties. Our results indicate that methylation of novel biomarkers in NPC could be used to enhance early detection approaches. Additionally, our functional studies reveal previously unknown tumor suppressor roles in NPC (Tables 2 and 3).

▶ This is one of the better articles that I have come across this year, as it emphasizes the potential impact that molecular testing in pathology can have in improving the quality of care for our patient population and the potential to enhance the ability of nasopharyngeal cancer early detection. All pathologists probably know 2 important facts about nasopharyngeal carcinoma (NPC): first, its association with Epstein-Barr virus and second, that most tumors respond well to radiation therapy except the keratinizing type, which tends to be more resistant. Over the years, the progress of more in-depth

TABLE 2.—Promoter Methylation Frequency for 11 Genes Analyzes in Nasopharyngeal Carcinoma

Gene	Frequency of Positivity Nasopharynegal Carcinoma	Controls	p	Cutoff	AUC (95% CI)	Sensitivity (%)	Specificity (%)
AIM1	15/50	2/28	0.002	1.85	0.61 (0.53–0.69)	30	92
APC	17/50	1/28	0.002	0.91	0.65 (0.57–0.72)	34	96
CALCA	22/50	2/28	0.001	0.91	0.68 (0.59–0.76)	40	92
DCC	23/46	1/27	0.01	2.49	0.77 (0.69–0.84)	50	96
DLEC	29/48	1/28	<0.0001	2.2	0.73 (0.65–0.81)	60	96
DLC1	21/48	0/27	<0.0001	2.3	0.71 (0.64–0.77)	43	100
ESR	13/50	1/28	0.01	1.61	0.61 (0.54–0.68)	26	96
FHIT	22/50	6/28	0.05	2.1	0.38 (0.28–0.49)	44	21
KIF1A	28/50	1/28	<0.0001	1.61	0.76 (0.68–0.83)	56	96
PGP9.5	32/50	2/28	<0.0001	2.3	0.78 (0.70–0.86)	66	96
TIG1	15/50	5/28	0.28	1.59	0.43 (0.43–0.53)	26	92
All genes	50/50	12/28	<0.0001		0.78 (0.69–0.87)	100	57

p values from two sided Fisher's exact test. AUC (area under the curve) and cutoffs derived from non parametric ROC curves.

TABLE 3.—Sensitivity and Specificity of Different Combinations of Methylation Markers

Gene Combinations	AUC	Sensitivity (%)	Specificity (%)
PGP9.5, ESR, DCC, AIM1, and KIF1A	0.87 (0.78–0.95)	92	82
PGP9.5, DLC1, DLEC	0.84 (0.73–0.96)	84	85
PGP9.5, DLEC, DCC, KIF1A	0.89 (0.86–0.96)	90	89
DLEC, DCC, KIF1A, AIM1	0.88 (0.81–0.96)	92	85
PGP9.5, KIF1A	0.85 (0.77–0.92)	78	92
PGP9.5, DLC1	0.85 (0.77–0.92)	78	92
PGP9.5, DCC	0.86 (0.78–0.96)	84	89
DLEC, KIF1A	0.87 (0.80–0.93)	78	96
PGP9.5, KIF1A, DLEC	0.88 (0.81–0.95)	84	92
AIM1, DCC	0.79 (0.70–0.88)	70	89
DCC, DLC1	0.81 (0.73–0.88)	66	96
KIF1A, DCC, DLEC	0.89 (0.82–0.96)	86	92

AUC is area under the curve derived from nonparametric ROC curves.

understanding of NPC has been somewhat limited in its impact, and patients continue to present usually in advanced disease stages when cervical lymph node metastasis has been established. This article sought and demonstrated novel methylated genes that have been tested in other tumors but not in NPC and showed that they can potentially be used to screen and identify patients with NPC with increased sensitivity and specificity. One of the nice aspects of this study is that it confirmed that those methylated genes were also more prevalent in the Southern Chinese population, thus providing a nice evidence-based molecular correlation with a fact that was observed for years when considering the race-related prevalence of NPC among population of Asian descent. Larger studies and more testing are certainly required to affirm the practicality/impact of this study, but it provided an exciting start for that effort that hopefully institutions at least in places of high-NPC prevalence may be willing to adopt and try.

M. S. Said, MD, PhD

Cavitating Otosclerosis: Clinical, Radiologic, and Histopathologic Correlations

Makarem AO, Hoang T-A, Lo WWM, et al (House Ear Inst, Los Angeles, CA; UCLA Med Ctr; St Vincent Med Ctr, Los Angeles, CA)
Otol Neurotol 31:381-384, 2010

Background.—Despite the high prevalence of otosclerosis and its having long been a subject of scrutiny, cavitary changes in otosclerosis are rare and not well known. Here, we describe and introduce into the literature the unusual histologic and radiologic findings of cavitation and its possible clinical relevance in patients with advanced cochlear otosclerosis.

Methods.—Cases with clinical otosclerosis and presence of cavitation were selected from our temporal bone collection and correlated with premortem imaging and clinical manifestations.

Results.—Two cases of cochlear otosclerosis presented with a clinical syndrome possibly attributed to the existence of a cavity within the otosclerotic foci.

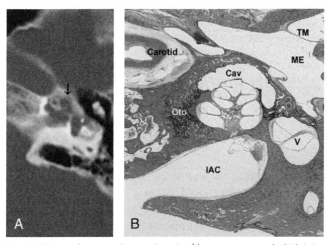

FIGURE 3.—*A*, Computed tomography reveals pericochlear cavities, one of which is in a periapical location. *B*, Histologic section of right temporal bone of another patient with comparable disease shows substantial otosclerosis foci (*Oto*) with a large cavity (*Cav*) capping (anterior and lateral to) the apex of the cochlea. FN indicates facial nerve; IAC, internal auditory canal; ME, middle ear; TM, tympanic membrane; V vestibule. H&E ×8. (Reprinted from Makarem AO, Hoang T-A, Lo WWM, et al. Cavitating otosclerosis: clinical, radiologic, and histopathologic correlations. *Otol Neurotol.* 2010;31:381-384.)

Conclusion.—Cavitating otosclerosis is a not well-known occurrence in patients with advanced cochlear otosclerosis, and it is a possible cause of a "third window" syndrome and surgical complications (Fig 3).

▶ Otosclerosis is a highly prevalent cause of conductive and/or sensorineural hearing loss in humans that is caused by specific bone remodeling abnormality (formation of soft, spongy, immature, vascularized bone) that can involve the stapedial annular ligament fixing the stapes (conductive hearing loss) or spreading to the cochlea and labyrinth (sensorineural hearing loss). The measles virus infection has been proposed as an etiological agent as well as genetic, autoimmune, and inflammatory causes. Otosclerosis is a diagnosis not usually made in biopsies in the usual practice of surgical pathology and is usually made on correlation of clinical/hearing test analysis and operative findings of the otologist, although histologic analysis of the ankylosed stapes ossicular bone footplate can, on occasions, differentiate between otosclerosis and nonotosclerosis stapedial fixation causes (nonstapedial causes include annular ligament calcifications, middle ear granulomas, amyloidosis, hemosiderosis, globular fibrosis, etc). Usually, the description of widespread disease involvement in otosclerosis has been limited histopathologically to examining postmortem temporal bone specimens, and on occasions, animal models have been tried (eg, knockout mice). This article introduces the findings on a rare disease complication that involves cavity formation within the temporal bone (cavitating otosclerosis) that can result in a potential connection to the membranous labyrinth, thus producing a third-window effect and adding to the list of previous recognized causes of that effect (basically causing sound energy away from the basilar membrane) and can also be a cause of failure of electrode placement in cochlear implants and cerebrospinal fluid (CSF) connection/gush. The weakness of the article—although it presents an interesting picture illustrating the histopathologic findings of the cavities forming in the pericochlear regions, which can be appreciated radiologically in the temporal bone in the living patient—is that it missed an opportunity to offer suggestions, possible explanations, or questions into the mechanisms of formation of the cavities. It importantly pointed out, though, as mentioned, the other important arm of the finding, which deals with the clinical implications of the cavity formation. Could it be, for example, inferred from the existing literature that the remodeling in the pericochlear areas in a continuously active disease focus eventually results in less bone deposition with more loose vascularized connective tissue areas that eventually breaks down with little to no bone deposition? Is the presence of CSF leaks and connections in some of these cavities, as illustrated in the article, a possible contributing factor? Could it be that elevated bone turnover enzymes locally like alkaline phosphatase or bone resorption enzymes like parathyroid hormone (PTH) (altered response to PTH has been observed in otosclerosis; it is also known that PTH causes osteitis fibrosa cystica in thicker bones) is an explanation of the continuous and excessive bone resorption in these cavities? Is that all false and unlikely? Are there better explanations? Certainly the article opens more questions that require an explanation into the nature of these cavities with its reported clinical implications.

For further reading, I recommend the review articles by Schrauwen and Van Camp[1] and Stankovic and McKenna.[2]

M. S. Said, MD, PhD

References

1. Schrauwen I, Van Camp G. The etiology of otosclerosis: a combination of genes and environment. *Laryngoscope.* 2010;120:1195-1202.
2. Stankovic KM, McKenna MJ. Current research in otosclerosis. *Current Opin Otolaryngol Head Neck Surg.* 2006;14:347-351.

Expression of p53, p16^{INK4A}, pRb, p21$^{WAF1/CIP1}$, p27^{KIP1}, cyclin D1, Ki-67 and HPV DNA in sinonasal endophytic Schneiderian (inverted) papilloma
Altavilla G, Staffieri A, Busatto G, et al (Univ of Padua, Italy; Dept of Clinical Pathology, Cittadella, Padua, Italy)
Acta Otolaryngol 129:1242-1249, 2009

Conclusions.—Human papilloma virus (HPV) was associated with sinonasal inverted papilloma (SIP) in 14/20 (70%) patients with a prevalence of HPV 6/11; alterations of the cell cycle proteins were statistically significant.

Objectives.—We investigated SIPs relationships between HPV infection and aberrant expression of cell cycle proteins.

Materials and Methods.—Twenty SIPs were evaluated for p53, p16^{INK4a}, pRb, p21^{WAF1}, p27^{Kip1}, cyclin D1 and Ki-67 expression by immunohistochemistry. HPV was investigated by polymerase chain reaction (PCR).

Results.—HPV DNA was detected in 14/20 patients with inverted papillomas (IPs) (70%). The majority of tumours showed strong p16, p21, p27, pRb and cyclin D1 staining and little or no p53 expression. Tumours harbouring dysplasia were significantly more likely to be p53-positive and exhibit upregulated p21 and p27, and showed altered intensity and distribution of reactive cells into and through the epithelium. Dysplastic epithelium was strongly reactive for p16 and the MIB 1 labelling index was almost 20%. These findings were associated with expression of p53 in the same zones. Comparing the p53 reactivity with the presence of HPV DNA, SIPs were stratified as follows: HPV+p53−, 12 (63.15%); HPV+p53+, 2 (10.52%); HPV−p53+, 3 (15.78%) and HPV−p53−, 2 (10.52%). Statistical analysis showed that HPV presence correlated with p53-positive immunostaining ($p = 0.045$) (Fig 2 and Table 2).

▶ Cervical cancers in women have a proven human papilloma virus (HPV)-related etiology through HPV oncogenes disruption (mainly E6 and E7 genes) of the cell cycle. Many head and neck cancers have found a strong candidate in HPV for providing an etiologic agent for the development of head and neck lesions including squamous cell carcinoma. One of these lesions is inverted Schneiderian nasal papillomas, which have had many proposed

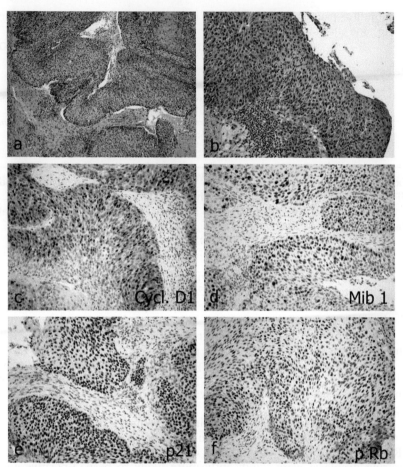

FIGURE 2.—Schneiderian inverted papillomas with squamous dysplasia (a and b) showing irregular distribution of the cyclin D1, p21 and pRb reactivity through all the cell layers (c, e and f). The proliferative marker MIB 1 is also found in the superficial nuclei (d). (Reprinted from Altavilla G, Staffieri A, Busatto G, et al. Expression of p53, p16[INK4A], pRb, p21[WAF1/CIP1], p27[KIP1], cyclin D1, Ki-67 and HPV DNA in sinonasal endophytic Schneiderian (inverted) papilloma. *Acta Otolaryngol.* 2009;129: 1242-1249. Reprinted by permission of Taylor and Francis Group.)

etiologies, with HPV seeming to be one of its strongest contenders. Although some studies have been done before on HPV relationship to Schneiderian inverted papillomas, this study tries to characterize some of the cell cycle protein alterations associated with HPV-associated inverted nasal papillomas in a similar fashion to those previously examined in cervical cancer. Although no prognostic values were observed on the analysis of these proteins, the alteration of the cell cycle proteins was statistically significant and HPV presence was correlated to the presence of p53 expression in inverted papillomas harboring dysplasia of the metaplastic squamous epithelium lining with those inverted papillomas harboring no dysplasia showing little or no expression as

TABLE 2.—SIPs: Morphological and Immunohistochemical Findings and Presence of HPV

Case no.	Dysplasia	Epithelium	HPV	p21	p27	p16	pRB	Cyclin D1	P53	Mib-1	Mib-1 (%)
1	No	Squamous	+	+	+	+	+	+	−	+	27
2	No	Squamous	+	+	+	+	+	+	−	+	30
3	No	Onco-transitional	+	+	+	+	+	+	−	+	8
4	No	Squamous	+	+	+	+	+	+	−	+	43
5	No	Onco-transitional	−	−	−	ND	ND	ND	ND	ND	ND
6	No	Squamous focally respiratory	+	+	+	+	+	+	−	+	20
7	No	Transitional	+	+	+	+	ND	+	−	+	4
8	No	Squamous	+	+	+	+	+	+	−	+	6.5
9	No	Squamous	+	+	+	+	+	+	−	+	8
10	No	Squamous-respiratory	−	+	+	+	+	+	+	+	24
11	No	Squamous	+	+	+	+	+	+	−	+	30
12	No	Squamous-respiratory	+	+	+	+	ND	+	−	+	9
13	No	Squamous	−	−	+	ND	ND	+	−	+	9
14	No	Squamous-respiratory	+	+	+	+	+	+	−	+	24
15	No	Squamous	−	+	+	ND	+	+	−	+	50
16	No	Squamous	−	+	+	+	+	+	+	+	40
17	No	Squamous	+	−	−	+	ND	ND	−	+	22
18	Yes (low grade)	Squamous	+	+	+	+	+	+	+	+	20
19	Yes (high grade)	Squamous-transitional	+	+	+	+	+	+	+	+	40*
20	Yes CSNCinv (high grade)	Squamous	−	+	+	+	+	+	+	+	40*

ND, no data; +, positive; −, negative.
*90% in dysplastic area.

mentioned above. This observation of p53 relation to severe dysplasia was previously investigated by a number of investigators in the literature,[1-3] and it seems from the current analysis of the other cell cycle proteins that p53 remains, at least until now, one of the better markers for potential dysplastic/cancerous transformation in sinonasal papillomas.

M. S. Said, MD, PhD

References

1. Buchwald C, Lindeberg H, Pederson BL, Franzmann MB. Human papilloma virus and p53 expression in carcinomas associated with sinonasal papillomas: a Danish Epidemiologic study 1980-1998. *Laryngoscope.* 2001;111:1104-1110.
2. Katori H, Nozawat A, Tsukuda M. Relationship between p21 and p53 expresssion, human papilloma virus infection and malignant transformation in sinonasal-inverted papilloma. *Clin Oncol (R coll Radiol).* 2006;18:300-305.
3. Caruana SM, Zweibel N, Cocker R, McCormick SA, Eberle RC, Lazarus P. p53 alteration and human papilloma virus infection in paranasal sinus cancers. *Cancer.* 1997;79:1320-1328.

Intercalated Duct Lesions of Salivary Gland: A Morphologic Spectrum From Hyperplasia to Adenoma

Weinreb I, Seethala RR, Hunt JL, et al (Univ Health Network, Toronto, Ontario, Canada; Univ of Pittsburgh Med Ctr, PA; Cleveland Clinic Foundation, OH)
Am J Surg Pathol 33:1322-1329, 2009

Intercalated duct lesions (IDLs) are rare, poorly understood and not well-studied lesions that have been associated with a small number of epithelial-myoepithelial carcinomas (EMC) and basal cell adenomas. To examine the nature of IDLs and their association with salivary gland tumors, we reviewed 34 lesions in 32 patients. The IDLs were stained with CK7, estrogen receptors (ER), progesterone receptors, lysozyme, S100, calponin, and CK14. The patients ranged in age from 19 to 80 years (mean 53.8) with a 1.7:1 female predominance. The majorities of IDLs were parotid lesions (82%), were small and nodular (average size 3.1 mm) and showed 3 architectural patterns: hyperplasia (20), adenoma (9), and hybrid forms (5). In 59% of cases, IDLs were seen in conjunction with another salivary gland tumor, most commonly basal cell adenoma (8 cases), followed by EMC (3 cases). One case showed a combination of intercalated duct hyperplasia and basal cell adenoma. The IDLs stained diffusely with CK7 (100%) and S100 (73%) and focally for ER (91%) and lysozyme (100%). Calponin and CK14 highlighted a thin myoepithelial cell layer around all ducts (100%). Normal intercalated ducts were also consistently positive for CK7 and lysozyme, and focally for ER, but were S100 negative. In summary, IDLs have a variety of patterns ranging from hyperplasia to adenoma with hybrid lesions and share morphologic and immunophenotypic features with normal intercalated

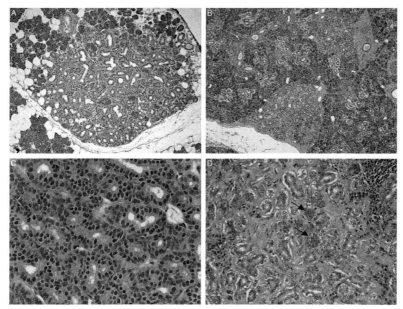

FIGURE 1.—A, Unifocal intercalated duct hyperplasia showing irregular edges. B, A multifocal lesion in the submandibular gland. C, Note the lack of atrophy and inflammation in the surrounding gland. The ductal proliferation in IDLs consisted of small ducts with minimal intervening stroma and inconspicuous myoepithelial cells. D, Intercalated duct hyperplasia containing acinic cells (arrows) in the center of the lesion and stromal hyalinization. This case was associated with focal lymphoid aggregates in the adjacent gland (upper right corner). Also note the presence of clear myoepithelial cells around the ducts. (Reprinted from Weinreb I, Seethala RR, Hunt JL, et al. Intercalated duct lesions of salivary gland: a morphologic spectrum from hyperplasia to adenoma. *Am J Surg Pathol.* 2009;33:1322-1329.)

ducts. There is an association with basal cell adenomas and EMC, which lends credence to their role as a putative precursor lesion (Figs 1 and 2).

▶ This is an interesting article that deals with and describes the rare and under-reported lesions of the intercalated ducts of salivary glands and includes 34 cases from 3 institutions (Cleveland Clinic, the University of Pittsburgh, and the University Health Network in Toronto). This article provides important descriptions about the range of morphologies of intercalated duct lesions that are not clear in the literature because of the scarcity of these lesions and provides a nice reasonably comprehensive reference that aids in understanding these lesions (Figs 1 and 2) and in considering them in the differential diagnosis of the more bland appearing salivary gland tumors (eg, polymorphous low-grade carcinoma). One of the interesting aspects of the article is the demonstration that the lesions, although occurring mainly in the parotid gland in most reported cases and in this series, are seen in other salivary gland locations (the submandibular gland and minor salivary glands of the oral cavity or buccal mucosa) and seen in a variety of other salivary gland tumors, mainly basal cell adenoma and epithelial-myoepithelial carcinoma and, to a lesser extent, mucoepidermoid carcinoma, acinic cell carcinoma,

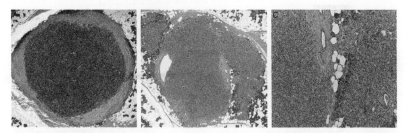

FIGURE 2.—A, Intercalated duct adenoma showing a thick capsule. B, Hybrid lesion demonstrating areas identical to adenomas but with irregular edges outside the capsule that resembled hyperplasia. C, High power of 2B showing the adenomatous area on the left with extension beyond the capsule of the hyperplasia-like area on the right. The hyperplasia-like area shows identical ducts and contains acinic cells. (Reprinted from Weinreb I, Seethala RR, Hunt JL, et al. Intercalated duct lesions of salivary gland: a morphologic spectrum from hyperplasia to adenoma. *Am J Surg Pathol.* 2009;33:1322-1329.)

Warthin tumor, as well as pleomorphic adenomas among others, sometimes in a hybrid fashion. These associations, the authors suggested, may be because of the fact that these small lesions may be precursors to some of these neoplasms. This is an interesting thought—not sufficiently explored before—on the discussion of the etiologies and origins of many salivary gland tumors.[1] Additional molecular studies may help determine if there is a coincidental relationship of 2 lesions colliding together or if there are true molecular similarities between intercalated duct lesions and some of the associated salivary gland tumors.

M. S. Said, MD, PhD

Reference

1. Yu GY, Donath K. Adenomatous ductal proliferation of the salivary gland. *Oral Surg Oral Med Oral Pathol Oral Radiol Endod.* 2001;91:215-221.

Molecular genotyping of papillary thyroid carcinoma follicular variant according to its histological subtypes (encapsulated *vs* infiltrative) reveals distinct *BRAF* and *RAS* mutation patterns
Rivera M, Ricarte-Filho J, Knauf J, et al (Memorial Sloan-Kettering Cancer Ctr, NY)
Mod Pathol 2010 [Epub ahead of print]

The follicular variant of papillary thyroid carcinoma usually presents as an encapsulated tumor and less commonly as a partially/non-encapsulated infiltrative neoplasm. The encapsulated form rarely metastasizes to lymph node, whereas infiltrative tumor often harbors nodal metastases. The molecular profile of the follicular variant was shown to be close to the follicular adenoma/carcinoma group of tumors with a high *RAS* and very low *BRAF* mutation rates. A comprehensive survey of oncogenic mutations in the follicular variant of papillary thyroid carcinoma according to its encapsulated and infiltrative forms has not been performed. Paraffin tissue from 28 patients with encapsulated and 19 with infiltrative

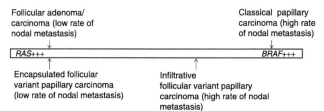

FIGURE 5.—*BRAF* and *RAS* mutational patterns of follicular variant of papillary thyroid carcinoma according to its encapsulated and infiltrative subtypes. The mutational pattern of encapsulated follicular variant of papillary thyroid carcinoma is similar to follicular adenoma/carcinoma, whereas infiltrative follicular variant of papillary thyroid carcinoma has a *BRAF* and *RAS* genotype in between follicular adenoma/carcinoma and classical papillary carcinoma, although closer to the latter. The mutational patterns of encapsulated and infiltrative follicular variant of papillary thyroid carcinomas parallel their lymph node metastatic rate. (Reprinted from Rivera M, Ricarte-Filho J, Knauf J, et al. Molecular genotyping of papillary thyroid carcinoma follicular variant according to its histological subtypes (encapsulated *vs* infiltrative) reveals distinct *BRAF* and *RAS* mutation patterns. *Mod Pathol.* 2010 [Epub ahead of print]. Reprinted by permission from Macmillan Publishers Ltd: Modern Pathology, copyright 2010.)

follicular variant were subjected to mass spectrometry genotyping encompassing the most significant oncogenes in thyroid carcinomas: 111 mutations in *RET, BRAF, NRAS, HRAS, KRAS, PIK3CA, AKT1* and other related genes. There was no difference in age, gender, tumor size and angioinvasion between encapsulated or infiltrative tumors. Infiltrative carcinomas had a much higher frequency of extrathyroid extension, positive margins and nodal metastases than encapsulated tumors ($P < 0.05$). The *BRAF 1799T> A* mutation was found in 5 of 19 (26%) of the infiltrative tumor and in none of the encapsulated carcinomas ($P = 0.007$). In contrast, *RAS* mutations were observed in 10 of 28 (36%) of the encapsulated group (5 *NRAS_Q61R*, 3 *HRAS_Q61*, 1 *HRAS_G13C* and 1 *KRAS_Q61R*) and in only 2 of 19 (10%) of infiltrative tumors ($P = 0.09$). One encapsulated carcinoma showed a *PAX8/PPARγ* rearrangement, whereas two infiltrative tumors harbored *RET/PTC* fusions. Encapsulated follicular variant of papillary thyroid carcinomas have a molecular profile very close to follicular adenomas/carcinomas (high rate of *RAS* and absence of *BRAF* mutations). Infiltrative follicular variant has an opposite molecular profile closer to classical papillary thyroid carcinoma than to follicular adenoma/carcinoma (*BRAF> RAS* mutations). The molecular profile of encapsulated and infiltrative follicular variant parallels their biological behavior (ie, metastatic nodal and invasive patterns) (Fig 5).

▶ This is an interesting article in that its conclusion of a similar molecular profile—between encapsulated follicular variant of papillary carcinoma and follicular adenoma/carcinoma and its different profile infiltrative follicular variant—supports the continuous debate over the reclassification of the encapsulated variant of papillary carcinoma and whether it should be more appropriately included under the same criteria that govern follicular neoplasms, capsular and/or vascular invasion being the more significant behavior predictor. This is certainly a provocative suggestion that is on the minds of a number of investigators and has merit based on the evidence presented in the article and would most significantly alter the management of this particular type of papillary carcinoma, saving patients an unnecessary morbidity associated with postoperative radioactive iodine treatment. Rosai,[1] in an article early in 2010, has asked the same question about the dilemma in classifying the encapsulated follicular variant of papillary carcinoma and about how the architectural pattern of growth, nuclear features, immunohistochemical profile, and finally molecular profile can lead to different classification conclusions between inclusion into follicular neoplasms or papillary carcinoma. Baloch et al,[2] in a very recent comparative study of the encapsulated classic and follicular variant of papillary carcinoma, concluded the very low mortality of both variants and that the follicular encapsulated variant were less prone to capsular/vascular invasion or extrathyroidal spread and nodal metastasis than the classic encapsulated variant. In conclusion, there is certainly a consequential growing debate that puts into question the classification of the encapsulated follicular variant of papillary thyroid carcinoma and whether it should be regarded as a carcinoma in the papillary group or should be considered as a follicular neoplasm where vascular and/or capsular invasion is the measure of considering it a carcinoma.

M. S. Said, MD, PhD

References

1. Rosai J. The encapsulated follicular variant of papillary thyroid carcinoma: back to the drawing board. *Endocr Pathol.* 2010;21:7-11.
2. Baloch Z, Shafique K, Flannagan M, Livolsi V. Encapsulated classic and follicular variant of papillary thyroid carcinoma: a comparative clinicopathologic study. *Endocr Pract.* 2010;24:1-26.

Nasopharyngeal mucoepidermoid carcinoma: A review of 13 cases
Zhang X-m, Cao J-z, Luo J-w, et al (Cancer Hosp of Chinese Academy of Med Sciences (CAMS) and Peking Union Med College (PUMC), Beijing, People's Republic of China)
Oral Oncol 46:618-621, 2010

Nasopharyngeal mucoepidermoid carcinoma (MEC) is an extremely rare entity. To date, there is little published about its clinical characteristics and treatment outcomes. Between 1997 and 2009, 13 cases of MEC were confirmed and treated at the department of Radiation Oncology, Cancer Hospital of Chinese Academy of Medical Sciences (CAMS) and Peking Union Medical College (PUMC). Nasal obstruction, bleeding and hearing loss were the most common presentations, whereas, neck mass, headache and cranial nerve palsy were uncommon. Tumors remained stable after either primary radiation therapy or post-operative radiation therapy for the residual, though the majority of them were high or high-intermediate grade tumors. Five patients, who received either primary surgery or salvage surgery, had positive surgical margins, however, all are alive with stable disease except one old patient died of heart failure. The

TABLE 1.—Clinical Parameters, Treatment Modalities and Outcomes

No.	Age/Sex	T/N	Grading	Symptoms	Primary Treatment	Adjuvant Treatment	Response to Therapy	Fllow-Up/Status
1	48/Female	T2N0	High/intermediate	Nasal obstruction/hearing loss	RT(50Gy)	NO	SD to RT Decline operation	8M/DWD
2	38/Female	T2N0	High	Nasal obstruction/bleeding	RT(76Gy+15Gy by brachytherapy+15Gy by SRT)	S(NP)	SD to RT S(−)	64M/lost F/U
3	56/Male	T1N0	High	Bleeding/tinnitus	RT(50Gy)	S(NP)	SD to RT S(+)	69M/AWND
4	40/Female	T2N0	High	Nasal obstruction/bleeding	RT(50Gy)	S(NP)	SD to RT S(−)	66M/AWND
5	29/Male	T2N2	High	Bleeding	RT(70Gy)	S(NP+N)	SD to RT S(−)	16M/AWND
6	43/Female	T2N0	High	Bleeding/hearing loss	RT(50Gy)	S(NP)+SRT(30Gy)	SD to RT S(+) SRT(+)	10M/AWD
7	41/Female	T2N0	High	Nasal obstruction	RT(70Gy)+SRT(5Gy)	NO	CR after RT DM after 3m SD after CT	63M/AWD
8	44/Female	T2N0	High	Bleeding	RT(50Gy)	S(NP)	SD to RT S(−)	45M/AWND
9	38/Male	T3N0	High/intermediate	Bleeding/Headache	S(NP)	RT(70Gy)	S(−)	80M/AWND
10	48/Female	T1N0	Low	Nasal obstruction/bleeding	S(NP)	NO	S(−)	43M/AWND
11	64/Female	T2N1	Unspecified	Nasal obstruction/bleeding	S(NP+N)	RT(70Gy)	S(NP+) SD to RT	24M/DWHF
12	49/female	T3N0	High	Nasal obstruction/Tinnitus	S(NP)	RT(70Gy)	S(+) SD to RT	42M/AWD
13	48/Male	T2N0	High	Nasal obstruction/Tinnitus	S(NP)	CT(DDP 1 cycle) RT(70Gy)	S(−) PD after 36m(T4N0) Re-S(NP)(+) SRT(30Gy)(+)	36M/AWD

NP – nasopharynx, N – neck, RT – radiation therapy, S – surgery, (+) – residual tumor, (−) – no residual tumor, CT – chemotherapy, SRT – stereotactic radiotherapy, CR – complete remission, PD – progression of disease, SD – stable disease, DM – distant metastasis, DWD – died with disease, DWHF – died with heart failure, AWND – alive with no evidence of disease, AWD – alive with disease, F/U – follow-up.

overall median survival of our patients was 43 months, ranging from 8 to 80 months. Based on the present results, we recommend that primary surgery should be the standard of care for all non-metastatic tumors regardless of histopathologic grade, and post-operative radiation therapy should be considered under the circumstances of positive surgical margins, macroscopic residual tumors, and high grade carcinomas (Table 1).

▶ This is an interesting and informative article reporting mostly the clinical findings and treatment outcomes in 13 cases of nasopharyngeal mucoepidermoid-type carcinoma from China, which is an extremely rare occurrence in any country—even in China, considering the number of its population (1.4 billion in 2010). In 2001, a review article by Kuo and Tsang[1] from Taiwan reported 15 cases of salivary gland-type carcinomas in the nasopharynx (NP), which included 8 mucoepidermoid carcinomas also with follow-up information, and in their review the authors found that 5 of the 8 mucoepidermoid carcinomas were also positive for Epstein-Barr virus (EBV) and suggested that the oncogenesis of most salivary gland-type NP carcinomas, including NP mucoepidermoid carcinoma, can also be related to EBV as shown in conventional NP carcinoma types. Although this article mentions the grades of mucoepidermoid carcinomas in their analysis, it missed the chance for doing EBV analysis on those cases, which could have supported the findings of the other review papers, and related the importance of EBV as an initiating factor in different cancer types of nasopharyngeal cancers. This could be particularly relevant when considering the findings of the article in that the surgical approach is the method of choice for primary treatment for NP mucoepidermoid carcinoma followed by adjuvant postoperative radiation for the larger and high-grade tumor in contrast to the conventional types of NP carcinomas in which radiation treatment is a primary treatment modality with few exceptions, and it may have elaborated on the fact that a common etiologic factor like EBV may result in different types of carcinomas with different treatment modalities not dependent on the initiating/etiologic factor.

M. S. Said, MD, PhD

Reference

1. Kuo TT, Tsang NM. Salivary gland type nasopharyngeal carcinoma. a histologic, immunohistochemical, and Epstein-Barr Virus study of 15 cases including a psammomatous mucoepidermoid carcinoma. *Am J Surg Pathol.* 2001;25:80-86.

Outcomes of Pediatric Patients with Malignancies of the Major Salivary Glands

Kupferman ME, de la Garza GO, Santillan AA, et al (MD Anderson Cancer Ctr, Houston, TX; Univ of Texas Health Science Center at San Antonio; et al)
Ann Surg Oncol 2010 [Epub ahead of print]

Background.—To report the outcomes and early to long term treatment complications among pediatric patients with major salivary gland malignancies treated at a single institution.

Materials and Method.—This study was a retrospective case review set at a tertiary referral cancer center. Patients less than 19 years of age with a diagnosis of a major salivary gland malignancy were identified at the M. D. Anderson tumor database between 1953 and 2006.

Results.—A total of 61 patients were identified, with equal gender distribution. The majority of tumors arose in the parotid gland (83%), and the most common pathology was mucoepidermoid carcinoma (46%). Lymphatic metastasis was identified in 37% of patients, nearly all with mucoepidermoid carcinoma. Although 65% of patients had prior treatment elsewhere, more than 75% of patients underwent surgical resection at our institution. External beam radiation was used in 45% of patients, with an average dose of 58.6 Gray. Average patient follow-up was 153 months. The overall survival rate was 93% at 5 years, and 26% developed a recurrence. A second primary was identified in 2 patients. Permanent facial paresis was noted in 7 patients (12%) and xerostomia in 1 patient (4%).

Conclusions.—Survival of pediatric patients with major salivary gland carcinomas is favorable. Adverse outcomes were best predicted by tumor grade, margin status, and neural involvement. Radiation therapy is beneficial for locoregional control of disease, with acceptable long-term

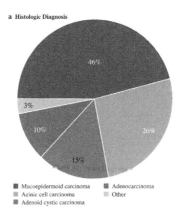

FIGURE 1.—a Distribution of pediatric major salivary gland tumors by histology. (Reprinted from Kupferman ME, de la Garza GO, Santillan AA, et al. Outcomes of pediatric patients with malignancies of the major salivary glands. *Ann Surg Oncol.* 2010;[Epub ahead of print], with kind permission from Springer Science+Business Media: Annals of Surgical Oncology.)

TABLE 3.—Univariate Analysis of DFS and OS ($n = 54$)

	DFS	OS
Gender	NS	NS
Age > 14 years	0.04	0.02
Non-Caucasian	<0.01	0.02
Tumor location	NS	NS
Tumor size (>2 cm)	0.08	NS
Nodal stage (N+)	NS	0.02
Multimodality therapy	NS	NS
Extent of primary surgery	NS	NS
Extracapsular spread	NS	0.05
Close\positive margins	NS	0.04
Histological type	NS	NS
Tumor grade (high)	<0.01	<0.01
Perineural invasion	0.04	NS
Lymphovascular invasion	NS	NS

treatment sequelae, and without a significant risk for developing second primary tumors. Survivorship issues need to be addressed in this patient population into adulthood (Fig 1a, Table 3).

▶ Experience with salivary gland tumors in the pediatric population among pathologists is variable. This is a significant retrospective study of malignant salivary gland tumors collected from 61 pediatric patients over a span of 53 years by MD Anderson Cancer Center, and it provides valuable data in this area. In addition to the outcome data it provides as listed above in the abstract, it notes a number of interesting pathologic facts. In this context, it was very interesting to note that after mucoepidermoid carcinoma as the most common salivary gland malignancy, it was acinic cell carcinoma that constituted the second most common malignant salivary gland tumor in this children series with 26% points. These findings confirm what was previously reported by Shapiro et al[1] in 2006 and contradict previous literature that considers acinic cell carcinoma a very rare pediatric salivary gland tumor constituting only 4% of malignant salivary gland tumors. Another significant fact for the pathologists was the unique findings that patients older than 14 years have higher prevalence of more aggressive histologies that is similar to the clinical behavior seen in the adult population. The article in general provides useful data for the clinicians in the management and outcome of malignant salivary gland malignancies.

M. S. Said, MD, PhD

Reference

1. Shapiro NL, Bhattacharyya N. Clinical characteristics and survival in major salivary gland malignancies in children. *Otolaryngol Head Neck Surg.* 2006; 134:631-634.

Prognostic factors of recurrence in salivary carcinoma ex pleomorphic adenoma, with emphasis on the carcinoma histologic subtype: a clinicopathologic study of 43 cases
Katabi N, Gomez D, Klimstra DS, et al (Memorial Sloan-Kettering Cancer Ctr, NY)
Hum Pathol 41:927-934, 2010

Carcinoma ex pleomorphic adenoma is a rare salivary gland neoplasm, especially when the malignant component is only intracapsular/minimally invasive. Moreover, only few studies have assessed the behavior of carcinoma ex pleomorphic adenoma according to the histologic subtype. Forty-three cases of carcinoma ex pleomorphic adenoma were identified over a 27-year period and subjected to a detailed histopathologic analysis. There were 13 intracapsular/minimally invasive and 30 widely invasive carcinomas. There were 15 myoepithelial carcinomas, 25 salivary duct carcinomas, 2 adenocarcinomas not otherwise specified, and 1 carcinosarcoma. There was a trend toward a higher frequency of myoepithelial carcinomas in widely invasive tumors (13/30, 43%) than in intracapsular/minimally invasive (2/13, 15%) carcinoma ex pleomorphic adenoma ($P = .095$). Adequate follow-up was available for 38 patients. Vascular invasion and distant metastases correlated with decreased disease-free survival and disease-specific survival ($P < .05$), whereas the extent of invasion and the presence of a high mitotic rate or atypical mitoses correlated with decreased disease-free survival only ($P < .05$). There was a trend toward worse disease-free survival and disease-specific survival in patients with myoepithelial carcinoma ($P = .08$). Within the intracapsular/minimally invasive carcinoma ex pleomorphic adenoma group, both myoepithelial carcinoma (2/2, 100%) had metastatic disease, whereas only 1 of 11 nonmyoepithelial carcinoma relapsed ($P = .038$). Vascular invasion, high mitotic rate, and histologic subtype were found to correlate with recurrence in carcinoma ex pleomorphic adenoma. Patients with intracapsular/minimally invasive tumor have a more favorable outcome than patients with widely invasive neoplasm, but intracapsular/minimally invasive carcinoma ex pleomorphic adenoma can recur and cause death. The presence of myoepithelial carcinoma subtype increases the risk of recurrence in carcinoma ex pleomorphic adenoma, especially within the group of intracapsular/minimally invasive tumors.

▶ A number of previous case studies and review articles dealt with the topic of carcinoma ex pleomorphic adenoma and commented on its evolution from noninvasive (so-called in situ or intracapsular [IC] stage) to minimally invasive (MI) (1.5 mm or less beyond the capsule) to more widely invasive. This study of 43 cases of carcinoma ex pleomorphic adenoma, in addition to reinforcing many of the well-established facts about these type of tumors, points out 2 findings that are probably not well recognized/reported about this entity. The first is that the categorization of a carcinoma ex ploemorphic adenoma as IC/MI does not guarantee a definitively favorable course once surgically removed as 3 of their 12 cases reported in this category recurred or developed distant metastasis. The second is reinforcing the sometimes unpredictable and underrecognized potential for aggressive behavior and less favorable prognosis of myoepithelial carcinoma ex pleomorphic adenoma. Some articles in the past have mentioned the potential difficulty in diagnosing and predicting the biological behavior myoepithelial carcinoma ex pleomorphic adenoma if judged only by histologic appearance (ie, appearing with bland histology yet showing aggressive clinical behavior). Its potential for recurrences, aggressive behavior, and less favorable overall prognosis remain somewhat underappreciated by a good section of the practicing pathologists. The strength of this article comes from the question that the conclusions put from the management point of view to the clinicians and oncologists, which is the ultimate goal of any good scientific inquiry. As all cases of IC/MI that were myoepithelial carcinoma ex pleomorphic adenoma (2 cases) developed metastatic disease, should this fact preempt a more aggressive treatment modality (adjuvant therapy of chemo/radiation etc) than surgical resection alone, which has been the main stay of management for this general category, particularly when we also consider the unpredictable behavior of myoepithelial carcinoma? Or should a more aggressive close follow-up at least suffice for these patients until more case analysis and follow-ups are available? Certainly both questions are valid points of further inquiry in the light of these findings. More discussion, analysis, case reports, and awareness of these cases will certainly help answer them correctly.

For further reading on the subject, I suggest articles by Brandwein et al and Savera et al.[1,2]

M. S. Said, MD, PhD

References

1. Brandwein M, Huvos AG, Dardick I, Thomas MJ, Theise ND. Noninvasive and minimally invasive carcinoma ex mixed tumor: a clinicopathologic and ploidy study of 12 patients with major salivary gland tumors of low (or no) malignant potential. *Oral Surg Oral Med Oral Pathol Oral Radiol Endod.* 1996;81:655-664.
2. Savera AT, Solman A, Huvos AG, Klimstra DS. Myoepithelial carcinoma of the salivary glands: a clinicopathologic study of 25 patients. *Am J Surg Pathol.* 2000;24:761-774.

Thyroid Tumor Marker Genomics and Proteomics: Diagnostic and Clinical Implications
Carpi A, Mechanick JI, Saussez S, et al (Univ of Pisa, Italy; Mount Sinai School of Medicine, NY; Univ of Mons, Belgium)
J Cell Physiol 224:612-619, 2010

Two systems biology concepts, genomics and proteomics, are highlighted in this review. These techniques are implemented to optimize the use of thyroid tumor markers (TTM). Tissue microarray studies can produce genetic maps and proteomics, patterns of protein expression of TTM derived from preoperative biopsies and specimens. For instance, papillary and medullary thyroid cancers harbor *RAS, RET,* and *BRAF* genetic mutations. Follicular thyroid cancers harbor translocations and fusions of certain genes (PAX 8 and PPAR-gamma). Proteomic analysis from various tissue sources can provide useful information regarding the overall state of a thyroid cancer cell. Understanding the molecular events related to these genetic and protein alterations can potentially clarify thyroid cancer pathogenesis and guide appropriate molecular targeted therapies. However, despite the realization that these emerging technologies hold great promise, there are still significant obstacles to the routine use of TTM. These include equivocal thyroid nodule tissue morphologic interpretations, inadequate standardization of methods, and monetary costs. Interpretative shortcomings are frequently due to the relative scarcity of cellular material from fine-needle aspiration biopsy (FNAB) specimens. This can be rectified with large needle aspiration biopsy (LNAB) techniques and is exemplified by the favorable performance of galectin-3 determinations on LNAB specimens (Fig 1, Tables 1 and 2).

▶ This is an interesting review article that summarizes most of the recent and more impressive advances in the molecular field in thyroid pathology, including

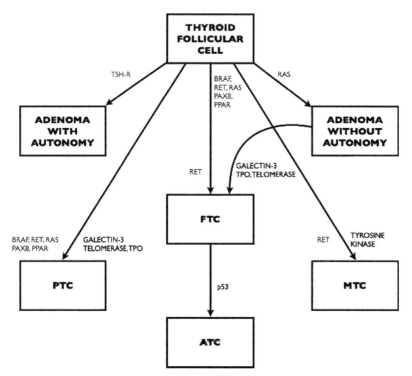

FIGURE 1.—Thyroid tumor markers derived from genomic and proteomic methods. The gray markers are derived from genomic methods; the black markers are derived from proteomic methods. See Table 1 for a more complete list of markers. (Reprinted from Carpi A, Mechanick JI, Saussez S, et al. Thyroid tumor marker genomics and proteomics: diagnostic and clinical implications. *J Cell Physiol.* 2010;224:612-619.)

TABLE 1.—Molecular Markers of Thyroid Tumors Derived from Genomic and Proteomic Methods (Modified from J.I. Mechanick and A. Carpi, 2008)

(a) Papillary thyroid cancer (PTC)
Pathogenesis
    Abnormal mitogenic signaling to the nucleus via the RET/RAS/BRAF–MAPK pathway
    Epigenetic inactivation (abnormal promoter methylation) of tumor suppressor, *RASSF1A*, and *TSH-R* gene
    Galectin-3 promotes K-Ras signaling to Raf and PI3K, which affects apoptosis
    CD44v6 encodes membrane glycoproteins affecting tumors
    Metallothionein 1G oncosuppression
Molecular markers
    RET/PTC1 > *RET/PTC3*, *TRK* rearrangements, *BRAF* (T1799A, V600E), *RAS* activating mutations, ↑ c-met, EGF-R expression, E-cadherin downregulation, galectin-3, CD44v6, P27^{KIP1}, cyclin D1, p53 inactivation, β-catenin, periostin gene expression, H4-PTEN mutation, SAGE: PTPRC + LIMD2 in LN, MDM4 alterations, IL 13, CD 10, trisomy 17, telomerase
(b) Follicular variant of PTC
Pathogenesis
    There is a greater tendency toward encapsulation compared with conventional PTC leading toward more hematogenous spread and pulmonary metastasis
Molecular markers
    BRAF (A1802G, K601E) mutations, E-cadherin, RAS mutations, PPARγ overexpression, *RET/PTC3* rearrangement, *PAX8–PPARγ* rearrangement, 6-gene model (*SYNGR2, LSM7, KIT, Hs.296031, c21orf4*, and *Hs.24183*); molecular expression signature (CSNK1G 2, HLA-DQB1, MT1X, RAB 23)
(c) Follicular thyroid cancer
Pathogenesis
    Vascular and capsular invasion
Molecular markers
    Aneuploidy, loss of heterozygosity, *RAS* mutations, *PAX8–PPARγ* rearrangement, 3-gene model (*cyclin D2, PCSK2, PLAB*), *hTERT* gene expression, *HMGA2* upregulation, reduced expression of *FZD-1* gene, QRT protein, telomerase
(d) Hurthle cell thyroid cancer
Pathogenesis
    Large deletions and point mutations in mtDNA inhibits apoptosis, increases HIF-1, and increases angiogenesis
    Subsequent *RET/PTC* rearrangements and/or *BRAF* mutations induce malignant transformation and loss of NIS function
Molecular markers
    Overexpression of *PRC, NRC1, TFAM, GRIM-19* downregulation
(e) Medullary thyroid cancer
Pathogenesis
    Arises from parafollicular CTN producing C-cells
    Tyrosine kinase RET signaling cascade
Molecular markers
    CTN, CEA, RET protooncogene, *pRb, p53, PTEN, p27Kip1, p18-INK4c* mutations, loss of heterozygosity in VHL tumor suppressor locus, reduced MMP-2/TIMP-2 expression
(f) Anaplastic thyroid cancer
Pathogenesis
    Undifferentiated, multistep carcinogenesis involving p53
    E$_2$ is proapoptotic in ATC (but growth promoting in PTC)
    Overexpression of gene cluster
    Deregulation of miRNAs
    Thyroid cancer derived from fetal thyroid (stem) cells
    Anaplastic transformation
Molecular markers
    Panel: TG, Bcl-2, MIB-1, apo E overexpression, RXRγ expression, PLK1 kinase expression, miRNA overexpression, onfFN overexpression, E-cadherin, p53, β-catenin, TOPO-II, VEGF

---

the genomic and proteomic findings in an up-to-date fashion, discusses the practicality and the limitations on some of these techniques (Tables 1 and 2), and points out the currently used/available tumor thyroid markers in most

TABLE 2.—Proteomics Techniques and Thyroid Tumor Markers (Modified from K. Krause et al., 2009)

Study Source	Main Technique	Principal Finding
Thyroid tissue (Brown LM et al., 2006)	2D gel electrophoresis	31 proteins differentially expressed in PTC and NT (S100 A6 protein 6.5-fold higher in PTC)
Thyroid tissue (Netea-Maier RT et al., 2008)	2D gel electrophoresis	FTC > FA, histone H2B, cytokeratin 7, FTC < FA, cytokeratin 8 78-kDa, glucose-regulated protein, calreticulin, annexin A3, β-actin
Serum (Moretz WH et al., 2008)	SELDI-TOF-MS	Serum expression patterns allowing discrimination between PTC vs. benign nodules
Serum (Wang JX et al., 2006)	SELDI-TOF-MS	Serum expression pattern allowing discrimination between: (1) PTC vs. healthy; (2) PTC vs. benign nodules; (3) different stages of PTC; (4) different pathological types of thyroid cancer
Cell culture (Arcinas A et al., 2009)	Glycoprotein denaturation, digestion, solid-phase extraction, and ESI-MS/MS analysis identification	An average of 150 glycoproteins per cancer cell line (papillary, follicular, Hurthle, anaplastic) were identified. Some glycoproteins are specific of differentiated or anaplastic thyroid tumors

advanced institutions (Fig 1). The article gains extra value in that the authors are from 3 different countries and probably put the current state of the advances in that field around the world into a more global perspective and a shared experience. No doubt that the use of new molecular methods will enhance the diagnostic and prognostic information that can influence the patient treatment options and outcomes. The authors particularly mention the importance of the selective use of these markers in the preoperative selection of patients who will undergo operative procedures and the richness of data that can help institutions implement these markers into their preoperative selection as well as mentioning the limitations of the use of these markers in gathering follow-up information as many of these still lack the evidence-based information from the postoperative period. One of the limitations that many of us face as we try to practically implement many of these techniques is definitely the tissue collection, particularly in thyroid pathology as most of the preoperative morphologic assessment of thyroid lesions depend mainly on fine-needle aspiration techniques and suggest the use of the large-needle aspiration biopsy as an effective method of preoperative tissue collection.

Probably one of the important tasks in the immediate future of various institutions based on the findings in this article is to gather the information presented by different institutions to determine the practicality, pitfalls, prognostic information, and different information that can help at some stage to provide a standard—or state of the art, if you like—for the use of these markers instead of the variable selective use/experience in different institutions and to provide more long-term prognostic information as it relates to these markers.

The article contains a good reference list for many of the essential articles in the molecular thyroid pathology field.

M. S. Said, MD, PhD

Tumor-Associated Lymphocytes and Increased FoxP3+ Regulatory T Cell Frequency Correlate with More Aggressive Papillary Thyroid Cancer
French JD, Weber ZJ, Fretwell DL, et al (Univ of Colorado Denver, Aurora)
J Clin Endocrinol Metab 95:2325-2333, 2010

Context.—Ten to 30% of patients with papillary thyroid cancer (PTC) develop recurrent disease and may benefit from innovative adjuvant therapies. Immune-based therapies are under investigation to treat many types of cancer. The role of the immune system in PTC is poorly understood.

Objective.—We investigated whether tumor-associated lymphocytes (TAL), in the absence of background thyroiditis (LT), contribute to disease severity. We hypothesized that the type of lymphocytes associated with PTC would correlate with parameters of disease.

Design.—This retrospective study analyzed archived PTC samples for the presence of TAL and/or LT. A group of patients with TAL was evaluated for lymphocyte subsets by immunohistofluorescence.

Patients and Setting.—One hundred PTC patients were analyzed for LT and TAL, and 10 PTC patients with TAL were assessed for lymphocyte subsets at University of Colorado Hospital.

Main Outcome.—We assessed correlations between disease and the presence of TAL, LT, and lymphocyte subset frequency.

Results.—Patients with TAL exhibited higher disease stage and increased incidence of invasion and lymph node metastasis compared with patients without lymphocytes or with LT. CD4$^+$ T cell frequency correlated with tumor size ($r = 0.742$; $P = 0.017$). FoxP3$^+$ regulatory T cell (Treg) frequency correlated with lymph node metastases ($r = 0.858$; $P = 0.002$), and CD8 to Treg ratio correlated inversely with tumor size ($r = -0.804$; $P = 0.007$).

Conclusions.—TAL and high Treg frequency in primary thyroid tumors correlates with more aggressive disease. Future prospective studies may identify Treg frequency as a predictive factor in PTC, and the suppressive effects of Treg should be considered in the design of immune-based therapies.

▶ The role of immune-based therapies in the treatment of thyroid cancer particularly in patients with advanced-stage papillary thyroid carcinoma (PTC) is yet to be fully explored. Lymphocytes are frequently found within and surrounding primary thyroid tumors; however, the role of the immune response in thyroid cancers remains poorly defined. In this recent study by French et al, PTC patients with tumor-associated lymphocytes (TALs) were shown to have more severe disease compared with patients with no lymphocytic infiltration or with concurrent thyroiditis. Specifically, patients with TAL display more invasive tumors and a higher incidence of lymph node metastases. Upon closer examination of lymphocyte subsets by immunohistofluorescence, CD4$^+$ T cells, CD8$^+$ T cells, and CD20$^+$ B cells were found in association with PTC at varying frequencies. Correlation analysis with disease parameters showed that an increased relative frequency of CD4$^+$ T cells was associated with larger tumor size. Costaining for the FoxP3 transcription factor revealed that CD4$^+$ FoxP3$^+$ regulatory T cells (Tregs) were present in all samples to varying degrees. As in many other types of cancer, Treg frequency was shown to correlate with worse prognosis. Specifically, higher levels of Tregs were found in patients with extensive lymph node metastasis, and CD8:Treg ratio showed a strong inverse correlation with tumor size. These data suggest that the immune response to PTC is insufficient and may even promote disease progression. Future prospective studies are necessary to determine the prognostic value of Treg frequency. These studies will undoubtedly encourage additional investigation into the role of the immune response in PTC and may support the use of immune-based therapies for patients with advanced disease.

M. S. Said, MD, PhD

12 Cytopathology

Atypia in fine needle aspirates of breast lesions

The Tran PV, Lui PCW, Yu AMC, et al (The Chinese Univ of Hong Kong; et al)
J Clin Pathol 63:585-591, 2010

Background.—The atypical category is controversial in fine needle aspiration cytology (FNAC) of the breast; most are benign, but a significant number are malignant. To date, no morphological criterion has been found to be consistent in predicting malignancy.

Aims.—To evaluate specific cytological parameters and assess their usefulness in predicting histological outcome in a cohort of atypical breast FNAC, in order to establish a set of objective criteria in defining 'high risk' atypical breast FNAC.

Methods.—A retrospective review of 98 cases of atypical breast FNAC with histological correlation was undertaken. The cytological preparations were evaluated for cellularity, percentage of epithelial cell cluster and single epithelial cells, nuclear atypia, nucleus:cytoplasm ratio, percentage of bipolar nuclei, and the presence of stromal fragments, histiocytes and necrosis.

Results.—66 of 98 cases (67.35%) showed benign histology and 32 cases (32.65%) showed malignant histology. Compared with the malignant group, the benign group had significantly lower patient age ($p=0.05$), higher bipolar nuclei ($p<0.0001$), less degree of nuclear pleomorphism ($p<0.0001$), lower nucleus: cytoplasm ratio ($p<0.0001$), lower cellularity ($p=0.05$) and less necrosis ($p<0.001$). There was no difference in the percentage of epithelial clusters and single cells, or the presence of stromal fragments and histiocytes.

Conclusions.—The presence of nuclear pleomorphism, high nucleus: cytoplasm ratio, epithelial cell atypia, low number of bipolar nuclei and necrosis are useful parameters to predict malignancy in atypical FNAC of the breast. Assessment of these factors in atypical FNAC may be helpful in predicting cancer risk and subsequent management decision making.

▶ A challenge for a cytopathologist in breast fine-needle aspiration is in recognizing that cytologic atypia is suggestive of a malignant process and cannot simply be ignored.[1,2] Tran and colleagues evaluated the presence of individual cytologic features and their association with malignancy. Studies of this type always leave me wondering if individual criterion alone can be useful for a definitive diagnosis. A regression analysis evaluating multiple simultaneous features would have been a better study design. In this study, all the criteria identified as indicating a benign lesion are rather obvious and are already reported in the cytology literature. The difficulty is recognizing that these features are present in a real practice fine-needle aspiration. In my view, these studies are better performed using a root cause analysis method to determine why the diagnosis of atypia was made in the first place instead of a more definitive diagnosis. This type of investigation would provide more insight as to the appropriate scenarios in which an indeterminate diagnosis should be rendered.

S. S. Raab, MD

References

1. Lim CJ, Al-Masri H, Salhadar A, Xie HB, Gabram S, Wojcik EM. The significance of the diagnosis of atypia in breast fine-needle aspiration. *Diagn Cytopathol.* 2004; 31:285-288.
2. Al-Kaisi N. The spectrum of the "gray zone" in breast cytology. *Acta Cytol.* 1994; 38:898-908.

Cytodiagnosis through use of a *z*-axis video by volunteer observers: a promising tool for external quality assessment
Yamashiro K, Tagami M, Azuma K, et al (Hokkaido Cancer Ctr, Shiroishi-ku, Sapporo, Japan; Hokkaido Cancer Society, Sapporo, Japan; Sapporo Med Univ Hosp, Japan; et al)
Cytopathology 2010 [Epub ahead of print]

Objective.—This study examined whether cytological diagnosis through the use of a video, which shows the changing depth of focus in the microscopic field, described as a *z*-axis video, is useful compared with a still image.

Methods.—From 17 cytology preparations of fine needle aspiration of the breast, we made six *z*-axis videos per case. A frame exhibiting the characteristic features was then extracted from each video and saved as a representative still image. One hundred and twenty-eight volunteer cytotechnologists were randomly divided into two groups of video observers and still image observers. The participants were asked to make a diagnosis of benign, indeterminate, suspicious or malignant without having any clinical information other than the age of the patient. Diagnoses were categorized as 'recommended' or 'unacceptable' according to degree of correlation with histology.

Results.—The number of definitive diagnoses of 'benign' or 'malignant' were increased in video observers, and indeterminate or suspicious categories were decreased ($P = 0.013$). The distribution of diagnostic categories in three of the 17 cases was significantly different; the distribution in the remaining cases was similar between the two groups. The *z*-axis video observers may have selected the definite diagnoses with confidence because they observed valuable microscopic findings by 'focusing through observation'. The average number of 'recommended' diagnoses by individual observers was significantly higher in the video observer group than in the still image observer group ($P = 0.016$). In contrast, the average number of 'unacceptable' diagnoses was significantly lower ($P = 0.019$).

Conclusions.—A z-axis video is easy to obtain and is therefore expected to become a powerful diagnostic modality for the external quality assessment of clinical cytology and even in the field of primary cytodiagnosis.

▶ A problem in telecytology has been the inability to interpret 3-dimensional groups using methods that only capture 2-dimensional images. Newer technologies capture the third dimension, known as the z-plane, for cytological interpretation.[1] When using whole-slide images, images from multiple z-planes must be captured so the cytotechnologist or cytopathologist can freely zoom in and out to examine the different z-planes. When using 2-dimensional captured images, images must still be captured from the different z-planes and viewed as a video of the different z-planes, as reported by Yamashiro et al.[2] The authors provide evidence that simply viewing a 2-dimensional image is not sufficient to render a quality diagnosis, and videos incorporating the different z-planes are necessary to render a more determinate diagnosis. The question is how telecytology will be used in actual practice. If telecytology is used only as a tool for immediate assessment of adequacy, a nondefinitive diagnosis may be acceptable and 2-dimensional images may be sufficient. If telecytology is used to render definitive final diagnoses, then including multiple z-planes is the first step in determining the equivalence of telecytology and microscopic cytology. Studies have focused on overall accuracy of telecytology for different specimen types but have not examined large numbers of classic pitfalls, difficult or rare cases, or sampling-related problems. The accuracy of telecytology for these types of cases needs to be compared with the accuracy of general cytology prior to wide acceptance.

S. S. Raab, MD

References

1. Marsan C, Vacher-Lavenu MC. Telepathology: a tool to aid in the diagnosis and quality assurance in cervicovaginal cytology. *Cytopathology.* 1995;6:339-342.
2. Yamashiro K, Kawamura N, Matsubayashi S, et al. Telecytology in Hokkaido Island, Japan: results of primary telecytodiagnosis of routine cases. *Cytopathology.* 2004;15:221-227.

Automatic Failure in Gynecologic Cytology Proficiency Testing: Results From the College of American Pathologists Proficiency Testing Program
Moriarty AT, Crothers BA, Bentz JS, et al (AmeriPath Indiana, Indianapolis; Walter Reed Army Med Ctr, Washington, DC; Univ of Utah, Salt Lake City; et al)
Arch Pathol Lab Med 133:1757-1760, 2009

Context.—Automatic failure in gynecologic cytology proficiency testing occurs when a high-grade lesion or carcinoma (HSIL+, Category D) is misinterpreted as negative for intraepithelial lesion or malignancy (Category B).

Objectives.—To document the automatic failure rate in 2006 and 2007 from the College of American Pathologists proficiency testing program (PAP PT) and compare them to projected values from 2004.

Design.—Identify automatic failures from PAP PT in 2006 and 2007 and compare the rates of failure regarding participant and preparation type to validated slides in the College of American Pathologists Interlaboratory Comparison Program in 2004.

Results.—There were 65 264 participant responses for HSIL+ slides included in this analysis from 2006 and 2007. Overall, 1% (666 of 65 264) of the HSIL+ responses were classified as negative, resulting in automatic failure for the participant. There were significantly fewer automatic failures in 2007 as compared with either 2006 or projected from 2004 data ($P < .001$). Conventional preparations had a lower automatic failure rate than liquid-based preparations but only for 2006. Both pathologists and cytotechnologists interpreting liquid-based preparations faired better than projected from 2004 data.

Conclusions.—The automatic failure rate in PAP PT is lower than expected based on 2004 data from the College of American Pathologists Interlaboratory Comparison Program. Automatic failures are a relatively small component (1% or less) of proficiency testing failures. The rate of automatic failure decreased from 2006 to 2007 and may be due to loss of poor performers in the testing pool, the test-taking environment, or removal of less robust slides from the program.

▶ As we already know, proficiency testing in gynecologic cytology is controversial. A component of this controversy lies in the fact that proficiency testing for cytology actually is a measure of individual competency, and many believe that the test is fundamentally not a good test.[1,2] Can a 10-slide test really determine if a cytotechnologist or a cytopathologist is competent? The causes of individual test failure are several, and Moriarty et al report the frequency of testing failure secondary to diagnosing a high-grade squamous intraepithelial lesion (HSIL) or cancer as benign. This frequency is extremely low (< 1%) indicating that most failures result from errors in 2 or more test challenges. Some argue that flaws in the testing system (eg, poor slide quality) could also contribute to this error, and to my knowledge, there are little published data examining the real causes of testing failure. If the most important end point of Papanicolaou testing is HSIL detection and only 1% of participants fail because of this miss, these participants are failing because of less important

reasons. To improve cytology proficiency testing, more formal methods of eval-
uative science need to be applied. Otherwise, it is unclear if the test is flawed or
if the test truly measures poor performance.

S. S. Raab, MD

References

1. Clinical Laboratory Improvement Amendments of 1988 Final Rule. *Fed Regist.* 1992;57:7001-7186.
2. Crothers BA, Moriarty AT, Faitheree L, et al. Appeals in Gynecologic Cytology Proficiency Testing (PT): review of 2006 PT from the College of American Pathologists (CAP). *Arch Pathol Lab Med.* 2009;133:44-48.

Telecytopathology for Immediate Evaluation of Fine-Needle Aspiration Specimens
Alsharif M, Carlo-Demovich J, Massey C, et al (Med Univ of South Carolina, Charleston)
Cancer Cytopathol 118:119-126, 2010

Background.—On-site evaluation of fine-needle aspiration (FNA) specimens by a pathologist is essential to obtain adequate samples and provide a preliminary diagnosis. Distance from the laboratory can make this difficult. The authors present their experience with on-site evaluation using telecytopathology.

Methods.—Dynamic images of cytology smears were captured and pro-cessed with a Nikon digital camera system for microscopy and transmitted via Ethernet. A pathologist accessed the real-time images on a computer and interpreted them while communicating with on-site operators over the telephone. Sample adequacy and accuracy of preliminary diagnosis were compared with those obtained by regular on-site evaluation.

Results.—A total of 429 telecytopathology cases and 363 conventional on-site cases were compared. Specimens were mainly from the pancreas, gastrointestinal tract, liver, and lymph nodes. Adequacy rate was 94.0% for telecytopathology and 97.7% for conventional cases. Preliminary diag-noses of unsatisfactory, adequate (defer), negative/benign, atypical, neoplasm, suspicious, and positive for malignancy were 6.3%, 13.5%, 14.9%, 17.9%, 7.2%, 8.6%, and 31.5% for telecytopathology and 3.9%, 30.6%, 21.5%, 9.6%, 5.0%, 5.2%, and 24.2% for conventional cases. Preliminary and final diagnoses were discrepant in 7 (1.8%) of 371 telecytopathology cases, and in 8 (3.1%) of 252 conventional cases. Difficulty was encountered in some cases in distinguishing pancreatic endocrine neoplasm from lymphoid proliferations, and low grade pancre atic tumors from chronic pancreatitis via telecytopathology.

Conclusions.—On-site evaluation of FNA specimens via telecytopa-thology assures sample adequacy and accurate preliminary diagnosis compared with the conventional method. It allows pathologists to use their time more efficiently and makes on-site evaluations at remote locations possible.

▶ Previous studies have examined the use of telepathology for frozen section interpretation.[1] This work by Alsharif et al is a natural extension of telepathology's immediate feedback in surgical pathology to cytopathology. Immediate interpretation affects the quality of the specimen, immediate patient management, and potentially patient centeredness. In many practice settings, clinicians perform their own fine-needle aspiration, and the specimen is of low quality. Poor quality specimens are a cause of diagnostic error and increased system costs secondary to delays in management and to repeat testing. If telecytology could improve system costs by improving quality, theoretically, the system would have fewer errors and lower costs. In this study, telecytology was evaluated in a single system and shown to be effective. The next and important step will be the evaluation of telecytology in the outpatient setting and in clinician offices. The ability of these sites to produce quality slides and send images will be complex and will require education and training. Pathology practices that could master these details could have a tremendous outreach business that would improve the quality of care.

S. S. Raab, MD

Reference

1. Baak JP, van Diest PJ, Meijer GA. Experience with a dynamic inexpensive video-conferencing system for frozen section telepathology. *Anal Cell Pathol.* 2000;21: 169-175.

Cervical cancer screening in Mediterranean countries: implications for the future
Syrjänen K, Di Bonito L, Gonçalves L, et al (Turku Univ Hosp, Finland; U.C.O. Anatomia Patologica, Trieste, Italy; Hospital do Espírito Santo E.P.E, Évora, Portugal; et al)
Cytopathology 2010 [Epub ahead of print]

Prompted by feedback from the 34th European Congress of Cytology (ECC), the practice of including a special symposium in the programme was continued in the 35th ECC in Lisbon (2009) by arranging a satellite symposium entitled 'Cervical Cancer Screening in the Mediterranean Countries'. Because of the importance to the future of this discipline, it was felt appropriate to summarize the highlights of this symposium here. Cervical cancer prevention strategies in the countries participating in the symposium (Portugal, Spain, Italy, Croatia, Greece and Turkey) appear to be highly variable. As yet, none of these countries can demonstrate a fully implemented national screening programme, but all are in different phases of designing and/or setting up such a programme, which is important. At present, the time-honoured concept of cervical cancer prevention by Pap smear screening is under review, because prophylactic human papillomavirus (HPV) vaccines demonstrate a potential to prevent the vast majority (albeit not all) of cases of cervical cancer in the foreseeable future. Cervical cancer screening is still needed in this emerging era of HPV vaccination, but clearly the existing screening strategies must be modified to provide a cost-effective combination of vaccination and screening. If the currently evaluated new screening strategies, such as HPV testing followed by cytology triage, become a reality, there is the likelihood that the Pap test will have only a secondary role, subordinate to HPV testing. Supporters of this scenario claim that Pap test performance will deteriorate in vaccinated populations. Reduced positive predictive value (PPV), due to lower disease prevalence, is inevitable, however, and this would also affect HPV tests. Any decline in sensitivity and specificity depends on human performance, and as such is avoidable by taking appropriate preventive measures. As clinical cytologists, we should focus attention on minimizing the risk to the Pap test of falling sensitivity because of unfamiliarity with abnormal cells, and also of reduced specificity if the fear of missing significant disease leads to overcalling of benign abnormalities.

▶ In my practice, the number of yearly Papanicolaou tests has decreased to the point that we are overstaffed with cytotechnologists. More women are undergoing high-risk human papillomavirus (HR HPV) testing as a primary method of screening, and the long-term effect this will have on laboratory Pap test volumes and quality is unclear. In this review article by Syrjänen et al, some of the challenges in maintaining high cytology laboratory screening metrics (eg, sensitivity and specificity) are discussed. Currently, cytology laboratories in the United States track epithelial abnormality rates but are not well equipped to measure overall sensitivity and specificity, let alone take actions to maintain high performance. This situation is similar to when HR HPV testing began to be performed for women who had a Pap test of atypical squamous cells of undetermined significance (ASC-US). Prior to Bethesda 2001, the early data indicated that approximately 50% of women who had ASC-US would be HR HPV positive.[1,2] More recent data indicate that this positivity frequency has dropped with one possible explanation being the increased over diagnosis of ASC-US. Overcalling of epithelial cell abnormalities could continue with the trend of switching HR HPV testing as the primary test with Pap testing as the second arm of triage.

S. S. Raab, MD

References

1. Gustafsson L, Pontén J, Zack M, Adami H-O. International incidence rates of cervical cancer after introducing cytological screening. *Cancer Causes Control*. 1997;8:755-763.
2. Coleman D, Day N, Douglas G, et al. European guidelines for quality assurance in cervical cancer screening. Europe against cancer programme. *Eur J Cancer*. 1993; 29A:S1-38.

The role of laboratory processing in determining diagnostic conclusiveness of breast fine needle aspirations: conventional smearing versus a monolayer preparation

Wauters CAP, Kooistra B, Strobbe LJA (Canisius Wilhelmina Ziekenhuis, Nijmegen, The Netherlands)
J Clin Pathol 62:931-934, 2009

Aim.—To compare breast fine needle aspiration (FNA) specimens prepared by conventional smearing (CS) versus monolayer preparation (MP), with respect to the conclusiveness of the cytopathological diagnosis.

Methods.—From 1992 to 1996, aspirators prepared aspirates themselves by direct smearing onto 2–4 slides. From 1999 to 2003, aspirate preparation was performed in the laboratory, creating a MP, using a Hettich cytocentrifuge. FNA diagnoses were categorised into inadequate (C1), benign (C2), atypical (C3), suspicious for malignancy (C4) and malignant (C5). The reference standard constituted histological follow-up. A conclusive FNA diagnosis was defined as C2 in lesions benign on follow-up and C5 in lesions malignant on histology.

Results.—From 1992 to 1996, 692 aspirates were processed by CS, whereas from 1999 to 2003, 1301 aspirates were processed by MP. More FNA were ultrasound-guided in the MP group (85.6% versus 21.5%, p<0.001). When compared with CS, MP-prepared FNA had conclusive diagnoses significantly more often (72.8% versus 58.5%, p<0.001). This effect remained significant when corrected for the difference in ultrasound guidance (adjusted odds ratio 1.7, 95% confidence interval 1.3 to 2.2, p<0.001), and was larger for malignant lesions than for benign lesions (51.7% versus 79.9%, p<0.001).

Conclusion.—Patients presenting with breast lesions can more often be offered a same-day, conclusive cytopathological diagnosis when FNA are prepared by a manual MP processing technique.

▶ The processes in a single-stop breast clinic may be organized in several ways. As Wauters et al briefly describe, the goal is to provide integrated clinical, radiologic, pathologic, oncologic, and surgical services. For the pathology services, the diagnoses need to be rapid and accurate. In the description of single-stop services provided by Wauters and colleagues, the radiologists perform the aspirates, fix the specimens (either smears or placed in solution for monolayer preparations), and then send the material to the laboratory for additional preparation and analysis. I believe that better fine-needle aspiration specimens are obtained when an immediate interpretation is provided, and this would necessitate smears being immediately prepared. Although Wauters et al reported that monolayer preparations surpassed smear preparations in terms of the ability to render a conclusive diagnosis, monolayer preparations still had inconclusiveness of a whopping 27.2%. This indicates that specimen quality is an important issue in their single-stop clinic and that this problem needs to be fixed first. The data indicate that with poor quality specimens, monolayer preparations may be superior to smear preparations. In the United States, the goal would be to develop more single-stop clinics, and this would require the reorganization of pathology services. This reorganization would necessitate the assignment of cytopathologists to perform immediate interpretation to improve specimen adequacy, or we would end up with the same problem presented by Wauters et al (ie, poor quality specimens).[1,2]

S. S. Raab, MD

References

1. Layfield LJ, Bentz JS, Gopez EV. Immediate on-site interpretation of fine-needle aspiration smears: a cost and compensation analysis. *Cancer.* 2001;93:319-322.
2. Joseph L, Edwards JM, Nicholson CM, Pitt MA, Howat AJ. An audit of the accuracy of fine needle aspiration using a liquid-based cytology system in the setting of a rapid access breast clinic. *Cytopathology.* 2002;13:343-349.

Thyroid Bed Fine-Needle Aspiration: Experience at a Large Tertiary Care Center
Bishop JA, Owens CL, Shum CH, et al (The Johns Hopkins Hosp, Baltimore, MD)
Am J Clin Pathol 134:335-339, 2010

Fine-needle aspiration (FNA) of thyroid bed (TB) lesions is a common diagnostic modality in monitoring patients for recurrent cancer after a thyroidectomy. To elucidate the value of TB FNA, we reviewed our experience at The Johns Hopkins Hospital, Baltimore, MD. We identified 57 TB FNA specimens from 50 patients. Of the patients, 36 were being followed up for papillary carcinoma, 7 for medullary carcinoma, 4 for follicular carcinoma (1 also had papillary carcinoma), and 1 for poorly differentiated neuroendocrine carcinoma; 3 had previous benign diagnoses. TB FNA yielded diagnostic material in 49 of 57 cases. Of 37 malignant or atypical FNA samples, 32 had surgical follow-up; 30 of 32 were confirmed malignant. The FNA result was benign in 12 of 57, including 6 cases of benign thyroid and 1 case of parathyroid tissue. Immunohistochemical staining was contributory in 5 of 57 cases. TB FNA is a highly reliable tool for diagnosing recurrent thyroid carcinoma. Residual benign thyroid and parathyroid tissue are potential pitfalls; awareness of these and judicious use of immunohistochemical staining can prevent misdiagnoses.

▶ Clinicians at my institution perform a number of thyroid bed fine-needle aspirations every year, and I think that these aspirates may be quite challenging.[1,2] The work by Bishop et al provides a single institutional account of this practice. The article touches upon several of the pitfalls that deserve greater emphasis. First, the thyroid bed may contain normal thyroid tissue not removed during previous surgery. If thyroid tissue is admixed with lymphocytes, a lymphocytic thyroiditis in residual thyroid or recurrence of a thyroid tumor in a lymph node should be considered. Second, normal structures in the thyroid bed may mimic thyroid tissue; 1 example is parathyroid tissue. Thus, simply identifying epithelial tissue does not mean that tumor is present. Third, some thyroid gland tumors may appear virtually indistinct from normal thyroid tissue. Such tumors include well-differentiated follicular carcinomas or papillary carcinomas that lack typical cytologic features such as nuclear pseudoinclusions or metaplastic cytoplasm. Last, poor quality specimens may be exceedingly difficult to interpret and may consist of blood or only rare tissue fragments. These specimens may be interpreted as benign rather than less than optimal or nondiagnostic. The optimal diagnosis is achieved through coordination among the clinical, cytology, and radiology teams that communicate regarding findings and possible interpretations. In our practice, we sometimes ask (depending on the clinical scenario and presumed preaspiration risk) for a separate aspirate for TG wash for additional correlation. If no epithelial material is seen on the cytology specimen and the TG wash is positive, we know that the cytology specimen was nondiagnostic.

S. S. Raab, MD

References

1. Shin JH, Han BK, Ko EY, Kang SS. Sonographic findings in the surgical bed after thyroidectomy: comparison of recurrent tumors and nonrecurrent lesions. *J Ultrasound Med.* 2007;26:1359-1366.
2. Krishnamurthy S, Bedi DG, Caraway NP. Ultrasound-guided fine-needle aspiration biopsy of the thyroid bed. *Cancer.* 2001;93:199-205.

Malignancy Risk for Fine-Needle Aspiration of Thyroid Lesions According to The Bethesda System for Reporting Thyroid Cytopathology
Jo VY, Stelow EB, Dustin SM, et al (Univ of Virginia, Charlottesville; et al)
Am J Clin Pathol 134:450-456, 2010

Fine-needle aspiration (FNA) is an important test for triaging patients with thyroid nodules. The 2007 National Cancer Institute Thyroid Fine-Needle Aspiration State-of-the-Science Conference helped instigate the recent publication of *The Bethesda System for Reporting Thyroid Cytopathology.* We reviewed 3,080 thyroid FNA samples and recorded interpretations according to the proposed standardized 6-tier nomenclature, and pursued follow-up cytology and histology. Of the 3,080 FNAs, 18.6% were nondiagnostic, 59.0% were benign, 3.4% were atypical follicular lesion of undetermined significance (AFLUS), 9.7% were "suspicious" for follicular neoplasm (SFN), 2.3% were suspicious for malignancy (SM), and 7.0% were malignant. Of 574 cases originally interpreted as nondiagnostic, 47.9% remained nondiagnostic. In 892 cases, there was follow-up histology. Rates of malignancy were as follows: nondiagnostic, 8.9%; benign, 1.1%; AFLUS, 17% (9/53); SFN, 25.4%; SM, 70% (39/56), and malignant, 98.1%. Thus, classification of thyroid FNA samples at the University of Virginia Health System, Charlottesville, according to The Bethesda System yields similar results for risk of malignancy as reported by others. Universal application of the new standardized nomenclature may improve interlaboratory agreement and lead to more consistent management approaches.

▶ In the past year, we have begun to see publications on the utility of the Bethesda System for Reporting Thyroid Cytopathology. The data by Jo et al showing the relationship of risk to malignancy and diagnostic category generally are not surprising. I think the more informative data linking the histopathologic category of neoplasia (ie, follicular neoplasm and Hürthle cell neoplasm) with cytopathologic category would be more informative. After all, would not we like to see data on the percentage of neoplasms seen in follow-up for the Bethesda System category of "suspicious" for follicular neoplasm? It would be good to know the frequency of nonneoplastic lesions in this category, as most of these lesions are excised. Another interesting finding in this article is that the unsatisfactory frequency is high, which has been previously reported following the use of standardized reporting for the interpretation of poor quality specimens. The rather shocking news is that almost 20% of patients who have a thyroid gland fine-needle aspiration have an uninterpretable specimen and almost 10% of patients who have an uninterpretable specimen have an underlying malignancy. The underlying causes resulting in poor quality specimens are system related, but need to be fixed to improve the care delivery model of thyroid fine-needle aspiration.[1,2]

S. S. Raab, MD

References

1. Baloch ZW, LiVolsi VA, Asa SL, et al. Diagnostic terminology and morphologic criteria for cytologic diagnosis of thyroid lesions: a synopsis of the National Cancer Institute Thyroid Fine-Needle Aspiration State of the Science Conference. *Diagn Cytopathol.* 2008;36:425-437.
2. Cibas ES, Sanchez MA. The National Cancer Institute thyroid fine-needle aspiration state-of-the-science conference: inspiration for a uniform terminology linked to management guidelines. *Cancer.* 2008;114:71-73.

A Weakly Positive Human Papillomavirus Hybrid Capture II Result Correlates With a Significantly Lower Risk of Cervical Intraepithelial Neoplasia 2,3 After Atypical Squamous Cells of Undetermined Significance Cytology

Jarboe EA, Venkat P, Hirsch MS, et al (Brigham and Women's Hosp and Harvard Med School, Boston, MA)
J Low Genit Tract Dis 14:174-178, 2010

Objective.—The Hybrid Capture II assay (hc2; QIAGEN, Inc) for high-risk human papillomavirus (hrHPV) is an in vitro nucleic acid hybridization assay using chemiluminescence for the qualitative detection of hrHPV DNA in cervical samples. Results are reported as a ratio of relative light units (RLUs) to a cutoff value based on a positive control. Specimens with RLU ratios of 1.0 or higher are scored positive for hrHPV. We tested the hypothesis that hrHPV positives with low-positive RLU ratios (1–10) had a lower prevalence of cervical intraepithelial neoplasia 2,3 (CIN 2,3) on histologic follow-up.

Materials and Methods.—Relative light unit ratios for 388 consecutive hrHPV-positive cervical cytologic specimens interpreted as atypical squamous cells of undetermined significance (ASCUS) were reviewed. Individual RLU ratios were compared with outcome histologic diagnosis in cases with colposcopic follow-up and tissue sampling (biopsy and/or endocervical curettage; $n = 236$).

Results.—Of 236 cases with histologic follow-up, 63 had RLU ratios in the range of 1 to 10; of these, 53 (84.1%) were negative for CIN, 7 (11.1%) had CIN 1, 1 (1.6%) had CIN of uncertain grade, and 2 (3.2%) had CIN 2,3. The difference in CIN 2,3 outcome between RLU ratios of 1 to 10 (3.2%) versus over 10 (17.3%) was significant ($p = .0047$). The difference in prevalence of CIN 1 was not significant ($p = .67$).

Conclusions.—An RLU ratio of 10 or less was associated with a significantly lower prevalence of CIN 2,3 on biopsy outcome after a Pap test result of ASCUS. The much lower prevalence of underlying CIN 2,3 in patients who are weakly HPV-positive may justify modification of the management algorithm for this subset of women with ASCUS.

▶ In grading high-risk human papillomavirus (hrHPV) test results with Hybrid Capture II assay on women with atypical squamous cells of undetermined significance (ASC-US), our laboratory uses the cutoffs of negative, equivocal, and positive. In this study, Jarboe et al report cutoffs of negative, low positive, and positive. Jarboe et al reported that < 3.2% of those women who had low positive results had cervical intraepithelial neoplasia 2,3 on histologic follow-up, indicating that this category of lesions is of low risk. The supposed consequence would be that this category of women would not need colposcopy with biopsy.[1,2] Individual laboratories would need to verify these results in their own patient populations, but if it held true in our laboratory, we could begin to interpret negative hrHPV and equivocal hrHPV results as of lower risk. The more important predictor for a laboratory is overall ASC-US with positive and negative results, which would indicate if that laboratory possibly overcalls ASC-US.

S. S. Raab, MD

References

1. Wright TC Jr, Massad LS, Dunton CJ, Spitzer M, Wilkinson EJ, Solomon D. 2006 consensus guidelines for the management of women with abnormal cervical screening tests. *J Low Genit Tract Dis.* 2007;11:201-222.
2. Arbyn M, Buntinx F, Van Ranst M, Paraskevaidis E, Martin-Hirsch P, Dillner J. Virologic versus cytologic triage of women with equivocal Pap smears: a meta-analysis of the accuracy to detect high-grade intraepithelial neoplasia. *J Natl Cancer Inst.* 2004;96:280-293.

A Shandon PapSpin liquid-based gynecological test: A split-sample and direct-to-vial test with histology follow-up study

Rimiene J, Petronytė J, Gudleviciene Z, et al (Vilnius Univ, Lithuania)
Cytojournal 7:2, 2010

Background.—Studies for liquid-based Papanicolaou (Pap) tests reveal that liquid-based cytology (LBC) is a safe and effective alternative to the conventional Pap smear. Although there is research on ThinPrep and Sure-Path systems, information is lacking to evaluate the efficiency and effectiveness of systems based on cytocentrifugation. This study is designed to determine the sensitivity and specificity of the Shandon PapSpin (ThermoShandon, Pittsburgh, Pennsylvania, USA) liquid-based gynecological system. We used split-sample and direct-to-vial study design.

Materials and Methods.—2,945 women referred to prophylactic check-up were enrolled in this study. Split sample design was used in 1,500 women and residual cervical cytology specimen from all these cases was placed in fluid for PapSpin preparation after performing conventional smear. The direct-to-vial study was carried out in another cohort of 1,445 women in whom the entire cervical material was investigated using only the PapSpin technique. Follow up histological diagnoses for 141 women were obtained from both study arms following 189 abnormal cytology cases. 80 LBC cases from the split sample group and 61 LBC cases in the direct-to-vial group were correlated with the histology results. The sensitivity and secificity of the conventional smear and PapSpin tests in both study arms were compared.

Results.—In the split sample group, conventional smears showed a higher proportion of ASC-US (atypical cells undetermined significance): 31 (2.1%) *vs* 10 (0.7%) in PapSpin ($P = 0.001$). A higher proportion of unsatisfactory samples was found in the conventional smear group: 25 (1.7%) *vs* 6 (0.4%) cases ($P = 0.001$). In the split sample group, the sensitivity of the conventional and PapSpin tests was 68.7% *vs* 78.1%, and the specificity 93.8% *vs* 91.8%, respectively. In the direct to vial group Pap-Spin sensitivity was 75.9% and specificity 96.5%. The differences in sensitivity and specificity were not significant. The positive predictive values for the conventional and PapSpin methods were not different in the split sample group: 88.0% *vs* 86.2% and 95.7% in the direct-to-vial group. Also, no differences were found for negative predictive value (82.1, 86.8% and 80.0% respectively).

Conclusions.—PapSpin showed good qualitative results in both study arms, even after the material splitting in the first study arm, and is a good alternative to the conventional Pap smear. Additionally, the Pap-Spin method offers several advantages such as the opportunity to prepare duplicate slides, option for HPV DNA testing and cell block preparations from residual material. Microscopic evaluation of thinner cell preparations is less time consuming than the conventional Pap smears.

▶ In the United States, the market for liquid-based Papanicolaou testing currently is dominated by SurePath and ThinPrep.[1,2] In Canada, Europe, and elsewhere, other Pap testing methods, including conventional Pap testing, are used more frequently. Rimiene et al report the use of a centrifugation method of Pap testing developed by ThermoShandon. I believe that these data essentially show equivalent or slightly improved performance metrics for the PapSpin method. The question in the United States is whether this technology will actually penetrate an already saturated market. I think the competition is welcome, but the degree of ultimate acceptance will strongly depend on cost and other metrics, such as usability. I think that the use of a new Pap test method necessarily will require the ability to perform conjoint high-risk human papillomavirus testing. The use of the cell block preparation, also offered by the PapSpin method, is unique, although it needs to be effectively adopted in practice. As cervical cancer screening is switching to a different paradigm, the Pap test method that ultimately will become used will need to mesh well with a changing model.

S. S. Raab, MD

References

1. Khalbuss WE, Rudomina D, Kauff ND, Chuang L, Melamed MR. SpinThin, a simple inexpensive technique for preparation of thin-layer cervical cytology from liquid-based specimens: data on 791 cases. *Cancer.* 2000;90:135-142.
2. Weynand B, Berlière M, Haumont E, et al. A new, liquid-based cytology technique. *Acta Cytol.* 2003;47:149-153.

BD FocalPoint Slide Profiler Performance With Atypical Glandular Cells on SurePath Papanicolaou Smears
Chute DJ, Lim H, Kong CS (Univ of Virginia, Charlottesville; Stanford Univ, CA)
Cancer Cytopathol 118:68-74, 2010

Background.—The FocalPoint Slide Profiler is an automated cervical cytology screening system that is approved for primary screening. It identifies up to 25% of slides as requiring No Further Review. However, few studies have evaluated FocalPoint performance with glandular abnormalities.

Methods.—Sixty-six SurePath Papanicolaou (Pap) tests with a diagnosis of atypical glandular cells were identified. A total of 172 Pap tests with a diagnosis of "endometrial cells present" were included as controls. Follow-up histology was abnormal if diagnosed as high-grade squamous intraepithelial lesions, adenocarcinoma in situ, carcinoma, or complex endometrial hyperplasia. The FocalPoint software ranked each case into

1 of 7 categories: quintiles 1 (high risk) through 5 (low risk), No Further Review, and Process Review.

Results.—A total of 215 slides were qualified for review; 38 (57.6%) atypical glandular cells cases were abnormal on follow-up biopsy, and 27 (71.1%) atypical glandular cells with abnormal follow-up qualified for review; no cases were classified No Further Review, and 9 (33%) were ranked in quintile 1. Twenty-three (82.1%) atypical glandular cells with benign follow-up were qualified for review; 3 (11%) cases were classified No Further Review, and 4 (17%) were ranked in quintile 1. There was a statistically significant difference between the ranking of benign atypical glandular cells cases, abnormal atypical glandular cells cases, and control cases ($P = .03$). However, when collapsed into No Further Review versus all other quintiles, the differences were not significant ($P = .20$).

Conclusions.—The Focal-Point Slide Profiler did not classify glandular lesions with abnormal follow-up in the No Further Review category. However, these cases were not preferentially ranked in quintile 1. FocalPoint-screened slides need to be carefully reviewed for glandular abnormalities, regardless of the quintile ranking.

▶ The diagnosis of the Papanicolaou test for glandular cell abnormalities has never been straightforward as long as I can remember. These data by Chute et al indicate that the automated screener BD FocalPoint Slide Profiler also finds Pap tests previously diagnosed as atypical glandular cells (AGCs) as a challenge. I think a weakness in this study was that the controls chosen by Chute et al were Pap tests diagnosed as negative for intraepithelial lesion or malignancy (NILM), endometrial cells present. I do not think that these are particularly challenging glandular abnormality cases, perhaps compared with false-negative Pap tests that had glandular abnormalities on follow-up or Pap tests that were diagnosed as AGC by a cytotechnologist and downgraded to NILM by a cytopathologist. The underlying problem with glandular disease is that cytotechnologists and cytopathologists are not standardized in their approach to diagnosis. Although criteria for AGC are published, these criteria are not well understood or applied. Reproducibility of AGC diagnoses is poor, as practitioners do not agree with each other. Thus, it is not surprising that an automated screener also would rank these lesions by different degrees of risk.[1,2]

S. S. Raab, MD

References

1. Sherman ME, Dasgupta A, Schiffman M, Nayar R, Solomon D. The Bethesda Interobserver Reproducibility Study (BIRST); a web-based assessment of the Bethesda 2001 System for classifying cervical cytology. *Cancer.* 2007;111:15-25.
2. Confortini M, Di Bonito L, Carozzi F, et al. Interlaboratory reproducibility of atypical glandular cells of undetermined significance: a national survey. *Cytopathology.* 2006;17:353-360.

Non-mycosis fungoides cutaneous T-cell lymphoma: reclassification according to the WHO-EORTC classification

Weaver J, Mahindra AK, Pohlman B, et al (Cleveland Clinic Taussig Cancer Inst, OH)
J Cutan Pathol 37:516-524, 2010

Background.—Non-mycosis fungoides (non-MF) primary cutaneous T-cell lymphomas (PCTCL) are heterogeneous and divided into subgroups by the World Health Organization-European Organization for Research and Treatment of Cancer (WHO-EORTC) classification of cutaneous lymphomas. We report the first North American series to examine the applicability of the classification, compare our findings with the predominant European literature and confirm the significance of separation into the indolent and aggressive groups.

Methods.—Forty-four non-MF PCTCL cases with available tissue for phenotyping, adequate clinical staging information and follow-up were reclassified according to the WHO-EORTC classification.

Results.—Non-MF PCTCL had a longer overall survival (OS) (13.8 years) compared with secondary cutaneous T-cell lymphoma (SC-TCL) (2.5 years). Primary cutaneous anaplastic large cell lymphoma (PC-ALCL) had the most favorable outcome (OS 14.1 years), whereas secondary and primary peripheral T-cell lymphoma, unspecified had the shortest OS (2.5 and 2.4 years, respectively). Primary cutaneous CD4+ small/medium-sized pleomorphic T-cell lymphoma (CTLCD4) appeared to have a favorable course.

Conclusions.—Most non-MF PCTCL can be classified according to the WHO-EORTC classification. The relative frequencies are similar to European experience. Non-MF PCTCL is a heterogeneous group with a favorable outcome compared to SC-TCL, especially PC-ALCL and CTLCD4. Separation of non-MF PCTCL into indolent and aggressive groups appears clinically significant and may provide direction for therapeutic decisions.

▶ In addition to historical controversy surrounding the classification of lymphomas in general, classification of cutaneous lymphomas, with the further requirement of interdisciplinary synchronization, has been especially vexing. Yet with the publication of the World Health Organization/European Organization for Research and Treatment of Cancer (WHO/EORTC) classification for cutaneous lymphomas in 2005,[1] we have arrived at an auspicious age. This new unified classification has made the clinical course of the disease the principal attribute by placing all of the lymphomas into 1 of 2 overarching groups, indolent and aggressive. Despite the advantages, few studies utilizing the unified classification have been published thus far. In this study, the authors review the nonmycosis fungoides primary cutaneous T-cell experience from the Cleveland Clinic applying the WHO/EORTC classification. They include 44 cases, a significant number, given the infrequent occurrence of these tumors. Their findings stress the importance of differentiating primary cutaneous lesions form secondary cutaneous involvement as they found striking differences in overall survival between these 2 groups (13.8 vs 2.5 years). Although, the "cutaneous T-cell lymphoma, unspecified" categories did not show significant survival differences between primary and secondary involvement. The results of their study also validate the WHO/EORTC designations of indolent and aggressive categories, finding both statistically and clinically significant differences between these groups. This type of exploration of the classification system provides important insight and increases the pathologist's ability to classify skin lymphomas in a clinically meaningful manner.

J. Wisell, MD

Reference

1. Burg G, Kempf W, Cozzio A, et al. WHO/EORTC classification of cutaneous lymphomas 2005: histological and molecular aspects. *J Cutan Pathol.* 2005;32: 647-674.

13 Hematolymphoid

A Novel Flow Cytometric Antibody Panel for Distinguishing Burkitt Lymphoma From CD10+ Diffuse Large B-Cell Lymphoma
Schniederjan SD, Li S, Saxe DF, et al (Emory Univ School of Medicine, Atlanta, GA; et al)
Am J Clin Pathol 133:718-726, 2010

Rapid and accurate differential diagnosis between Burkitt lymphoma (BL) and CD10+ diffuse large B-cell lymphoma (DLBCL) is imperative because their treatment differs. Recent studies have characterized several antigens differentially expressed in these 2 types of lymphoma. Our goal was to determine whether use of these markers would aid in the differential diagnosis of BL vs CD10+ DLBCL by flow cytometric immunophenotyping (FCI). Twenty-three cases of CD10+ B-cell lymphomas with available cryopreserved samples were identified (13 BL and 10 CD10+ DLBCL). Multiparameter FCI was performed using the following antibodies: CD18, CD20, CD43, CD44, and CD54 and isotype controls. Expression of CD44 and CD54 was detected at a significantly lower level in BL compared with CD10+ DLBCL ($P = .001$ and $P = .01$, respectively). There was not a significant difference in expression of CD18 and CD43. Our data show that expression of CD44 and CD54 differs significantly between BL and CD10+ DLBCL.

▶ Differentiating between Burkitt lymphoma (BL) and diffuse large B-cell lymphoma (DLBCL) can occasionally be a difficult proposition for the pathologist, as these entities may have much histologic and phenotypic overlap. Choice of the correct chemotherapeutic regimen rides on making this distinction correctly. Cytogenetic information is probably the most useful information in making this distinction for problematic cases, especially the results of fluorescence in situ hybridization assays looking for the translocations of the *MYC* gene that are seen in BL. Depending on how rapidly these results are available, the pathologist may or may not have to make a preliminary distinction without genetic information. If a preliminary distinction must be made, he or she must use histologic features, immunohistochemical findings, and clinical information to try to arrive at the correct diagnosis. As around half of the cases of DLBCL and essentially all cases of BL are positive for CD10, flow cytometry panels, as currently used, are often not useful in making this distinction.

In their article, Schniederjan et al look for additional phenotypic markers that could be assessed by flow cytometry in an effort to separate these 2 entities. They report that the 2 markers not yet in routine use in diagnostic flow cytometry, CD44 and CD54, are differentially expressed by these 2 entities. CD44 is usually negative in BL and is usually moderately to strongly expressed in CD10-positive DLBCL. CD54 is usually more strongly expressed by CD10-positive DLBCL. Unfortunately, there is much overlap between the levels of expression of CD54, making it of questionable use, and there are rare cases of CD44-positive BL and CD44-negative DLBCL. Thus, these findings provide additional information arguing for or against BL or DLBCL but are not by themselves definitive.

J. T. Schowinsky, MD

Cytoplasmic Expression of Nucleophosmin Accurately Predicts Mutation in the Nucleophosmin Gene in Patients With Acute Myeloid Leukemia and Normal Karyotype
Luo J, Qi C, Xu W, et al (Univ Health Network, Toronto, Canada)
Am J Clin Pathol 133:34-40, 2010

Mutations in the nucleophosmin (NPM1) exon 12 resulting in delocalization of NPM1 into the cytoplasm occur in 50% to 60% of acute myeloid leukemia cases with a normal karyotype (AML-NK). As recent studies suggest such patients have a favorable prognosis and there are discordant reports of the immunohistochemical detection of cytoplasmic NPM1 (NPMc+) for predicting *NPM1* gene mutations, we correlated the immunohistochemical detection of NPMc+, *NPM1* gene mutations, and prognosis in 57 cases of AML-NK. All 31 NPMc+ cases (54% of total) had *NPM1* mutations, but none of the 26 nucleus-restricted (NPMc−) cases (46% of total) had *NPM1* mutations ($P < .0001$). *NPM1* mutations were correlated with FLT3–internal tandem duplication (ITD) ($P = .0062$), absence of CD34 ($P = .0001$), and absence of CD7 ($P = .041$). There was a favorable survival outcome in AML-NK cases that were *NPM1* mutated and FLT3-ITD nonmutated. Our data confirm that cytoplasmic NPM1 immunoreactivity predicts *NPM1* mutations and warrants inclusion in the routine diagnostic and prognostic workup of AML.

▶ Genetic findings are playing an increasingly larger role in the categorization and treatment of acute myeloid leukemia (AML). Much of the work done over the previous decades has focused on AML with recurrent cytogenetic abnormalities by karyotyping. Many of these abnormalities now exist as distinct entities in the WHO classification scheme for AML. However, around half of the new cases of AML have a normal karyotype, and these cases (known as AML-NK) display variable behaviors; thus, genetic clues were sought to try to predict how these AML-NK cases would behave. The most important finding in this regard has been mutations of the *FLT3* gene, especially the *FLT3*-ITD (internal tandem duplication) mutation, which carries a relatively unfavorable prognosis. Testing for *FLT3* mutations has now become routine in the workup of new AML diagnoses. The mutational status of the nucleophosmin gene

(*NPM1*) is now considered the second most important piece of genetic information in the work-up of AML-NK. *NPM1* mutations carry a relatively good prognosis, especially if they are not accompanied by the *FLT3*-ITD mutation.

In their article, Luo et al describe a method of determining *NPM1* mutational status by immunohistochemistry (IHC). The mutated NPM1 protein accumulates abnormally in the cytoplasm. Thus, they evaluated for cases showing cytoplasmic localization of *NPM1* by IHC, instead of the usual nuclear localization. In the 57 cases reported, their findings by IHC correlated perfectly with the gold standard of determining *NPM1* mutational status by reverse transcriptase-polymerase chain reaction. This is welcome news, as this suggests that the practicing pathologist will now have a surrogate method that may deliver information to the clinician more quickly regarding *NPM1* mutational status and that may also allow for the determination of this status in cases where quality specimen material may not be available for molecular analysis. As the authors note in their discussion, now we are just left waiting for an immunohistochemical surrogate for *FLT3* status.

J. T. Schowinsky, MD

14 Techniques/Molecular

Chromosomal abnormalities determined by comparative genomic hybridization are helpful in the diagnosis of atypical hepatocellular neoplasms
Kakar S, Chen X, Ho C, et al (Univ of California, San Francisco; et al)
Histopathology 55:197-205, 2009

Aims.—To explore the utility of cytogenetic abnormalities in the distinction of hepatic adenoma (HA) and well-differentiated hepatocellular carcinoma (HCC).

Methods and Results.—Array-based comparative genomic hybridization (CGH) was used to determine chromosomal abnormalities in 39 hepatocellular neoplasms: 12 HA, 15 atypical hepatocellular neoplasms (AHN) and 12 well-differentiated HCC. The designation of AHN was used in two situations: (i) adenoma-like neoplasms ($n = 8$) in male patients (any age) and women >50 years and <15 years old; (ii) adenoma-like neoplasms with focal atypical features ($n = 7$). CGH abnormalities were seen in none of the HAs (0/12), eight (53%) AHNs and 11 (92%) HCCs. The number and nature of abnormalities in AHN was similar to HCC with gains in 1q, 8q and 7q being the most common. Although follow-up information was limited, recurrence and/or metastasis were observed in three AHNs (two with abnormal, one with normal CGH).

Conclusions.—Adenoma-like neoplasms with focal atypical morphological features or unusual clinical settings such as male gender or women outside the 15–50 year age group can show chromosomal abnormalities similar to well-differentiated HCC. Even though these tumours morphologically mimic adenoma, they can recur and metastasize. Determination of chromosomal abnormalities can be useful in the diagnosis of AHN (Table 1).

▶ Definitive distinction between hepatocellular adenoma (HA) and well-differentiated hepatocellular carcinomas (HCCs) can be very difficult based on histologic grounds alone. This article investigates the utility of comparative genomic hybridization (CGH) in cases where either clinical or histologic features are atypical. HCCs have shown fairly consistent chromosomal abnormalities including gains of 8q, 1q, and 7q as well as loss of 16q, while HAs usually show genomic stability. Table 1 highlights how some lesions with both atypical clinical and histologic features were found to have abnormal CGH results, several of which are also typically found in HCC. Drawbacks of this study include the limited clinical follow-up and sample size for each

TABLE 1.—Clinical and Cytogenetic Characteristics of Atypical Hepatocellular Neoplasms (AHN)

		Age/Gender	CGH Results	Chromosomal Abnormalities	Follow-up
AHN adenoma-like	1	43/M	Normal	None	NA
	2	27/M	Normal	None	NA
	3	54/F	Normal	None	NA
	4	57/M	Normal	None	NA
	5	3/F	Abnormal	Gains: 7q, 18p, 19p	NA
	6	48/M	Abnormal	Gains: 1q, 7p, 7q, 8q	Recurred as HCC
	7	53/F	Abnormal	Gains: 1q, 7p, 7q, 8p, 8q, 11p, 20q Losses: 4q, 14q	Recurrence 3 years later*
	8	55/F	Abnormal	Gains: 1q, 7p, 7q, 8p Losses: X	NA
AHN with atypia	1	33/M	Normal	None	Metastasized 3 years later
	2	57/F	Normal	None	NA
	3	57/M	Normal	None	No evidence of disease
	4	51/F	Abnormal	Gains: 19p, 23p, 23q Losses: 21 q	No evidence of disease
	5	39/M	Abnormal	Gains:1p, 1q, 2p, 7p, 8p, 8q, 11q, 20q Losses: 4q, 7q	NA
	6	27/F	Abnormal	Gains: 1q, 7p, 7q, 8q Losses: 8p	NA
	7	26/M	Abnormal	Gains: 20q	NA

CGH, comparative genomic hybridization; AHN, atypical hepatocellular neoplasm; NA, not available; HCC, hepatocellular carcinoma.
*Three hypervascular tumours detected on imaging at recurrence. Histological confirmation has not been done.

diagnostic category. Immunohistochemical/molecular analysis for β-catenin has also been suggested as a predictor of so called malignant transformation of HA. As CGH becomes increasingly available for clinical use, an argument may be made for its use in atypical hepatocellular lesions. If CGH is not available, selected fluorescence in situ hybridization probes for the earliest molecular changes in HCC including chromosomes 1 and 8 may be another viable approach.

M. L. Smith, MD

Classification of Inflammation Activity in Ulcerative Colitis by Confocal Laser Endomicroscopy
Li C-Q, Xie X-J, Yu T, et al (Shandong Univ, Jinan, China; et al)
Am J Gastroenterol 105:1391-1396, 2010

Objectives.—The assessment of inflammation activity in ulcerative colitis (UC) includes endoscopy and histology. Confocal laser endomicroscopy (CLE) combines real-time endoscopy and histology. This study was aimed at evaluating the application of CLE in the assessment of inflammation activity in UC.

Methods.—In total, 73 consecutive patients with UC who visited Qilu Hospital for colonoscopy surveillance underwent CLE. Inflammation activity was first assessed by the colonoscopy Baron score, then by CLE with a 4-grade classification of crypt architecture, as well as by analysis of microvascular alterations and fluorescein leakage. Targeted biopsy samples were taken for histological analysis. Stored CLE images were subjected to post-CLE objective assessment.

Results.—Both assessment of crypt architecture and fluorescein leakage with CLE showed good correlations with histological results (Spearman's rho, both $P < 0.001$). CLE seemed to be more accurate than conventional white-light endoscopy for evaluating macroscopical normal mucosa. More than half of the patients with normal mucosa seen on conventional white-light endoscopy showed acute inflammation on histology, whereas no patients with normal mucosa or with chronic inflammation seen on CLE showed acute inflammation on histology. Assessment of microvascular alterations by CLE showed good correlation with histological findings ($P < 0.001$). On post-CLE objective assessment, subjective architectural classifications were supported by the number of crypts per image ($P < 0.001$) but not fluorescein leakage results by gray scale ($P = 0.194$).

Conclusions.—CLE is reliable for real-time assessment of inflammation activity in UC. Crypt architecture, microvascular alterations, and fluorescein leakage are promising markers in CLE evaluation (Tables 3-5).

▶ This article studies a new technique in the evaluation of patients with ulcerative colitis (UC) and should gain the attention of the pathology community.

TABLE 3.—Confocal Laser Endomicroscopy (CLE) Crypt Architecture Assessment in Relation to Histology Findings

| | Histology (Geboes Index) | | |
CLE Crypt Architecture	≤3 (%)	>3 (%)	Total Number of Patients (%)
CLE A	7 (100)	0 (0)	7 (100)
CLE B	14 (100)	0 (0)	14 (100)
CLE C	2 (7)	27 (93)	29 (100)
CLE D	0 (0)	23 (100)	23 (100)
Total number of patients	23 (32)	50 (68)	73 (100)

TABLE 4.—Confocal Laser Endomicroscopy (CLE) Microvascular Alteration Assessment by Histology Findings

| | Histology (Geboes Index) | | |
CLE Microvascular Alterations	≤3 (%)	>3 (%)	Total Number of Patients (%)
None	19 (59)	13 (41)	32 (100)
Mild to moderate	4 (33)	8 (67)	12 (100)
Severe	0 (0)	29 (100)	29 (100)
Total number of patients	23 (32)	50 (68)	73 (100)

TABLE 5.—Fluorescein Leakage into Crypt Lumen (FLIL) by Histology Findings

| | Histology (Geboes Index) | | |
FLIL	≤3 (%)	>3 (%)	Total Number of Patients (%)
No	18 (64)	10 (36)	28 (100)
Yes	5 (11)	40 (89)	45 (100)
Total number of patients (%)	23 (32)	50 (68)	73 (100)

Using the recently described method of confocal laser endomicroscopy (CLE), the authors demonstrate correlation between features found on CLE at the time of endoscopy and eventual histologic assessment of UC activity. CLE assesses 3 key features including crypt architecture, microvascular alteration, and fluorescein leakage. Fluorescein leakage is a surrogate marker for intraepithelial inflammation. Histologic activity was graded using the Geboes Index in which a score of > 3 indicates intraepithelial neutrophils. Using crypt architectural changes alone, only 2 of 73 patients would have been misclassified as not having activity when histologic samples showed activity (false negatives) (Table 3). Microvascular alterations and fluorescein leakage showed much less correlation with many more incorrect classifications (Tables 4 and 5). As endoscopists develop the capability of identifying mucosal inflammation and disease activity, pathologists must continue to identify ways to add value to the care of UC patients.

M. L. Smith, MD

Comparison of fluorescent *in situ* hybridization *HER-2/neu* results on core needle biopsy and excisional biopsy in primary breast cancer
Apple SK, Lowe AC, Rao PN, et al (UCLA Ctr for the Health Sciences)
Mod Pathol 22:1151-1159, 2009

HER-2/neu status is critical for the therapy for breast carcinoma. Fluorescent *in situ* hybridization for gene amplification and immunohistochemical stains for protein expression are widely used methods to detect *HER-2/neu* status. Multiple studies have shown fluorescent *in situ* hybridization and immunohistochemical stain results to have high concordance rates. To our knowledge, a comparison between fluorescent *in situ* hybridization results for core needle biopsy and the subsequent excisional biopsy specimens has not yet been studied. We retrospectively evaluated the fluorescence *in situ* hybridization and immunohistochemical results in both the breast core needle and the excisional biopsy of 125 patients with invasive breast carcinoma from 2002 to 2005. There was complete concordance with respect to both immunohistochemical and fluorescence *in situ* hybridization results for core needle biopsy and excisional biopsy specimens in 87% of the patients evaluated. Comparison of fluorescent *in situ* hybridization results of the 129 core needle biopsies to the 131

TABLE 2.—FISH Concordant and Discordant Data Between Core Needle and Excisional Biopsies

			Number of Patients	Patients (%)
Concordant	92%	Concordant negative	102	82%
		Concordant positive	13	10%
Discordant	8%	Discordant: CNB+/EXC−	6	5%
		Discordant CNB−/EXC+	4	3%
Total			125	100%

CNB, core needle biopsy; EXC, excisional biopsy; FISH, fluorescent *in situ* hybridization.

TABLE 3.—Immunohistochemical Stain Concordant/Discordant Data Between Core Needle and Excisional Biopsies

	No. of Patients	Patients (%)
Concordant negative	83	66%
Concordant positive	6	5.0%
Indeterminate	33	26%
Discordant CNB+/EXC−	0	0%
Discordant CNB−/EXC+	3	2%
Total	125	100%

CNB, core needle biopsy; EXC, excisional biopsy.

excisional biopsies of all 125 patients showed a concordance rate of 92%. The immunohistochemical stain results of the same core needle and excisional biopsies showed a concordance rate of 98%. Comparison of the immunohistochemical stain results with the fluorescent *in situ* hybridization results for all 260 cases examined showed 95% concordance. On the basis of our study, we observed that repeating *HER-2/neu* testing by immunohistochemical stain and/or fluorescent *in situ* hybridization methods on excisional biopsy is not unreasonable, in particular in cases of intratumoral heterogeneity, indeterminate/borderline *HER-2/neu* results and after neoadjuvant chemotherapy (Tables 2 and 3).

▶ This article provides data to answer the common clinical question as to whether *HER-2/neu* status should be reevaluated on excisional specimens after prior determination on core needle biopsies. Immunohistochemical (IHC) and fluorescent in situ hybridization (FISH) techniques are expensive, and repeating them unnecessarily for all cases of invasive ductal carcinoma of the breast would result in an extensive cost burden. Although 87% of patients remained classified correctly if *HER-2/neu* status was done on the core biopsy alone, 13% may be assigned to the incorrect treatment protocol. In the FISH analysis, both false positives and false negatives were identified. In the IHC analysis, only false negatives were recognized. IHC showed higher concordance than FISH testing, possibly secondary to the testing complexity involved

(Tables 2 and 3). Two patients showed complete discordance between the core needle biopsy and excisional specimen. Further analysis into these cases revealed that the *HER-2/neu* was negative in the biopsy and positive in the excision for both cases. Histologic examination showed prominent tumor heterogeneity with well-differentiated areas and poorly differentiated areas. Therefore, sampling bias may effect *HER-2/neu* status on biopsy specimens. It is also likely that biologically borderline cases contribute to lack of concordance, which supports the more recent 2007 guidelines for FISH reporting, which includes an equivocal range. Perhaps the most cost-effective protocol would be to perform *HER-2/neu* analysis on the excisional specimen alone, unless neoadjuvant treatment is required.

M. L. Smith, MD

Comparison of Single-Copy and Multicopy Real-Time PCR Targets for Detection of *Mycobacterium tuberculosis* in Paraffin-Embedded Tissue

Luo RF, Scahill MD, Banaei N (Stanford Univ School of Medicine, CA; Stanford Hosp and Clinics, Palo Alto, CA)
J Clin Microbiol 48:2569-2570, 2010

Real-time PCR can rapidly identify *Mycobacterium tuberculosis* in paraffin-embedded tissue in the absence of microbiological culture. In a comparison of single-copy and multicopy PCR targets in 70 tissue samples, the sensitivities were 26% and 54%, respectively, with 100% specificity. Sensitivity was 75% for newer samples and was not decreased for acid-fast bacillus (AFB) stain-negative specimens.

▶ Pathologists are frequently confronted with necrotizing granulomatous inflammation in a variety of different specimen types. Often these tissues are submitted without a clinical suspicion for infection and cultures are not performed. Fungal and acid-fast bacilli (AFB) stains are frequently ordered. Even if the AFB stain is positive, it is not specific for *Mycobacterium tuberculosis*. Different polymerase chain reaction (PCR) modalities have been developed for definitive diagnosis of *M tuberculosis*, but the sensitivity and specificity has not been rigorously studied. This study evaluates the sensitivity and specificity of *M tuberculosis* PCR using 2 different targets, single copy and multicopy, as well as a diverse group of tissue sources and ages. Positive culture was used as the gold standard. In samples less than 2 years old, the sensitivity was 75%. A trend toward increased sensitivity was seen in pulmonary samples, but it was not statistically significant. The multicopy target method showed a significantly higher sensitivity (54% vs 26%), and AFB stain status was not significant. Multicopy real-time PCR for *M tuberculosis* is a viable diagnostic option for paraffin-embedded tissues, particularly in specimens less than 2 years old, and possibility in pulmonary specimens.

M. L. Smith, MD

Do Liquid-Based Preparations of Urinary Cytology Perform Differently Than Classically Prepared Cases? Observations From the College of American Pathologists Interlaboratory Comparison Program in Nongynecologic Cytology

Laucirica R, Bentz JS, Souers RJ, et al (Baylor College of Medicine, Houston, TX; Univ of Utah, Salt Lake City; College of American Pathologists, Northfield, IL; et al)
Arch Pathol Lab Med 134:19-22, 2010

Context.—The cytomorphology of liquid-based preparations in urine cytology is different than classic slide preparations.

Objectives.—To compare the performance of liquid-based preparation specimens to classically prepared urine specimens with a malignant diagnosis in the College of American Pathologists Interlaboratory Comparison Program in Nongynecologic Cytology.

Design.—Participant responses between 2000 and 2007 for urine specimens with a reference diagnosis of high-grade urothelial carcinoma/carcinoma in situ/dysplasia (HGUCA), squamous cell carcinoma, or adenocarcinoma were evaluated. ThinPrep and SurePath challenges were compared with classic preparations (smears, cytospins) for discordant responses.

Results.—There were 18 288 pathologist, 11 957 cytotechnologist, and 8086 "laboratory" responses available. Classic preparations comprised 90% (n = 34 551) of urine challenges; 9% (n = 3295) were ThinPrep and 1% (n = 485) were SurePath. Concordance to the general category of "positive-malignant" was seen in 92% of classic preparations, 96.5% of ThinPrep, and 94.6% of SurePath challenges ($P < .001$). These results were statistically different for the exact reference interpretation of HGUCA ($P < .001$) but not for adenocarcinoma ($P = .22$). Cytotechnologists demonstrate statistically better performance for the general category of "positive-malignant" compared with pathologists for all urinary slide types and for the exact reference interpretation of HGUCA (94% versus 91.1%; $P < .001$) but not adenocarcinoma (96.3% versus 95.8%; $P = .77$) or squamous cell carcinoma (93.6% versus 87.7%; $P = .07$).

Conclusions.—Liquid-based preparations performed significantly better in urinary cytology challenges when evaluating malignant categories in the College of American Pathologists interlaboratory comparison program. The liquid-based preparation challenges also performed better for the exact reference interpretation of HGUCA, but no difference was observed for adenocarcinoma challenges. Cytotechnologists perform better than pathologists for all slide types, as well as those demonstrating HGUCA. These results suggest that liquid-based preparations facilitate a more accurate diagnosis than conventional preparations (Table 1).

▶ It is not surprising that liquid-based urine cytology showed better concordance for both pathologists and cytotechnologists when compared with more

TABLE 1.—Participant Concordance Rate for Urinary Challenges in the College of American Pathologists Interlaboratory Comparison Program in Nongynecologic Cytopathology by Slide Preparation Type and the General Category of "Positive-Malignant" ($P < .001$)

Performance	Classic, % (N = 34 551)[a]	SurePath, % (N = 485)	ThinPrep, % (N = 3295)
Concordance	92.0	94.6	96.5
Discordant	8.0	5.4	3.5

[a]Classic includes cytospin and concentrated direct smears.

conventional preparations, such as urine cytospins and smears (Table 1). Similar improved sensitivity has been identified in cervicovaginal preparations as well. The design of the study was primarily to compare urine concordance rates between different preparation techniques using data from the College of American Pathologists Interlaboratory Comparison Program in Nongynecologic Cytology. As a byproduct of using this existing data set, the concordance/discordance rates of pathologists and cytotechnologists could be compared. Interestingly, the cytotechnologists performed statistically significantly better than the pathologists when evaluating the general category of positive-malignant. There are several reasons why cytotechnologists may show better concordance, including more experience locating cells of interest, bias toward a positive result because they are trained to overcall as screeners, and their increased experience with liquid-based preparations. These data support the use of liquid-based preparations for urine cytology analysis and cytotechnologist involvement in screening.

M. L. Smith, MD

Fluorescence In Situ Hybridization (FISH) as an Ancillary Diagnostic Tool in the Diagnosis of Melanoma
Gerami P, Jewell SS, Morrison LE, et al (Northwestern Univ, Evanston, IL; Abbott Molecular Laboratories, Des Plaines, IL; et al)
Am J Surg Pathol 33:1146-1156, 2009

Although the clinical and pathologic diagnosis of some melanomas is clear-cut, there are many histopathologic simulators of melanoma that pose problems. Over-diagnosis of melanoma can lead to inappropriate therapy and psychologic burdens, whereas under-diagnosis can lead to inadequate treatment of a deadly cancer. We used existing data on DNA copy number alterations in melanoma to assemble panels of fluorescence in situ hybridization (FISH) probes suitable for the analysis of paraffin-embedded tissue. Using FISH data from a training set of 301 tumors, we established a discriminatory algorithm and validated it on an independent set of 169 unequivocal nevi and melanomas as well as 27 cases with ambiguous pathology, for which we had long-term follow-up data. An

TABLE 4.—Characteristics of Cohort 4

Case No.	Breslow Depth	Clark Level	Mitoses/ mm^2	Follow-up Time (mo)	Adverse Event	Time to Adverse Event (mo)	FISH Result
1	3.1 mm	IV	4	120	_		+
2	1.2 mm	IV	7	79	_		+
3	3.05 mm	IV	2	89	_		_
4	1.2 mm	IV	1	82	_		_
5	3.0 mm	IV	1	99	_		_
6	At least 1.3 mm	IV	3	79	_		_
7	1.0 mm	IV	<1	79	_		_
8	At least 3.3 mm	IV	<1	93	_		+
9	At least 1.1 mm	IV	<1	24	+/distant metastasis and DOD	24	+
10	At least 1.4 mm	IV	2	83	+/lymph node metastasis	21	+
11	1.25 mm	IV	<1	84	_		_
12	2.22 mm	IV	1	90	_		+
13	3.2 mm	IV	1	12	+/lymph node metastasis	12	+
14	At least 9.5 mm	V	5	103	+/lung metastasis	103	+
15	1.3 mm	IV	<1	36	+/lymph node metastasis	36	+
16	0.7 mm	IV	<1	105	_		_
17	0.5 mm	III	<1	105	_		_
18	3.5 mm	IV	2	65	_		_
19	1.3 mm	IV	2	122	_		_
20	2.35 mm	IV	1	103	_		_
21	1.45 mm	IV	<1	159	_		_
22	1.7 mm	IV	<1	60	_		_
23	0.65 mm	IV	<1	112	_		_
24	1.4 mm	IV	2	82	_		+
25	>16 mm	V	1	24	+/lymph node metastasis and distant metastasis with DOD	24	+
26	2 mm	IV	<1	82	_		+
27	4.2 mm	IV	6	60	_		_

DOD indicates died of disease; FISH, fluorescence in situ hybridization.

algorithm-using signal counts from a combination of 4 probes targeting chromosome 6p25, 6 centromere, 6q23, and 11q13 provided the highest diagnostic discrimination. This algorithm correctly classified melanoma with 86.7% sensitivity and 95.4% specificity in the validation cohort. The test also correctly identified as melanoma all 6 of 6 cases with ambiguous pathology that later metastasized. There was a significant difference in the metastasis free survival between test-positive and negative cases with ambiguous pathology ($P = 0.003$). Sufficient chromosomal alterations are present in melanoma that a limited panel of FISH probes can distinguish most melanomas from most nevi, providing useful diagnostic information in cases that cannot be classified reliably by current methods. As a diagnostic aid to traditional histologic evaluation, this assay can have significant clinical impact and improve classification of melanocytic neoplasms with conflicting morphologic criteria (Table 4).

▶ While many melanocytic lesions are easily classified as benign or malignant, cases of uncertain malignant potential do arise. Currently, morphologic features alone are not sufficient for definitive classification of some lesions, and disagreements among experts are not uncommon. Therefore, a tool for more precise classification of melanocytic lesions of uncertain malignant potential would be ideal. As with most molecular markers, additional studies have shown a high sensitivity and specificity for fluorescence in situ hybridization (FISH) in the classification of melanocytic lesions.[1] In addition to evaluating unequivocally benign and malignant melanocytic lesions, this study also investigates the possible utility of FISH on ambiguous melanocytic cases with long-term follow-up. In this study, only 1 trained technician evaluated each case. Subsequent studies have shown poor reproducibility in the scoring of FISH cases.[2] Twelve of the 27 ambiguous cases showed a positive FISH result (Table 4). No cases with ambiguous histology and evidence of metastatic disease on long-term follow-up showed a negative FISH result. Further investigation of melanocytic lesions with ambiguous or equivocal histology is required; however, these data suggest that a positive FISH result may increase suspicion for malignancy.

M. L. Smith, MD

References

1. Morey AL, Murali R, McCarthy SW, Mann GJ, Scolyer RA. Diagnosis of cutaneous melanocytic tumours by four-colour fluorescence in situ hybridisation. *Pathology.* 2009;41:383-387.
2. Gaiser T, Kutzner H, Palmedo G, et al. Classifying ambiguous melanocytic lesions with FISH and correlation with clinical long-term follow up. *Mod Pathol.* 2010; 23:413-419.

In Situ Evidence of *KRAS* Amplification and Association With Increased p21 Levels in Non–Small Cell Lung Carcinoma
Wagner PL, Perner S, Rickman DS, et al (Weill Med College of Cornell Univ, NY; et al)
Am J Clin Pathol 132:500-505, 2009

Recent advances in the characterization of the lung cancer genome have suggested that *KRAS* may frequently be amplified, although little is known regarding the significance of this finding. This is in contrast with activating mutations of *KRAS*, which occur in approximately 20% of non–small cell lung carcinomas (NSCLCs).

We used fluorescence in situ hybridization to provide direct evidence of *KRAS* amplification for the first time in clinical specimens. We detected amplification in 7 of 100 consecutive NSCLCs, with a concurrent activating *KRAS* mutation in 4 cases. *KRAS* amplification was associated with greater expression of p21 as assessed by quantitative immunohisto-chemical analysis ($P = .015$).

Our data indicate that a sizable subgroup of NSCLCs harbor *KRAS* amplification, some of which also contain point mutations, and suggest that an increased *KRAS* copy number may drive p21 overexpression. *KRAS* amplification may define a unique clinicopathologic subset of NSCLCs with potentially altered responsiveness to targeted therapies.

▶ This article describes a second mechanism by which increased *KRAS* activity can result in downstream phosphorylation of cell cycle proteins and ultimately unchecked cellular proliferation. While *KRAS* mutation is estimated in 20% of nonsmall cell lung cancers (NSCLCs), the incidence of *KRAS* amplification has not been previously studied. *KRAS* amplification was not limited to a particular subset of NSCLCs, being found in adenocarcinoma, squamous cell carcinoma, and large cell (undifferentiated) carcinoma. Although 4 of the 7 cases were found to have a concurrent *KRAS*-activating mutation, it is important to note that typical *KRAS* molecular testing being developed would not identify cases of *KRAS* amplification alone. *KRAS* may be similar to epidermal growth factor receptor (EGFR) in that EGFR may be either mutated or amplified and each type of molecular alteration has different predictive and prognostic features. One of the weaknesses of this study was the small number of *KRAS*-amplified tumors available for study. Further analysis on a larger cohort is necessary. For more on the molecular alterations involved in lung adenocarcinomas and *KRAS* involvement, I suggest the article by Ding et al.[1]

M. L. Smith, MD

Reference

1. Ding L, Getz G, Wheeler DA, et al. Somatic mutations affect key pathways in lung adenocarcinoma. *Nature*. 2008;455:1069-1075.

Long-Term Outcomes of Positive Fluorescence *In Situ* Hybridization Tests in Primary Sclerosing Cholangitis
Bangarulingam SY, Bjornsson E, Enders F, et al (Mayo Clinic, Rochester, MN)
Hepatology 51:174-180, 2010

Patients with primary sclerosing cholangitis (PSC) are at increased risk for developing cholangiocarcinoma (CCA). Fluorescence *in situ* hybridization (FISH) is a cytological test designed to enhance early CCA diagnosis. The long-term outcome of PSC patients with a positive FISH test (polysomy, trisomy/tetrasomy) are unclear. All PSC patients with at least one FISH test were identified and defined to have CCA if they had a positive tissue biopsy, positive cytology, or evidence of cancer in the explant after liver transplantation. A total of 235 PSC patients had at least one FISH test performed, and 56 patients had CCA on histopathology (n = 35) or cytology (n = 21). Overall, 120 of 235 (51%) of PSC patients

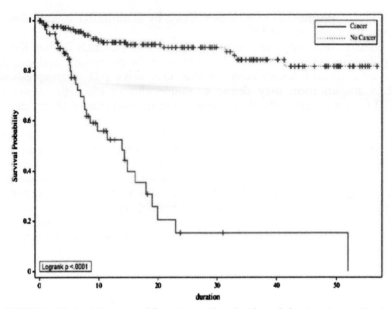

FIGURE 1.—Kaplan-Meier survival for patients with and without cholangiocarcinoma. (Reprinted from Bangarulingam SY, Bjornsson E, Enders F, et al. Long-term outcomes of positive fluorescence in situ hybridization tests in primary sclerosing cholangitis. *Hepatology.* 2010;51:174-180.)

tested for FISH were positive, but only one third of these positive patients had CCA. Sensitivity and specificity for FISH polysomy were 46% and 88%, and for trisomy/tetrasomy they were 25% and 67%, respectively. Survival analysis showed that patients with FISH polysomy had an outcome similar to patients with CCA; whereas FISH trisomy/tetrasomy patients had an outcome similar to patients with negative FISH tests. The FISH polysomy patients without cancer compared with those with CCA had lower serum bilirubin, lower carbohydrate antigen 19-9 (CA 19-9), lower Mayo risk score, and lower occurrence of dominant strictures.

Conclusion.—In PSC patients, the presence of a dominant stricture plus FISH polysomy has a specificity of 88% for CCA. Patients with FISH showing trisomy or tetrasomy have a similar outcome to patients with negative FISH. FISH testing should be used selectively in patients with other signs indicating CCA and not as a screening tool in all PSC patients undergoing endoscopic retrograde cholangiopancreatography (ERCP) (Figs 1 and 2).

▶ Patients with primary sclerosing cholangitis (PSC) are at increased risk for cholangiocarcinoma and have traditionally been screened for cancer using endoscopic retrograde cholangiopancreatography (ERCP) and a combination of biliary biopsies, brushings, and endoscopic fine needle aspiration. Florescence in situ hybridization (FISH) is increasingly being used in the work-up and screening of patients with biliary strictures for the diagnosis of

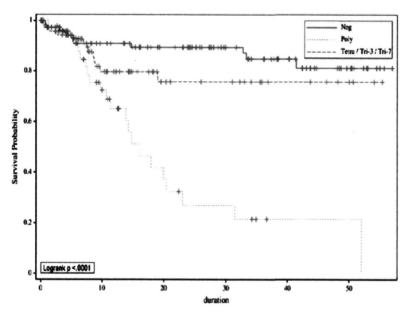

FIGURE 2.—Kaplan-Meier curve comparing survival of FISH polysomy, trisomy 3/7/tetrasomy, and FISH-negative PSC patients. (Reprinted from Bangarulingam SY, Bjornsson E, Enders F, et al. Long-term outcomes of positive fluorescence in situ hybridization tests in primary sclerosing cholangitis. *Hepatology.* 2010;51:174-180.)

cholangiocarcinoma. FISH used in biliary disease is based on the UroVysion platform, which uses probes for chromosomes 3, 7, 17, and band 9p21. Traditionally, any chromosomal abnormalities have been interpreted as positive by FISH. Three patterns of FISH reactivity are typically identified, including polysomy (greater than 2 copies of 2 or more chromosomes), tetrasomy (greater than 4 copies of all 4 chromosomes), and trisomy of chromosome 3 or 7. In this retrospective study, the authors evaluate the long-term outcome of patients with various types of chromosomal abnormalities. Fig 1 is a Kaplan-Meier survival curve for patients dichotomized into cancer or no cancer groups. Fig 2 is a similar survival curve grouping patients by FISH results: negative, polysomy, tetrasomy, and trisomy 3 or 7. The survival of patients with negative, tetrasomy, or trisomy 3 or 7 FISH patterns more closely resembles patients without cancer than those with cancer. Trisomies 3 and 7 have a very low sensitivity and specificity for cholangiocarcinoma. It is stressed that FISH may not be an appropriate cancer screening test for all patients with PSC and that clinical correlation with the presence or absence of a dominant stricture and type of FISH abnormality are important clinical aspects to consider.

M. L. Smith, MD

Molecular Testing for Lipomatous Tumors: Critical Analysis and Test Recommendations Based on the Analysis of 405 Extremity-based Tumors

Zhang H, Erickson-Johnson M, Wang X, et al (Sichuan Univ, Chengdu, China; Mayo Clinic, Rochester, MN; et al)
Am J Surg Pathol 34:1304-1311, 2010

Ancillary molecular testing has been advocated for diagnostic accuracy in the differentiation of lipomas from atypical lipomatous tumors/well-differentiated liposarcomas (ALT/WDL); however, the implications and specific indications for use are not well-established in the current literature. Herein, we extend previous findings by quantitatively evaluating the impact of molecular testing of lipomatous neoplasms in our routine clinical practice, how it modifies the historical perspective of their clinical course, and the effect of distinct surgical procedures in modulating the risk of local recurrence for these tumors after molecular classification. On the basis of these analyses, we suggest a specific set of basic recommendations for complementary molecular assessment in the diagnosis of lipomatous tumors. Four hundred and five lipomatous neoplasms located in the trunk and extremities were analyzed histologically and for the presence of 12q13-15 amplification on paraffin-embedded tissues by assessing *MDM2/CPM* amplification. Survival analyses were calculated with Kaplan-Meier and compared with the log-rank. Multivariate analysis was evaluated by the Cox regression method. The 405 tumors were histologically classified as ordinary lipoma (n = 324), intramuscular lipoma (n = 29), and ALT/WDL (n = 52). The level of agreement between the histologic diagnosis and the molecular diagnosis was high (96%) but pathologists showed a tendency to overestimate cytologic atypia and the diagnosis of ALT/WDL (precision, 79%; accuracy, 88%). Molecular assessment led to a major diagnostic reclassification in 18 tumors (4%). Eleven of the tumors histologically classified as ALT/WDL were reclassified as ordinary lipoma (n = 5) and intramuscular lipoma (n = 6); none of which recurred. Seven ordinary lipomas were reclassified as ALT/WDL, 6 of which were larger than 15 cm and deeply located; 2 recurred locally. After molecular data, the 5-year local recurrence rates for ordinary lipoma, intramuscular lipoma, and ALT/WDL were 1%, 12%, and 44%, respectively. Multivariate analyses after molecular assessment showed tumor type and type of resection to be associated with the risk of local recurrence. Complementary molecular testing refines the histologic classification of lipomatous tumors and better estimates the impact of surgical procedures on the risk of local recurrence. Pathologists tend to overestimate the degree of cytologic atypia and the indiscriminate use of molecular testing should be avoided, especially for extremity-based tumors. Molecular testing should be considered for "relapsing lipomas," tumors with questionable cytologic atypia (even if widely excised), or for large

TABLE 1.—Classification of Lipomatous Tumors Before and After Complementary Molecular Analysis for *CPM/MDM2*

After Molecular Analysis	Before Molecular Analysis			Total
	Lipoma	IM Lipoma	ALT/WDL	
IM Lipoma	0	29	6	35
Lipoma	317	0	5	322
ALT/WDL	7	0	41	48
Total	324	29	52	405

ALT/WDL indicates atypical lipomatous tumor/well-differentiated liposarcoma; IM, intramuscular.

TABLE 3.—Indications for Molecular Analysis for Lipomatous Tumors

Lipomatous tumors with equivocal cytologic atypia
Recurrent "lipomas"
Deep seated lipomatous tumors without cytologic atypia larger than 15 cm
Retroperitoneal (or intra-abdominal) lipomatous tumors without cytologic atypia*

*See Ref. 23.

lipomatous tumors (> 15 cm) without diagnostic cytologic atypia (Tables 1 and 3).

▶ The histologic differentiation between lipoma and atypical lipomatous tumor/well-differentiated liposarcoma is difficult and not an uncommon occurrence for the general surgical pathologist. Despite recent advances in molecular testing, several questions remain as to how to optimally evaluate these cases and when molecular testing may be useful. The specific molecular testing consisted of fluorescence in situ hybridization to identify amplification of carboxypeptidase M (*CPM*) and *MDM2* located on chromosome band 12q15. Amplification was defined as *CPM* or *MDM2* signals to CEP12 ratio of greater than or equal to 3, and the tumor was considered positive if greater than 10 of 100 cells showed amplification. Table 1 shows the effects of molecular analysis for *CPM/MDM2* on the classification. Histologic classification alone resulted in both false negative (2%) and false positive (3%) diagnoses. Based on the vast experience of the authors, indications for molecular analysis in lipomatous tumors are given and are based on tumor size, possible cytologic atypia, location, and recurrence status (Table 3). The most important finding for surgical pathologists is that we tend to overestimate cytologic atypia and in these cases, molecular testing may help guide optimal treatment.

M. L. Smith, MD

The Application of Cytogenetics and Fluorescence In Situ Hybridization to Fine-Needle Aspiration in the Diagnosis and Subclassification of Renal Neoplasms

Roh MH, Dal Cin P, Silverman SG, et al (Univ of Michigan Med School, Ann Arbor; Brigham and Women's Hosp, Boston, MA)
Cancer Cytopathol 118:137-145, 2010

Background.—Percutaneous fine-needle aspiration (FNA) cytology is an important diagnostic test for the evaluation and management of selected renal masses. Cytogenetic analysis of cytology specimens can serve as an adjunct for precise classification because certain tumors are associated with specific chromosomal aberrations. This study summarizes our experience with the application of conventional cytogenetics and fluorescence in situ hybridization (FISH) to renal FNA specimens.

Methods.—All percutaneous renal FNAs performed during 2005 through 2008 were identified from the electronic pathology database. Results of cytogenetic and FISH analyses were correlated with the final diagnoses of the renal FNAs.

Results.—A total of 303 renal FNAs were performed. During an onsite assessment, a portion of the cytology specimen was allocated for cytogenetic analysis in 74 cases. Karyotypic analysis or FISH was successful in 44 (59%) of these. Characteristic chromosomal abnormalities were observed in 27 cases. In 17 cases, a karyotype revealed a combination of trisomies/tetrasomies and in another 5 cases, FISH revealed trisomy 7 and 17, both of which are consistent with papillary renal cell carcinoma (RCC). Two cases showed 3p deletions consistent with clear cell RCC. Trisomy 3 was observed in 1 case of clear cell RCC. Monosomy 1 and 17 was observed in a case of papillary RCC comprised oncocytic cells. In 1 case of primary renal synovial sarcoma, FISH revealed a rearrangement at the *SYT* locus (18q11.2).

Conclusions.—Renal FNA specimens are amenable to analysis by cytogenetics and FISH in the diagnosis and subclassification of renal neoplasms (Table 3).

▶ Small needle core biopsies and fine-needle aspiration (FNA) specimens from renal neoplasms are increasingly being submitted for pathologic evaluation. Because of the small nature of some of the specimens and some of the differential diagnostic challenges, pathologists are often looking for ancillary testing to support initial morphologic interpretations. Unfortunately, immunohistochemical analysis for markers such as cytokeratin 7, CD117, renal cell carcinoma, vimentin, and alpha-methyl-Co A racemase often leads to equivocal or contradictory results. Therefore, other more definitive ancillary studies would be ideal. In this retrospective study, the authors evaluate the feasibility of cytogenetic analysis and fluorescence in situ hybridization (FISH) on percutaneous FNA biopsies from renal masses. Unfortunately, because of the retrospective design of the study, the cytogenetic and FISH results were used in conjunction with the morphologic analysis and immunohistochemical workup to arrive at

TABLE 3.—Common Cytogenetic Abnormalities in Different Subtypes of Renal Tumors and Number of Tumors From This Study That Exhibit These Abnormalities

Diagnosis/Cytogenetic Abnormality	No. (%)
Clear cell RCC	
3p deletion	2 (7)
Trisomy 3	1 (4)
Papillary RCC	
Combination of trisomies or tetrasomies (including chromosomes 3, 7, 12, 16, 17, and 20)	17 (63)
Trisomy or tetrasomy 7 and trisomy 17[a]	5 (18)
Chromophobe RCC	
Combination of monosomies (including chromosomes 1, 2, 6, 10, 13, 17, and 21)	0 (0)
Monosomy 1 and 17[a]	1 (4)[b]
Translocation RCC	
t(X;1) translocation	0 (0)
t(X;17) translocation	0 (0)
Synovial sarcoma	
t(X:18) translocation[a]	1 (4)
Total	27 (100)

FISH indicates fluorescence in situ hybridization; RCC, renal cell carcinoma.
Obtained by FISH.
In this case, the tumor comprised papillary clusters of oncocytic cells; the diagnosis rendered on the follow-up partial nephrectomy specimen was papillary RCC.

a final diagnosis. Thus, the study design does not allow for an investigation of the impact of cytogenetic and FISH testing on the overall diagnostic process. Nevertheless, it does introduce the concept of widespread cytogenetic and FISH testing for the evaluation of renal FNA specimens (Table 3). Additional prospective and blinded studies to evaluate the sensitivity and specificity of cytogenetic and FISH testing on renal mass FNA specimens are needed to justify not only the diagnostic utility but also the associated increase in cost.

M. L. Smith, MD

Visualization of FISH Probes by Dual-Color Chromogenic In Situ Hybridization

Hoff K, Jørgensen JT, Müller S, et al (Antibody Development, Dako Denmark, Glostrup; CMC Contrast, Copenhagen, Denmark)
Am J Clin Pathol 133:205-211, 2010

The overall purpose of the study was to demonstrate applicability of the DAKO dual-color chromogenic in situ hybridization (CISH) assay (DAKO Denmark, Glostrup) with respect to 4 fluorescence in situ hybridization (FISH) probes: *MYC (c-MYC)*, *FGFR*, *ERBB2 (HER2)*, and *TOP2A*. The study showed that the dual-color CISH assay can convert Texas red and fluorescein isothiocyanate (FITC) signals into chromogenic signals with an almost complete 1:1 conversion ratio. Agreement studies between the FISH assays for *HER2* and *TOP2A* and the corresponding CISH conversion assays showed 100% concordance (*k* values of 1.0) between the CISH and FISH methods for *HER2* and *TOP2A* status. The correlations of the gene copy number to centromere-17 ratios were similarly high, with a correlation coefficient (*r*) for *HER2* and *TOP2A* of more than 0.95. Owing to the relatively small number of specimens in this study, it is important that the data are confirmed in a larger study.

▶ Chromogenic in situ hybridization (CISH) is a relatively new method to recognize specific chromosomal abnormalities under bright field microscopy. The advantages of CISH over florescence in situ hybridization (FISH) are numerous and include the ability to evaluate and interpret the findings within a morphologic context under bright field microscopy, the lack of required specialized equipment and personnel (florescence microscopy stations and specialized technicians), and the lack of fluorescent signal fading over time. The conversion from FISH to CISH is shown conceptually in Fig 1 in the original article and is relatively simple, using alkaline phosphatase- and horseradish peroxidase-conjugated antibodies with specificity directed to Texas red conjugate and fluorescein isothiocyanate conjugate, respectively. Therefore, the red FISH probe becomes red and the green FISH probe becomes blue under light microscopy. Example figures given in the article highlight robust dot-to-dot conversion. Although they found a 100% correlation between FISH and CISH, the small sample size is one of the limitations of this study. Looking closely at the individual cases (Figs 2 and 3 in the original article), there are slight ratio variations which, given enough cases, would likely result in rare misclassified cases.

M. L. Smith, MD

Visualizing Hepatitis C Virus Infections in Human Liver by Two-Photon Microscopy
Liang Y, Shilagard T, Xiao S-Y, et al (Univ of Texas Med Branch Cancer Ctr; Univ of Texas Med Branch at Galveston)
Gastroenterology 137:1448-1458, 2009

Background & Aims.—Although hepatitis C virus (HCV) is a common cause of cirrhosis and liver cancer, efforts to understand the pathogenesis of HCV infection have been limited by the low abundance of viral proteins expressed within the liver, which hinders the detection of infected cells in situ. This study evaluated the ability of advanced optical imaging techniques to determine the extent and distribution of HCV-infected cells within the liver.

Methods.—We combined 2-photon microscopy with virus-specific, fluorescent, semiconductor quantum dot probes to determine the proportion of hepatocytes that were infected with virus in frozen sections of liver tissue obtained from patients with chronic HCV infection.

Results.—Viral core and nonstructural protein 3 antigens were detected readily in liver tissues from patients with chronic infection without confounding tissue autofluorescence. Specificity was confirmed by blocking with specific antibodies and by tissue colocalization of distinct viral antigens. Between 7% and 20% of hepatocytes were infected in patients with plasma viral RNA loads of 10^5 IU/mL or greater. Infected cells were in clusters, which suggested spread of the virus from cell to cell. Double-stranded RNA, a product of viral replication, was abundant within cells at the center of such clusters, but often scarce in cells at the periphery, consistent with more recent infection of cells at the periphery.

Conclusions.—Two-photon microscopy provides unprecedented sensitivity for the detection of HCV proteins and double-stranded RNA. Studies using this technology indicate that HCV infection is a dynamic process that involves a limited number of hepatocytes. HCV spread between cells is likely to be constrained by host responses.

▶ Although hepatitis C virus (HCV) was discovered over 20 years ago, efforts to visualize HCV infection within affected livers have not been consistently successful. In this very interesting article, the authors combine 2 different advanced techniques, quantum dot technology and 2-photon microscopy, to visualize HCV infection within hepatocytes of patients with chronic HCV infection. Quantum dots are small semiconducting crystals that emit much brighter for their size and have a flexible emission spectrum. Two-photon microscopy uses 2 photons instead of the typical 1 to excite a fluorophore. This technique decreases background florescence and photobleaching. Although only a small number of samples were involved (3 patients without HCV and 9 patients with HCV), the primary goal of the article is to describe the technique. Not only was specificity for HCV confirmed by use of a blocking antibody but also none of the non-HCV–infected tissues were positive, and colocalization with double-stranded RNA was verified. Although some have suggested that HCV may also infect lymphocytes or macrophages, none were identified. This methodology opens the door to morphologic visualization of HCV infection in the liver but requires verification by other investigators and on additional samples.

M. L. Smith, MD

PART II

LABORATORY MEDICINE

15 Laboratory Management and Outcomes

A Novel Class of Laboratory Middleware: Promoting Information Flow and Improving Computerized Provider Order Entry
Grisson R, Kim JY, Brodsky V, et al (Massachusetts General Hosp, Boston; et al)
Am J Clin Pathol 133:860-869, 2010

A central duty of the laboratory is to inform clinicians about the availability and usefulness of laboratory testing. In this report, we describe a new class of laboratory middleware that connects the traditional clinical laboratory information system with the rest of the enterprise, facilitating information flow about testing services. We demonstrate the value of this approach in efficiently supporting an inpatient order entry application. We also show that order entry monitoring and iterative middleware updates can enhance ordering efficiency and promote improved ordering practices. Furthermore, we demonstrate the value of algorithmic approaches to improve the accuracy and completeness of laboratory test searches. We conclude with a discussion of design recommendations for middleware applications and discuss the potential role of middleware as a sharable, centralized repository of laboratory test information (Fig 1).

▶ Laboratories have long recognized the importance of providing their customers with updated reliable information about their diagnostic testing services. Historically, this has been accomplished by using printed materials that laboratories have found challenging to keep up to date because of the ever-changing nature of laboratory policies, the test menu, specimen requirements, and reference ranges. An online laboratory manual has been shown to be a useful means for maintaining and distributing the latest laboratory information. The problem with the typical model of an online laboratory handbook is that it is separate from the laboratory information system (LIS) and thus requires significant maintenance and updating to remain current, especially considering how frequently laboratory test information changes. In addition to the laboratory handbook, numerous other clinical applications use laboratory test data. For example, inpatient and outpatient order entry systems are

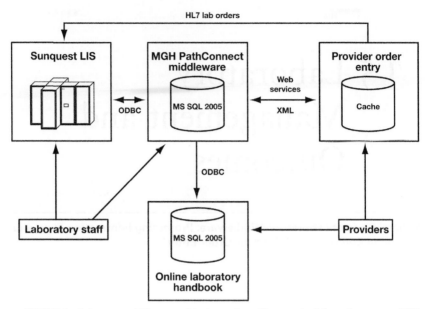

FIGURE 1.—Laboratory middleware and its interaction with enterprise information systems. HL7, Health Level Seven; LIS, laboratory information system; MGH, Massachusetts General Hospital; MS SQL 2005, Microsoft SQL Server 2005 database; ODBC, open database connectivity; XML, extensible markup language. (Reprinted from Grisson R, Kim JY, Brodsky V, et al. A novel class of laboratory middleware: promoting information flow and improving computerized provider order entry. *Am J Clin Pathol*. 2010;133:860-869, with permission from American Society for Clinical Pathology.)

important consumers of laboratory test information. There is an inherent update problem with the storage of laboratory test data in multiple places (eg, the LIS, laboratory handbook, and order entry systems) because there can be only one source of truth for laboratory testing and there is considerable cost in maintaining at least 3 separate repositories of laboratory test information. At a fundamental level, the single source of truth for the laboratory is the LIS. The LIS drives the test ordering and results reporting processes, and up-to-date order codes are required for the LIS to function properly and efficiently report results. With the continued progress toward electronic interfacing of provider order entry (POE) systems and LISs, there is a growing need for order entry applications to be in synchrony with the LIS. Such synchronization can be challenging because the group or groups responsible for POE systems are often outside the domain of pathology and have numerous other priorities and limited resources. In this report, the authors describe a novel application (Fig 1) that interacts with the LIS to enhance the ability of the LIS to support enterprise information flow. They demonstrate how this novel middleware application can be used to efficiently support an inpatient order entry system. They show that the use of the middleware, combined with order monitoring, permits rapid cycle improvement in an order entry system. In addition, they describe the usefulness of the middleware application to drive other key informatics tasks in the organization, such as producing the online laboratory handbook and providing a central point for cataloging laboratory knowledge.

M. G. Bissell, MD, PhD, MPH

Application of the Toyota Production System Improves Core Laboratory Operations
Rutledge J, Xu M, Simpson J (Seattle Children's Hosp, WA; et al)
Am J Clin Pathol 133:24-31, 2010

To meet the increased clinical demands of our hospital expansion, improve quality, and reduce costs, our tertiary care, pediatric core laboratory used the Toyota Production System lean processing to reorganize our 24-hour, 7 d/wk core laboratory. A 4-month, consultant-driven process removed waste, led to a physical reset of the space to match the work flow, and developed a work cell for our random access analyzers. In addition, visual controls, single piece flow, standard work, and "5S" were instituted.

The new design met our goals as reflected by achieving and maintaining improved turnaround time (TAT; mean for creatinine reduced from 54 to 23 minutes) with increased testing volume (20%), monetary savings (4 full-time equivalents), decreased variability in TAT, and better space utilization (25% gain). The project had the unanticipated consequence of eliminating STAT testing because our in-laboratory TAT for routine testing was less than our prior STAT turnaround goal.

The viability of this approach is demonstrated by sustained gains and further PDCA (Plan, Do, Check, Act) improvements during the 4 years after completion of the project.

▶ The clinical laboratory, like the US health care industry in general, is under pressure to improve quality and provide test results faster while decreasing costs. This is an ever-increasing and difficult task owing to rising test volume, increased test complexity, space constraints, and shortage of medical technologists. The authors' laboratory was faced with a similar mandate but also saw pressures to provide better service to a growing emergency department patient load, to accommodate the addition of 40 new hospital beds, and to provide not only faster results but also improved quality.

A bottleneck for their multidisciplinary laboratory was its central processing area and core laboratory (routine chemistry, hematology, coagulation, and urinalysis), which stood to be most affected by this increased demand and most susceptible to making mistakes under pressure. From past experience, their usual response to increased volume was to add technologists to the core laboratory; their core laboratory space would not easily accommodate more technologists. Moreover, their core service consisted of a large number of technologists trained to perform a broad spectrum of cross-disciplinary testing, predisposing to a lack of standardization. They sought to address these issues by the application of the Toyota Production System management principles. This system has been proposed as one that, if applied to health care, could reduce errors and waste. The Toyota Production System results in Lean manufacturing, a system by which value to the customer is achieved with less work expenditure.

In The Toyota Way, production principles embrace the totality of the Toyota management style and go far beyond the transfer of Lean manufacturing principles into the clinical laboratory. Some of these principles are just beginning to be applied to hospitals, a few clinical laboratories, and more recently, anatomic pathology. The authors used a consulting firm (ValuMetrix, Ortho-Clinical Diagnostics, Raritan, NJ) with experience in clinical laboratory operations to conduct a lean overhaul of their core laboratory. Selection of this method coincided with the hospital's adoption of similar methods as a new management philosophy; they therefore did not investigate other methods for their work. This report covers the project applied to their core laboratory and provides outcome measures 4 years after completion.

M. G. Bissell, MD, PhD, MPH

Applying Lean/Toyota Production System Principles to Improve Phlebotomy Patient Satisfaction and Workflow
Melanson SEF, Goonan EM, Lobo MM, et al (Brigham and Women's Hosp, Boston, MA)
Am J Clin Pathol 132:914-919, 2009

Our goals were to improve the overall patient experience and optimize the blood collection process in outpatient phlebotomy using Lean principles. Elimination of non–value-added steps and modifications to operational processes resulted in increased capacity to handle workload during peak times without adding staff. The result was a reduction of average patient wait time from 21 to 5 minutes, with the goal of drawing blood samples within 10 minutes of arrival at the phlebotomy station met for 90% of patients. In addition, patient satisfaction increased noticeably as assessed by a 5-question survey. The results have been sustained for 10 months with staff continuing to make process improvements.

▶ Despite the temporary tarnish the Toyota brand name has at the moment because of the recent recalls, the Toyota Production System with its Lean principles is nonetheless justly renowned. It emphasizes the elimination of waste and nonvalue-added steps in a setting of limited resources, for example, money, space, and human capital. Kaizen, which means continuous improvement, events are one method to apply Lean principles to a process or setting. Occurring over 4 days, a Kaizen event brings together front-line staff members who are experts in the process to brainstorm issues, identify solutions, and iteratively test ideas in the work area in real time. Successful tests are further refined and incorporated as part of the standard work. Applying theses principles in health care is a timely response to the tarnish our institutions have had from waste and medical errors.

Brigham and Women's Hospital (Boston, Massachusetts) is a 777-bed teaching affiliate of Harvard Medical School (Boston, Massachusetts) with approximately 46 000 admissions per year and 1 million outpatient visits. The clinical laboratory provides phlebotomy services for inpatients and outpatients. There are 5 onsite locations for outpatient blood draws. The primary outpatient phlebotomy area draws samples from an average of 190 patients and obtains 500 specimens per day during the week. It is staffed by 8 phlebotomists and operates between the hours of 7:30 AM and 6:00 PM.

The clinical laboratory leadership selected the main outpatient phlebotomy laboratory to undergo Lean process improvement through a Kaizen event owing to its large volume of patients and specimens and its direct impact on patient care. Our objectives were to improve patient satisfaction and reduce patient wait time. This article outlines the process, details its impact on workflow and patients, and offers suggestions for laboratories embarking on similar process improvement projects. This is one of the few articles describing the use of Lean principles in phlebotomy.

M. G. Bissell, MD, PhD, MPH

Educating Medical Students in Laboratory Medicine: A Proposed Curriculum
Smith BR, for the Academy of Clinical Laboratory Physicians and Scientists (Yale Univ School of Medicine, New Haven, CT; et al)
Am J Clin Pathol 133:533-542, 2010

As the 100th anniversary of the Flexner report nears, medical student education is being reviewed at many levels. One area of concern, expressed in recent reports from some national health care organizations, is the adequacy of training in the discipline of laboratory medicine (also termed clinical pathology). The Academy of Clinical Laboratory Physicians and Scientists appointed an ad hoc committee to review this topic and to develop a suggested curriculum, which was subsequently forwarded to the entire membership for review. The proposed medical student laboratory medicine curriculum defines goals and objectives for training, provides guidelines for instructional methods, and gives examples of how outcomes can be assessed. This curriculum is presented as a potentially helpful outline for use by medical school faculty and curriculum committees.

▶ Educational research data question the success of current laboratory medicine teaching in educating students to apply critical principles in practice. Attending physicians also show suboptimal ability to properly order diagnostic tests in various settings. Laboratory medicine procedural skills that may be commonly used in clinical practice, for example, urine microscopy, are often poorly assimilated by students. In a British survey, 18% to 20% of medical graduates described themselves as less than competent in using laboratory testing and more than 20% thought they were less than competent in all diagnostic approaches. Medical student exposure to transfusion medicine principles and practice has been a particular area of concern owing to the recognition that this is an area of suboptimal knowledge in most physician specialties, resulting in significant patient safety and cost issues. Based on these considerations and on the rapid pace of major advances that have occurred in laboratory medicine, it appeared prudent to attempt to develop some consensus on what should be included in the medical student curriculum for this discipline. It is critical to consider such a curriculum in the context of improved integration of the most modern scientific paradigms. Teaching modalities should be identified that are more effective in attaining the goal of educating students to truly apply what they learn in the practical clinical setting and also in encouraging them to develop appropriate habits for lifelong learning. Methods for inclusion of laboratory medicine principles during all stages of the medical student curriculum during all 4 years are critical to reap the benefits of integrated curricula, as is instruction in the use of electronic resources. The Academy of Clinical Laboratory Physicians and Scientists appointed an ad hoc committee to review this topic and to develop a suggested curriculum, which was subsequently forwarded to the entire membership for review. The proposed medical student laboratory medicine curriculum defines goals and objectives for training, provides guidelines for instructional methods, and gives examples of how outcomes can be assessed. This curriculum is presented as a potentially helpful outline for use by medical school faculty and curriculum committees.

M. G. Bissell, MD, PhD, MPH

Establishing Reference Intervals for Clinical Laboratory Test Results: Is There a Better Way?
Katayev A, Balciza C, Seccombe DW (Laboratory Corporation of America (LabCorp), Burlington, NC; Canadian External Quality Assessment Laboratory, Vancouver; Univ of British Columbia, Vancouver)
Am J Clin Pathol 133:180-186, 2010

Reference intervals are essential for clinical laboratory test interpretation and patient care. Methods for estimating them are expensive, difficult to perform, often inaccurate, and nonreproducible. A computerized indirect Hoffmann method was studied for accuracy and reproducibility. The study used data collected retrospectively for 5 analytes without exclusions and filtering from a nationwide chain of clinical reference laboratories in the United States. The accuracy was assessed by the comparability of reference intervals as calculated by the new method with published peer-reviewed studies, and reproducibility was assessed by the comparability of 2 sets of reference intervals derived from 2 different data sets. There was no statistically significant difference between the calculated and published reference intervals or between the 2 sets of intervals that were derived from different data sets. A computerized Hoffmann method for indirect estimation of reference intervals using stored test results is proved to be accurate and reproducible.

▶ In the modern environment when laboratories are struggling to stay profitable, not everyone is willing to budget the appropriate resources for a lengthy and expensive reference interval (RI) study. An alternative approach for establishing RIs is to do an indirect so-called a posteriori study of the patient data already collected and stored in the laboratory database. This is appealing because the data are readily available and will result in time and cost savings. A number of publications discuss this approach. Most of these studies were able to report clinically relevant and meaningful RIs. All of them used various sophisticated filters to exclude results from unhealthy subjects, and some used data from hospital laboratories and some from outpatient care settings or noninstitutionalized population study databases. Most of these studies used complex statistical algorithms to derive the final intervals. However, current guidelines do not endorse these methods as a primary approach for establishing RIs, mainly out of concern for the fact that most of the data may not come from reference or healthy subjects. This position may be justified for test results collected from hospitalized patients but is questionable when considering a very large number of results that have been collected in outpatient settings. Indeed, there is no disease with prevalence close to 50%. On the other hand, as discussed, the recommended direct sampling techniques are not without their own assumptions. The reliability of an RI study should be a function of its accuracy and reproducibility and have a direct relationship with the number of observations used and method standardization. Statistically, it is more robust to analyze thousands of measurements that may include some unhealthy subjects than 120 measurements that are assumed to be from healthy subjects. The main problem with most of the reported indirect studies is that they used statistical analyses designed for a direct sampling technique. Hoffmann, in his classic *JAMA* article from 1963, described a technique designed for indirect estimation of RIs using all available test results from a laboratory's database: "This statistical technique can be used for obtaining any normal values in medicine where a group of measurements are available and the mathematical assumptions are reasonable." Although his work has been widely cited, few authors have actually applied the Hoffmann method in their calculations. A notable exception is the manual of pediatric RIs by Soldin et al that is now in its sixth edition and published by American Association for Clinical Chemistry. This fundamental work was limited by the relatively small number of observations (typically 50-100) that were used and by the semimanual application of Hoffmann analysis of data, which added subjectivity to the calculations. The authors' goal in this study was to assess the reliability of the Hoffmann approach using a newly developed computer program designed to remove subjectivity from RI calculations.

M. G. Bissell, MD, PhD, MPH

Multiple Patient Samples of an Analyte Improve Detection of Changes in Clinical Status

Kroll MH (Boston Univ School of Medicine, MA)
Arch Pathol Lab Med 134:81-89, 2010

Context.—When comparing results over time, biologic variation must be statistically incorporated into the evaluation of laboratory results to identify a physiologic change. Traditional methods compare the difference in 2 values with the standard deviation (SD) of the biologic variation to indicate whether a "true" physiologic change has occurred.

Objective.—To develop methodology to reduce the effect of biologic variation on the difference necessary to detect changes in clinical status in the presence of biologic variation.

Design.—The standard test for change compares the difference between 2 points with the 95% confidence limit, given as $\pm 1.96 \cdot \sqrt{2} \cdot SD$. We examined the effect of multiple data pairs on the confidence limit.

Results.—Increasing the number of data pairs using the formula $1.96 \cdot \sqrt{2/n} \cdot SD$, where $n = $ number of data pairs, significantly reduces the difference between values necessary to achieve a 95% confidence limit.

Conclusions.—Evaluating multiple paired sets of patient data rather than a single pair results in a substantial decrease in the difference between values necessary to achieve a given confidence interval, thereby improving the sensitivity of the evaluation. A practice of using multiple patient samples results in enhanced power to detect true changes in patient physiology. Such a testing protocol is warranted when small changes in the analyte precede serious clinical events or when the SD of the biologic variation is large.

▶ Clinicians rely on laboratory tests to monitor the progression or remission of disease or to identify pathologic alterations in physiology that may precede clinical events. Monitoring quantitative laboratory results represents a crucial component in the assessment of response to therapy. Laboratories assist the physician's clinical decision making by providing empiric values and applicable reference intervals. Although population- and laboratory-based reference intervals are useful, clinicians frequently encounter changes in analyte values that remain within or outside the reference interval. Therefore, the clinician needs to discern the statistical significance of a change in analyte values, which can be achieved by using the patient as his own control. Didactic and clinical training teaches physicians to develop their judgment to assess whether serial tests represent a significant clinical change (physiologic, pathologic, or therapeutic)? An evidence-based medicine approach calculates the probability of significant change, presented as a confidence limit. The 95% confidence limit of a test is given as $\pm 1.96 \cdot \sqrt{2} \cdot SD$, where the SD refers to the biologic variation expressed as a standard deviation. The multiplier, 1.96 (Z), is determined by choosing an alpha value of .05 (other multipliers may be calculated for alpha, values of .1 or .01 as desired). If the absolute change in analyte value exceeds a 95% confidence limit, then the difference is considered statistically significant and likely represents a true change in patient physiology. Conversely, if the absolute change in analyte does not exceed the 95% confidence limit, then there is a greater than 5% probability that the change in analyte value is not due to a change in patient physiology but instead attributable to inherent biologic variation or laboratory analytic variation. Although this method of determining the significance of changing analyte values is satisfactory in cases where analytic and biologic variation is small compared with the measured values, it is limited to only 2 analyte values encompassing a discrete period of time (ie, 1 value at time A and a second at time B, the interval in question being from A to B). For many analytes and clinical situations—for example, B-natriuretic peptide (BNP) in heart failure—the biologic variation is so large that it reduces the efficiency of the test, resulting in poor discrimination and power. In such cases, the power of comparing 2 analyte values often remains insufficient to discern statistically significant change. Despite this obvious limitation, current literature concentrates on single difference comparison, avoiding the mechanics and implication of using multiple differences. Determining whether calculating multiple differences would narrow the width of the confidence interval and improving the power of the test require examination. The author investigated ways to arrange measuring multiple points to improve the power of the test, measured by demonstrating narrowing limits of detection for fixed confidence intervals. He hypothesized that the addition of one or more analyte measurements at the initial or later point of time could be statistically incorporated into the determination of the critical standard error to result in enhanced sensitivity to clinically significant physiologic change within the patient.

M. G. Bissell, MD, PhD, MPH

Neonatal Screening for Treatable and Untreatable Disorders: Prospective Parents' Opinions
Plass AMC, van El CG, Pieters T, et al (VU Univ Med Ctr, Amsterdam, Netherlands)
Pediatrics 125:e99-e106, 2010

Objective.—In the Netherlands, in 2007, the national newborn screening program was expanded from 3 to 17 disorders that met the World Health Organization's Wilson and Jungner screening criteria, especially regarding treatability. The decision of whether to add diseases to the program is generally based on experts' advice, whereas the opinion of those whom it concerns—prospective parents—remains unknown. In this study, we investigated the opinion of prospective parents concerning newborn screening for disorders that are incurable yet treatable to some extent or even untreatable.

Methods.—A structured questionnaire that consisted of 3 parts in which similar questions were posed about treatable, less treatable, and untreatable childhood-onset disorders was posted on the Web site of a national pregnancy fair.

Results.—A total of 1631 prospective parents filled out the questionnaire, 259 of whom were excluded. In contrast to current policy, respondents showed a positive attitude toward inclusion of less treatable (88%) or untreatable childhood-onset disorders (73%) within the national newborn screening program. Respondents who already had children at the time of completing the questionnaire were even more in favor of screening for especially untreatable disorders. The most important reason mentioned was to prevent a long diagnostic quest. Obtaining information to enable reproductive choices in future pregnancies was hardly mentioned.

Conclusions.—Prospective parents in the Dutch population seem interested in newborn screening for untreatable childhood-onset disorders; therefore, we argue that additional debate of pros and cons is needed among policy makers, health care professionals, and consumers.

▶ The decision of whether to add diseases to a newborn screening program has often been based on the advice of experts in various areas of medicine and primary care, health policy, law, ethics, etc, whereas the opinion of those it concerns—prospective parents—remains unknown. Recently, 2 Dutch-focus group studies were conducted. One was directed at parental opinions about the expansion of the newborn screening program; a divergence in attitude and preferences among the participants was found regarding screening for less treatable and untreatable diseases. Some participants said that benefits to the family, such as reproductive choice, certainty due to screening, or anticipation of the future, were sufficient criteria for neonatal screening. The other was held among representatives of several societal groups: prospective parents, the elderly, those who are familiar with a monogenetic hereditary disease (themselves or within their family), and those who are familiar with a multifactorial disease (themselves or within their family). The aim of this study was to explore whether the concerns and considerations of these prospective users regarding genetic screening criteria were similar to those expressed by the Health Council of the Netherlands and current screening policy. When discussing untreatable disorders, participants in some groups expressed the view that although they would not have screening for untreatable disorders themselves, they could see benefits if the screening were for their newborn child. This is an interesting finding given the overall reluctance to offer screening for untreatable disorders. Given these recent scientific and societal trends and the results of these qualitative studies, the aim of this study was to explore the opinion of a broader, less selected group of prospective users, namely future parents, on addition of category I (treatable disorders), category II (less treatable disorders), and category III (untreatable disorders) to the national newborn screening program, provided that a valid test were available.

M. G. Bissell, MD, PhD, MPH

Patient Misidentification in Laboratory Medicine: A Qualitative Analysis of 227 Root Cause Analysis Reports in the Veterans Health Administration
Dunn EJ, Moga PJ (Lexington VA Med Ctr, KY; VA Ann Arbor Healthcare System, MI)
Arch Pathol Lab Med 134:244-255, 2010

Context.—Mislabeled laboratory specimens are a common source of harm to patients, such as repeat phlebotomy; repeat diagnostic procedure, including tissue biopsy; delay in a necessary surgical procedure; and the execution of an unnecessary surgical procedure. Mislabeling has been estimated to occur at a rate of 0.1% of all laboratory and anatomic pathology specimens submitted.

Objective.—To identify system vulnerabilities in specimen collection, processing, analysis, and reporting associated with patient misidentification involving the clinical laboratory, anatomic pathology, and blood transfusion services.

Design.—A qualitative analysis was performed on 227 root cause analysis reports from the Veterans Health Administration. Content analysis of case reports from March 9, 2000, to March 1, 2008, was facilitated by a Natural Language Processing program. Data were categorized by the 3 stages of the laboratory test cycle.

Results.—Patient misidentification accounted for 182 of 253 adverse events, which occurred in all 3 stages of the test cycle. Of 132 misidentification events occurring in the preanalytic phase, events included wrist bands labeled for the wrong patient were applied on admission (n = 8), and laboratory tests were ordered for the wrong patient by selecting the wrong electronic medical record from a menu of similar names and Social Security numbers (n = 31). Specimen mislabeling during collection was associated with "batching" of specimens and printed labels (n = 35), misinformation from manual entry on laboratory forms (n = 14), failure of 2-source patient identification for clinical laboratory specimens (n = 24), and failure of 2-person verification of patient identity for blood bank specimens (n = 20). Of 37 events in the analytic phase, relabeling all specimens with accession numbers was associated with mislabeled specimen containers, tissue cassettes, and microscopic slides (n = 27). Misidentified microscopic slides were associated with a failure of 2-pathologist verification for cancer diagnosis (n = 4), and wrong patient transfusions were associated with mislabeled blood products (n = 3) and a failure of 2-person verification for blood products before release by the blood bank (n = 3). There were 13 events in the post analytic phase in which results were reported into the wrong patient medical record (n = 8), and incompatible blood transfusions were associated with failed 2-person verification of blood products (n = 5).

Conclusions.—Patient misidentification in the clinical laboratory, anatomic pathology, and blood transfusion processes were due to a limited set of causal factors in all 3 phases of the test cycle. A focus on these factors will inform systemic mitigation and prevention strategies.

▶ Specimen misidentification in laboratory medicine can have significant consequences for patients. Mislabeled tissue specimens will often result in harm to patients, such as undergoing unnecessary surgical or diagnostic procedures. In other cases, patients will be subjected to unnecessary diagnostic studies or experience significant delays in the treatment of medical conditions they never knew they had. Mislabeling specimens can lead to unnecessary hospitalizations or failure to treat unreported conditions. If a patient suffers no physical harm from specimen misidentification, the prospect of being subjected to additional procedures is not without risk. Such additional procedures, such as prostate biopsy, colonoscopy, fine-needle aspiration of the lung, phlebotomy, or other diagnostic testing, are not without risks that have associated opportunity costs to patients, families, the health care system, and society. The authors set 3 objectives for this study: The first was to develop an algorithm for the categorization of adverse events in laboratory medicine mapped to the 3 phases of the testing cycle. The second was to better understand how and why patient specimens can be misidentified in the laboratory. In the third objective, they considered potential solutions to reduce the probability of future recurrence of these adverse events. Specimen mislabeling during collection was associated with "batching" of specimens and printed labels ($n = 35$), misinformation from manual entry on laboratory forms ($n = 14$), failure of 2-source patient identification for clinical laboratory specimens ($n = 24$), and failure of 2-person verification of patient identity for blood bank specimens ($n = 20$). Of 37 events in the analytic phase, relabeling all specimens with accession numbers was associated with mislabeled specimen containers, tissue cassettes, and microscopic slides ($n = 27$). Misidentified microscopic slides were associated with a failure of 2-person pathologist verification for cancer diagnosis ($n = 4$), and wrong patient transfusions were associated with mislabeled blood products ($n = 3$) and a failure of 2-person verification for blood products before release by the blood bank ($n = 3$). There were 13 events in the postanalytic phase in which results were reported into the wrong patient medical record ($n = 8$), and incompatible blood transfusions were associated with failed 2-person verification of blood products ($n = 5$). Patient misidentification in the clinical laboratory, anatomic pathology, and blood transfusion processes were because of a limited set of causal factors in all 3 phases of the test cycle. A focus on these factors will inform systemic mitigation and prevention strategies.

M. G. Bissell, MD, PhD, MPH

Racial and Ethnic Disparities in Awareness of Genetic Testing for Cancer Risk

Pagán JA, Su D, Li L, et al (Univ of North Texas Health Science Ctr, Fort Worth; Univ of Texas–Pan American, Edinburg; et al)
Am J Prev Med 37:524-530, 2009

Background.—Racial and ethnic disparities in awareness of genetic testing for cancer risk are substantial.

Purpose.—This study assesses the relative importance of contributing factors to gaps in awareness of genetic testing for cancer risk across racial and ethnic groups.

Methods.—Data from the 2005 National Health Interview Survey (N = 25,364) were analyzed in 2009 to evaluate the contribution of demographic factors, SES, health status, nativity/length of residency in the U.S., personal/family history of cancer, and perceived cancer risk to racial and ethnic disparities in genetic testing awareness for cancer risk. The contribution of each factor was assessed using the Fairlie decomposition technique.

Results.—About 48% of non-Hispanic whites reported that they had heard about genetic testing, followed by 31% of blacks, 28% of Asians, and 19% of Hispanics. Education and nativity/length of residency in the U.S. explained 26% and 30% of the gap between whites and Hispanics, respectively. Education accounted for 22% of the white–black gap, with residential region explaining another 11%. Nativity/length of residency in the U.S. explained 51% of the white–Asian gap.

Conclusions.—The relative importance of factors contributing to racial and ethnic disparities in genetic testing awareness is specific to the particular groups under comparison. Diverse, culturally competent approaches are needed to improve awareness for different racial and ethnic groups.

▶ Genetic testing for cancer susceptibility is becoming more commonplace because of the availability of new tests as well as clinical guidelines for genetic counseling and testing. Not all demographic and socioeconomic groups, however, have benefited from the growing use of genetic counseling and testing for cancer susceptibility. In particular, racial and ethnic minorities display considerably less use of genetic counseling and testing for cancer risk than non-Hispanic whites. An important contributing factor to racial and ethnic disparities in the use of genetic tests for cancer susceptibility lies in differential levels of awareness of these tests across racial and ethnic groups. According to the 2000 National Health Interview Survey (NHIS), 49.9% of non-Hispanic whites aged ≥25 years reported having heard of genetic testing for increased cancer risk, compared with 32.9% of African Americans, 20.6% of Hispanics, 28% of Asians, and 32.3% of American Indians. One explanation for the lower awareness on the part of racial and ethnic-minority groups is that minorities, particularly Hispanics, are less exposed to health information through the health care system partially because of language barriers and acculturation factors. This explanation has been corroborated in other studies, suggesting that minority groups who are relatively more acculturated to the United States—as indicated by either nativity or English proficiency—are also relatively more likely to be aware of genetic testing for cancer risk. Besides language and acculturation, racial and ethnic disparities in genetic testing awareness might also result from differences in education, health insurance status, marital status, health, personal or family history of cancer, or other factors. This study uses survey data from the 2005 NHIS and applies logistic regression models and the Fairlie decomposition technique to better understand the multiple factors that may contribute to racial and ethnic differences in awareness of genetic testing for cancer risk.

M. G. Bissell, MD, PhD, MPH

Strategies for Improving the Collection of 24-Hour Urine for Analysis in the Clinical Laboratory: Redesigned Instructions, Opinion Surveys, and Application of Reference Change Value to Micturition

Tormo C, Lumbreras B, Santos A, et al (Hospital Universitario de Elche, Alicante, Spain; Universidad Miguel Hernandez, San Juan, Alicante, Spain)
Arch Pathol Lab Med 133:1954-1960, 2009

Context.—The preanalytic phase of 24-hour urine collection, before clinical analysis, requires the active participation of patients and usually takes place outside the laboratory.

Objective.—We verify whether distribution of adequate information to health care personnel and patients will result in fewer preanalytic incidents. We also determine the intraindividual biologic variability associated with micturition and the corresponding reference change value (RCV).

Design.—The intervention provided training for 24-hour urine collection to the health care personnel of the 20th health district of the Valencian community in Spain. The preanalytic incidents related to 24-hour micturition were estimated before and after the intervention. An opinion survey on the problems involved in urine collection was also conducted among patients. The Harris formula was used to calculate the RCV.

Results.—Before the intervention, 130 preanalytic incidents were recorded (11.5%) and after the intervention, 76 (8.6%) $(P = .04)$ were recorded. Of the 130 incidents recorded before the intervention, 63 (48.5%) involved omission to indicate the urine volume, and of the 76 incidents recorded after the intervention, only 1 (1.3%) $(P < .001)$ involved this omission. Forty of 302 patients (13.2%) surveyed reported problems and more than half (175; 57.9%) had to collect various urine samples sequentially. The RCV determined was 54.5% for a percentage of variation in volume of 24-hour urine (PVVI) of 19.0 ± 16.5%. Therefore, micturition associated with a PVVI > ± 54.5% suggests that 24-hour urine collection by the patient was incomplete. The results obtained when applying the RCV after the intervention showed that 6.3% of the 24-hour urine samples should be rejected.

Conclusions.—The percentage of preanalytic incidents was reduced by providing health care personnel with information and training. The percentage of variation in volume of 24-hour urine can be used to evaluate the variation in patients' micturition. Reference change value was shown to be useful when determining whether 24-hour urine was properly collected.

▶ In the case of 24-hour urine sample collection, the preanalytic problems associated with specimen collection in general are exacerbated because active participation of the patients is necessary. Most laboratories provide specific written instructions to reinforce the verbal explanations given to the patient and provide suitable containers for each type of determination to be conducted. These instructions should be clear, simple, and easily understood by all patients. The reality is that often patients do not give the 24-hour urine samples requested by the clinician to the staff in the hospital laboratory who knows the protocol to proceed with their handling. On other occasions, the samples are not collected under the right conditions or micturition is incomplete. On the other hand, satisfaction surveys together with the opinions of internal staff members (doctors and nurses, end users of the analytic results) or external customers (patients) are considered quality elements and are even deemed to be essential by those in charge of monitoring the quality control systems implemented in clinical laboratories. The results of these surveys and the opinions expressed are important tools for ongoing improvement of the laboratory. They provide information on the quality of the services rendered by the laboratory and include suggestions made by the interviewees for implementing improvement strategies. The aim of this study was to carry out an intervention among nonhospitalized patients (outpatients from external hospital surgery services and from public health centers) to determine whether the distribution of adequate information to staff responsible for collecting the 24-hour urine specimens, who then provide this information to patients, results in fewer preanalytic incidents. Furthermore, patient opinion surveys on the quality of information material were conducted. Based on these data, specific improvements may be proposed. Before the intervention, preanalytic incidents during urine collection were evaluated for a 1-month period and reported by laboratory personnel. One year later, after the implementation of the new recommendations, the number of preanalytic incidents was reevaluated. In addition, the aim was to capitalize on the micturition data of patients with preintervention incidents to determine the intraindividual biologic variability and thus predict the proper complete collection of 24-hour urine for each patient on the basis of their usual rate of micturition.

M. G. Bissell, MD, PhD, MPH

16 Clinical Chemistry

Δ⁹-Tetrahydrocannabinol (THC), 11-Hydroxy-THC, and 11-Nor-9-carboxy-THC Plasma Pharmacokinetics during and after Continuous High-Dose Oral THC

Schwilke EW, Schwope DM, Karschner EL, et al (Biomed Res Ctr, Baltimore, MD; et al)

Clin Chem 55:2180-2189, 2009

Background.—Δ⁹-Tetrahydrocannabinol (THC) is the primary psychoactive constituent of cannabis and an active cannabinoid pharmacotherapy component. No plasma pharmacokinetic data after repeated oral THC administration are available.

Methods.—Six adult male daily cannabis smokers resided on a closed clinical research unit. Oral THC capsules (20 mg) were administered every 4–8 h in escalating total daily doses (40–120 mg) for 7 days. Free and glucuronidated plasma THC, 11-hydroxy-THC (11-OH-THC), and 11-nor-9-carboxy-THC (THC COOH) were quantified by 2-dimensional GC-MS during and after dosing.

Results.—Free plasma THC, 11-OH-THC, and THCCOOH concentrations 19.5 h after admission (before controlled oral THC dosing) were mean 4.3 (SE 1.1), 1.3 (0.5), and 34.0 (8.4) µg/L, respectively. During oral dosing, free 11-OH-THC and THCCOOH increased steadily, whereas THC did not. Mean peak plasma free THC, 11-OH-THC, and THCCOOH concentrations were 3.8 (0.5), 3.0 (0.7), and 196.9 (39.9) µg/L, respectively, 22.5 h after the last dose. *Escherichia coli* β-glucuronidase hydrolysis of 264 cannabinoid specimens yielded statistically significant increases in THC, 11-OH-THC, and THCCOOH concentrations ($P < 0.001$), but conjugated concentrations were underestimated owing to incomplete enzymatic hydrolysis.

Conclusions.—Plasma THC concentrations remained >1 µg/L for at least 1 day after daily cannabis smoking and also after cessation of multiple oral THC doses. We report for the first time free plasma THC concentrations after multiple high-dose oral THC throughout the day and night, and after *Escherichia coli* β-glucuronidase hydrolysis. These data will aid in the interpretation of plasma THC concentrations after multiple oral doses.

▶ Δ⁹-Tetrahydrocannabinol (THC) is the primary psychoactive constituent of cannabis, the most commonly abused illicit drug. Although predominantly smoked, oral administration occurs during illicit use and licit pharmacotherapy. Oral synthetic THC (dronabinol) is Food and Drug Administration (FDA)-approved for treating nausea, vomiting, and anorexia, and there is strong interest in treatment with whole plant extracts containing THC and cannabidiol. Dronabinol also suppresses cannabis withdrawal and withdrawal-associated drug relapse. Peak THC concentrations are lower after oral than smoked administration, but conversely, 11-OH-THC/THC ratios are higher after oral than smoked drug. Cannabinoids undergo phase II metabolism with glucuronide and sulfate. There are few data on cannabinoid conjugate concentrations after smoked cannabis or oral THC. There is a single supplier for THC-glucuronide and no available 11-OH-THC-glucuronide and cannabinoid sulfate standards. Little is known about the proportions of ether and ester glucuronide conjugates in authentic specimens following oral or smoked cannabis. Furthermore, different hydrolysis efficiencies were reported for 3-glucuronidase from *Helix pomatia* and *Escherichia coli* and after alkaline hydrolysis. Finally, the stability of cannabinoid glucuronide and sulfate conjugates in authentic specimens after cannabis use is unknown. Most cannabinoid research requires frozen storage and specimen analysis after study completion. Rapid authentic plasma analysis without frozen storage has not been previously attempted. Cannabinoid glucuronides have been estimated by subtracting free cannabinoids from concentrations after enzyme or base hydrolysis. Available data do not differentiate among individual cannabinoid glucuronides or describe only 11-nor-9-carboxy-THC (THCCOOH) glucuronide. Knowing free and glucuronidated cannabinoid disposition after smoked and oral THC may improve interpretation of plasma cannabinoid concentrations in clinical and forensic investigations. Of several published human daily oral THC administration studies, none report plasma concentrations during continuous dosing. The authors previously described plasma cannabinoids after oral THC 3 times per day for 5 days, but the highest daily dose was 14.8 mg, much lower than single 20-mg doses prescribed for appetite stimulation. Another study determined only ^{14}C-labeled plasma THC concentrations before and after, not during, continuous dosing. In this study, the authors characterized free and glucuronidated plasma THC, 11-OH-THC, and THC COOH in daily cannabis users after self-administered smoked cannabis, after 20-mg oral THC, during 2 to 7 daily THC doses for 7 days, and for 22.5 hours after last THC dose. Authentic plasma specimens stored at 4°C were analyzed generally within 2 weeks.

M. G. Bissell, MD, PhD, MPH

25-Hydroxyvitamin D Levels Inversely Associate with Risk for Developing Coronary Artery Calcification

de Boer IH, Kestenbaum B, Shoben AB, et al (Univ of Washington, Seattle; et al)

J Am Soc Nephrol 20:1805-1812, 2009

Vitamin D deficiency associates with increased risk for cardiovascular events and mortality, but the mechanism driving this association is unknown. Here, we tested whether circulating 25-hydroxyvitamin D concentration associates with coronary artery calcification (CAC), a measure of coronary atherosclerosis, in the Multi-Ethnic Study of Atherosclerosis. We included 1370 participants: 394 with and 976 without chronic kidney disease (estimated GFR <60 ml/min per 1.73 m^2). At baseline, CAC was prevalent among 723 (53%) participants. Among participants free of CAC at baseline, 135 (21%) developed incident CAC during 3 yr of follow-up. Lower 25-hydroxyvitamin D concentration did not associate with prevalent CAC but did associate with increased risk for developing incident CAC, adjusting for age, gender, race/ethnicity, site, season, physical activity, smoking, body mass index, and kidney function. Further adjustment for BP, diabetes, C-reactive protein, and lipids did not alter this finding. The association of 25-hydroxyvitamin D with incident CAC seemed to be stronger among participants with lower estimated GFR. Circulating 1,25-dihydroxyvitamin D concentrations among participants with chronic kidney disease did not significantly associate with prevalent or incident CAC in adjusted models. In conclusion, lower 25-hydroxyvitamin D concentrations associate with increased risk for incident CAC. Accelerated development of atherosclerosis may underlie, in part, the increased cardiovascular risk associated with vitamin D deficiency.

▶ Vitamin D deficiency is associated with increased risks for cardiovascular disease (CVD) and death. Specifically, low circulating concentrations of 25-hydroxyvitamin D [25(OH)D] are associated with increased risks for mortality among incident hemodialysis patients and patients with stages 2 to 5 chronic kidney disease (CKD), cardiovascular events in the Framingham Offspring Study, myocardial infarction in the Health Professionals Follow-up Study, cardiovascular- and all-cause mortality among patients with acute coronary syndrome, and all-cause mortality in follow-up from the Third National Health and Nutrition Examination Survey (NHANES III). Observational studies among patients with CKD suggested that treatment with 1,25-dihydroxyvitamin D (calcitriol) reduces mortality. A meta-analysis of clinical trials, conducted predominantly among postmenopausal women, demonstrated a statistically significant 7% reduction in total mortality with cholecalciferol or ergocalciferol supplementation. Accelerated atherosclerosis may explain in part the associations of vitamin D deficiency with CVD and death. Low circulating 25 (OH) D concentration is associated with a number of established risk factors for atherosclerosis, including obesity, diabetes, hypertension, and dyslipidemia. Moreover, vitamin D seems to regulate additional biologic pathways implicated in the development of atherosclerosis. Calcitriol down regulates the renin angiotensin-aldosterone system in animal models and modulates immune cell function, enriching the antiatherogenic T helper-2 (Th2) lymphocyte population and reducing proinflammatory cytokine secretion. The presence of 1-α-hydroxylase in vascular smooth muscle cells, which converts 25 (OH) D to calcitriol, suggests that vitamin D may also have direct effects on the vascular wall, potentially including prevention of vascular calcification. The authors tested whether low circulating levels of 25 (OH) D are associated with prevalent and incident coronary artery calcium (CAC) in the Multi-Ethnic Study of Atherosclerosis (MESA), a community-based cardiovascular cohort study. 25 (OH) D concentration reflects total intake of vitamin D from cutaneous synthesis and dietary intake. CAC is a sensitive measure of subclinical coronary atherosclerosis and a strong risk factor for cardiovascular events. Serum concentrations of calcitriol (1,25-dihydroxyvitamin D), the most biologically potent metabolite of vitamin D, were additionally measured among participants with CKD.

M. G. Bissell, MD, PhD, MPH

A comparison between B-type natriuretic peptide, Global Registry of Acute Coronary Events (GRACE) score and their combination in ACS risk stratification
Ang DSC, Wei L, Kao MPC, et al (Univ of Dundee, UK)
Heart 95:1836-1842, 2009

Background.—In acute coronary syndrome (ACS), both the Global Registry of Acute Coronary Events (GRACE) score and B-type natriuretic peptide (BNP) predict cardiovascular events. However, it is unknown how BNP compares with GRACE and how their combination performs in ACS.

Methods.—The authors recruited 449 consecutive ACS patients and measured admission GRACE score and bedside BNP levels. The main outcome measure was all-cause mortality, readmission with ACS or congestive heart failure (defined as a cardiovascular event) at 10 months from presentation.

Results.—Of the 449 patients, 120 patients presented with ST-elevation myocardial infarction (MI) (27%). There were 90 cardiovascular events at 10 months. Both higher GRACE terciles and higher BNP terciles predicted cardiovascular events. There was a significant but only partial correlation between the GRACE score and log BNP (R = 0.552, p < 0.001). On multivariate analyses, after adjusting for the GRACE score itself, increasing BNP terciles independently predicted cardiovascular events (second BNP tercile adjusted RR 2.28 (95% CI 1.15 to 4.51) and third BNP tercile adjusted RR 4.91 (95% CI 2.62 to 9.22)). Patients with high GRACE score-high BNP were more likely to experience cardiovascular events at 10 months (RR 6.00 (95% CI 2.40 to 14.83)) compared to those with high GRACE score-low BNP (RR 2.40 (95% CI 0.76 to 7.56)).

Conclusion.—In ACS, most but not all of our analyses suggest that BNP can predict cardiovascular events over and above the GRACE score. The combined use of both the GRACE score and BNP can identify a subset of ACS patients at particularly high risk. This implies that both the GRACE score and BNP reflect somewhat different risk attributes when predicting adverse prognosis in ACS and their synergistic use can enhance risk stratification in ACS to a small but potentially useful extent.

▶ With the advent of new therapeutic approaches for the treatment of patients with acute coronary syndrome (ACS), the need for risk stratification is becoming increasingly important, especially to guide key management decisions. Recently, several risk scores have been developed to enable risk stratification on admission. The thrombolysis in myocardial infarction (TIMI) and platelet glycoprotein IIb/IIIa in unstable angina: Receptor Suppression Using Integrilin (PURSUIT) scores were developed with databases from large clinical trials of non-ST- segment Elevation -ACS (NSTE-ACS). The more recent Global Registry of Acute Coronary Events (GRACE) score represents patients across the entire spectrum of ACS and provides robust prediction of the cumulative 6-month risk of death or myocardial infarction (MI). Another widely acknowledged way of risk stratifying ACS patients that has gained much attention lately is the biomarker B-type natriuretic peptide (BNP): BNP and N-amino terminal fragment of the prohormone (NT proBNP) levels sampled up to 7 days after the onset of ACS has been shown to predict both short-term and long-term risk of death, reinfarctions, and new congestive heart failure (CHF). Previous studies have also demonstrated that BNP predicts mortality independent of certain elements of the GRACE score, such as age, ST deviation, and cardiac troponin. However, it is unknown how BNP and GRACE compare and whether adding BNP to the full GRACE score itself would enhance risk prediction in routine ACS patients. In this study, the authors sought to address this question. Most, but not all, of their analyses suggest that in a heterogeneous cohort of ACS patients, BNP predicts mortality and cardiovascular events over and above the GRACE score, which implies that BNP and GRACE reflect somewhat different risk attributes in ACS. In addition, they also demonstrated that both BNP and the GRACE score can be used synergistically to identify a subset of ACS patients who are at a particularly high risk of future cardiovascular events.

M. G. Bissell, MD, PhD, MPH

A modified low-cost colorimetric method for paracetamol (acetaminophen) measurement in plasma

Shihana F, Dissanayake D, Dargan P, et al (Univ of Peradeniya, Sri Lanka; NHS Foundation Trust, London, UK)
Clin Toxicol 48:42-46, 2010

Background.—Despite a significant increase in the number of patients with paracetamol poisoning in the developing world, plasma paracetamol assays are not widely available. The purpose of this study was to assess a low-cost modified colorimetric paracetamol assay that has the potential to be performed in small laboratories with restricted resources.

Methods.—The paracetamol assay used in this study was based on the Glynn and Kendal colorimetric method with a few modifications to decrease the production of nitrous gas and thereby reduce infrastructure costs. Preliminary validation studies were performed using spiked aqueous samples with known concentrations of paracetamol. Subsequently, the results from the colorimetric method for 114 stored clinical samples from patients with paracetamol poisoning were compared with those from the current gold-standard high-performance liquid chromatography method. A prospective survey, assessing the clinical use of the paracetamol assay, was performed on all patients with paracetamol poisoning attending the Peradeniya General Hospital, Sri Lanka, over a 10-month period.

Results.—The recovery study showed an excellent correlation ($r^2 > 0.998$) for paracetamol concentrations from 25 to 400 mg/L. The final yellow color was stable for at least 10 min at room temperature. There was also excellent correlation with the high-performance liquid chromatography method ($r^2 = 0.9758$). In the clinical cohort study, use of the antidote N-acetylcysteine was avoided in over a third of patients who had the plasma paracetamol concentration measured. The cost of consumables used per assay was $0.50 (US).

Conclusions.—This colorimetric paracetamol assay is reliable and accurate and can be performed rapidly, easily, and economically. Use of this assay in resource-poor clinical settings has the potential to have a significant clinical and economic impact on the management of paracetamol poisoning.

▶ Paracetamol (acetaminophen) is one of the most widely used analgesics/antipyretics worldwide. In patients presenting with paracetamol overdose, the current standard of care is to undertake a risk assessment based on measurement of the plasma paracetamol concentration and to compare this with a nomogram to establish the need for antidote treatment with N-acetylcysteine. In some circumstances, such as the absence of an assay service, risk assessment can be made on the history of the ingested dose; however, this generally leads to overtreatment of many patients who are at low risk of hepatotoxicity as there is a poor correlation between patients stated ingested dose of paracetamol and paracetamol concentration. In Sri Lanka, the incidence of paracetamol poisoning gradually increased over 5 years (2004-2008) from 2.8% to 6.4% (95% confidence interval = 2.3-4.9; $P < .001$). Although pesticide poisoning remains more common, paracetamol is now the most common drug in patients presenting with self-poisoning. Paracetamol poisoning is becoming more common in other areas of South Asia such as Nepal. In Sri Lanka and other areas of South Asia, laboratory facilities to determine plasma paracetamol concentrations are only available in a few private laboratories. As paracetamol assays are not widely available, risk assessment in patients presenting with paracetamol poisoning is based on the history of the dose ingested, and this results in a significant proportion of individuals having unnecessary treatment with the antidote. The plasma paracetamol concentration is also important in patients admitted with paracetamol poisoning with an uncertain history and/or in individuals who have coingested agents that cause drowsiness. The aim of this study was to assess and validate a low-cost colorimetric paracetamol assay that has the potential to be performed in small laboratories with restricted resources and to look at its impact on the management of a cohort of patients with paracetamol poisoning.

M. G. Bissell, MD, PhD, MPH

A Recipe for Proteomics Diagnostic Test Development: The OVA1 Test, from Biomarker Discovery to FDA Clearance

Fung ET (Vermillion, Inc, Fremont, CA)
Clin Chem 56:327-329, 2010

Background.—New technologies may be helpful in identifying biomarkers to facilitate the development of clinically relevant diagnostic tests. A recipe was developed to combine the basic ingredients of clinical research with appropriate analytical tools in the development of the OVA1 test.

Process.—Unmet clinical need was identified as the most important ingredient. Clinician surveys revealed an appropriate unmet clinical need. Biomarkers were then identified, relative to quality clinical samples and choice of technology. The last piece was a regulatory strategy. With these pieces in place, a multicenter clinical trial was conducted and the data used to develop a diagnostic tool.

Results.—The unmet clinical need related to ovarian tumor triage. Ovarian tumors are relatively common but few are malignant. Identifying malignant ones before surgery allows better preoperative management of all women and beneficial referral to specialist surgeons for women highly likely to have a malignancy. The latter group could then have the debulking and staging surgeries that optimally address ovarian tumors.

SELDI-TOF mass spectrometry has a throughput allowing hundreds of clinical samples to be assessed and was chosen for this quality. Clinical history was attached to the samples along with documentation of the handling history. Relatively large retrospective studies from multiple institutions were initially used to mitigate variations in analytical and clinical quality. Biomarkers identified from these sources were better than cancer antigen 125 (CA125) for detecting early-stage ovarian cancer. A mega-study of over 600 individuals from several institutions helped refine the biomarker search, eventually showing a combination of markers could discriminate between benign and malignant tumors. These markers were validated using samples obtained worldwide.

US Food and Drug Administration (FDA) clearance was chosen as the regulatory strategy for the test. Among the sites for the multicenter clinical trial were women's health clinics, primary care centers, and several academic medical centers where ovarian tumors are typically analyzed. This trial allowed independent validation of a specific marker algorithm in a prospective, real-life clinical setting. Both clinical and analytical data were required for the FDA submission. Application of the SELDI assays showed that the reproducibility of the platform was inadequate for routine clinical settings. Immunoassays for several components were run on a training set of data, with new prospective samples obtained to validate the assay. The immunoassays were better than the SELDI-based assays both clinically and in relation to analytical-performance metrics.

Conclusions.—The result of these efforts is an ovarian tumor triage test that can be combined with clinical assessment, including imaging and physical examination, to yield a sensitivity exceeding 90% and a negative predictive value of 90% in women with an ovarian tumor for whom surgery is planned. The score for the OVA1 test ranges from 0 to 10, with cutoffs of 5.0 for premenopausal women and 4.4 for postmenopausal women. The likelihood of malignancy is increased in women whose scores exceed these cutoff values. The final ovarian tumor triage test can assist physicians in deciding which patients should be referred to a gynecologic oncologist because they are highly likely to have a malignant tumor.

▶ Although diagnostic test development remains challenging, novel technologies, including proteomics, genomics, and microRNA analysis, provide opportunities to identify biomarkers that in principle could accelerate the development of new diagnostic tests. Unfortunately, the literature is littered with initial biomarker discoveries that have failed to reach the clinic. The authors sought to identify a recipe that combines the basic ingredients of clinical research with novel analytical tools to create a new diagnostic test. In their test kitchen, they understood that the most important ingredient is the unmet clinical need. Having made the decision to develop a test for ovarian cancer, they discussed with clinicians what they felt were the most pressing needs in this field. Their initial instinct was to pursue ovarian cancer screening, but in conversations with key opinion leaders, including Ian Jacobs (University College London), Bob Bast (MD Anderson), and Daniel Chan (Johns Hopkins University), they came to understand that because of the low prevalence of ovarian cancer, development of a screening test would require large studies that would exceed budget and time constraints. Additionally, because a positive initial result in a screening test would likely lead to pelvic surgery, the test would demand a level of clinical specificity that they were unlikely to achieve. However, their colleagues identified a critical unmet need in the area of ovarian tumor triage. Although ovarian tumors are relatively common, only a fraction of them are malignant. Being able to identify the malignant ones preoperatively would permit better preoperative management of women with ovarian tumors. In particular, women with a high likelihood of malignancy could benefit from referral to specialist surgeons (eg, gynecologic oncologists) who would be able to perform debulking and staging surgeries that form the basis of optimal care for ovarian cancer. Having identified the clinical question, they set about turning their attention to the identification of biomarkers. Numerous technologies exist for biomarker discovery, each with inherent advantages and disadvantages. These are examined in the article.

M. G. Bissell, MD, PhD, MPH

A Sensitive Cardiac Troponin T Assay in Stable Coronary Artery Disease

Omland T, for the Prevention of Events with Angiotensin Converting Enzyme Inhibition (PEACE) Trial Investigators (Akershus Univ Hosp, Lørenskog, Norway; et al)
N Engl J Med 361:2538-2547, 2009

Background.—In most patients with stable coronary artery disease, plasma cardiac troponin T levels are below the limit of detection for the conventional assay. The distribution and determinants of very low circulating troponin T levels, as well as their association with cardiovascular events, in such patients are unknown.

Methods.—We used a new, high-sensitivity assay to determine the concentration of cardiac troponin T in plasma samples from 3679 patients with stable coronary artery disease and preserved left ventricular function. Results of the assay were analyzed in relation to the incidence of cardiovascular events during a median follow-up period of 5.2 years.

Results.—With the highly sensitive assay, concentrations of cardiac troponin T were at or above the limit of detection (0.001 μg per liter) in 3593 patients (97.7%) and at or above the 99th percentile for apparently healthy subjects (0.0133 μg per liter) in 407 patients (11.1%). After adjustment for other independent prognostic indicators, there was a strong and graded increase in the cumulative incidence of cardiovascular death (adjusted hazard ratio per unit increase in the natural logarithm of the troponin T level, 2.09; 95% confidence interval [CI], 1.60 to 2.74; $P < 0.001$) and of heart failure (adjusted hazard ratio, 2.20; 95% CI, 1.66 to 2.90; $P < 0.001$) in this study group. Increased risk associated with higher levels of troponin T was evident well below the limit of detection of conventional cardiac troponin T assays and below the 99th percentile of values in a healthy population. There was no association between troponin T levels as measured with the highly sensitive assay and the incidence of myocardial infarction (adjusted hazard ratio, 1.16; 95% CI, 0.97 to 1.40; $P = 0.11$).

Conclusions.—After adjustment for other independent prognostic indicators, cardiac troponin T concentrations as measured with a highly sensitive assay were significantly associated with the incidence of cardiovascular death and heart failure but not with myocardial infarction in patients with stable coronary artery disease (Fig 2).

▶ Cardiac troponins T and I are components of the contractile apparatus of cardiomyocytes and are the preferred biochemical markers of myocardial necrosis in patients with suspected acute coronary syndromes. Among such patients, a strong association between elevated troponin levels and recurrent coronary ischemic events has been firmly established. It has been shown that even very small elevations in troponins are associated with an increased risk of an adverse outcome in patients with acute coronary syndromes. Moreover, among men clinically free of cardiovascular disease and in patients with recent

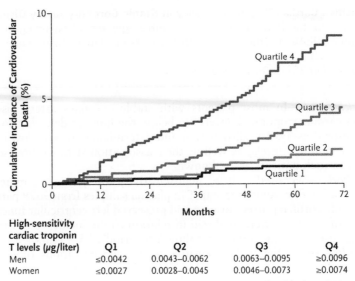

High-sensitivity cardiac troponin T levels (µg/liter)	Q1	Q2	Q3	Q4
Men	≤0.0042	0.0043–0.0062	0.0063–0.0095	≥0.0096
Women	≤0.0027	0.0028–0.0045	0.0046–0.0073	≥0.0074

FIGURE 2.—Incidence of cardiovascular death according to quartile of high-sensitivity cardiac troponin T level. (Reprinted from Omland T, for the Prevention of Events with Angiotensin Converting Enzyme Inhibition (PEACE) Trial Investigators. A sensitive cardiac troponin T assay in stable coronary artery disease. *N Engl J Med*. 2009;361:2538-2547. Copyright 2009, with permission from Massachusetts Medical Society. All rights reserved.)

acute coronary syndromes, levels of cardiac troponin greater than 0.01 microgram per liter have been associated with increased mortality. Thus, it seems plausible that cardiac troponin levels below the conventional limits of detection may further discriminate between subjects at high risk and those at low risk for future cardiovascular events. A highly sensitive assay for cardiac troponin T has recently been developed, permitting measurement of concentrations that are lower by a factor of 10 than those measurable with conventional assays. The authors hypothesized that with the highly sensitive assay, cardiac troponin T would be detectable in patients who had stable coronary artery disease without heart failure or left ventricular systolic dysfunction and that these levels would be associated with the risk of future cardiovascular events (Fig 2).

M. G. Bissell, MD, PhD, MPH

Association of Very Highly Elevated C-Reactive Protein Concentration with Cardiovascular Events and All-Cause Mortality

Hamer M, Chida Y, Stamatakis E (Univ College London, UK)
Clin Chem 56:132-135, 2010

Background.—The clinical relevance of very highly increased high-sensitivity C-reactive protein (hsCRP) concentrations (>10 mg/L) is incompletely understood. We examined the association between very highly increased hsCRP and risk of incident cardiovascular disease (CVD) events and all-cause mortality.

Methods.—We recruited 5248 participants free from overt CVD and acute infection [mean age 53.5 (SD 12.4) years, 55.5% women] from the Scottish Health Survey, a representative sample of communitydwelling adults. hsCRP and other conventional risk factors were measured at baseline.

Results.—Over an average of 7 years' follow-up, there were a total of 259 incident CVD events (including myocardial infarction, coronary artery bypass, percutaneous coronary angioplasty, stroke, heart failure) and 357 all-cause deaths. Very highly increased hsCRP was associated with CVD events after adjustment for Framingham risk score (FRS), body mass index (BMI), central obesity, and hormone replacement therapy (HRT) (hazard ratio 2.40, 95% CI 1.51–3.81) and also with all-cause death (hazard ratio 3.64, 95% CI 2.57–5.15). With the addition of CRP scores to the conventional Framingham model, 7.4% of participants were reclassified into a high-risk (>20% FRS) CVD category. Very highly increased hsCRP was also associated with several modifiable risk factors, including smoking, HDL cholesterol, and central obesity.

Conclusions.—hsCRP > 10 mg/L was a stronger predictor of clinical events than a conventional cut point of 3 mg/L. Very highly increased hsCRP may provide clinically meaningful prognostic information.

▶ The utility of high-sensitivity C-reactive protein (hsCRP) as a disease biomarker, especially in relation to cardiovascular disease (CVD) risk, has been extensively studied. Debate continues about the clinical utility of different hsCRP cut points. A hsCRP concentration of 3 to 10 mg/L has been established to identify high-risk individuals, although the relevance of very highly increased hsCRP concentrations (> 10 mg/L) is incompletely understood: some physicians consider it to represent nonspecific inflammation and therefore to lack positive predictive value. Data from the Women's Health Study demonstrated that very high concentrations of hsCRP (> 10 mg/L) provided important prognostic information on CVD risk, although these findings were not replicated in the Framingham Offspring Study. The aim of this study was to examine the association between very highly increased hsCRP (> 10 mg/L) and risk of CVD events and all-cause mortality. For these analyses, the authors used data from the Scottish Health Survey (SHS), which is a periodic survey (typically every 3-5 years) that draws a nationally representative sample of the general population living in households. They combined data from the 1998 and 2003 SHS in adults aged 30 to 95 years old, as described. The surveys were linked to a patient-based database of CVD hospital admissions and deaths (Information Services Division, Edinburgh, Scotland) to perform prospective analyses on CVD events. Participants gave full informed consent to participate in the study, and ethics approval was obtained from the London Research Ethics Council. The SHS is funded by the Scottish Executive, although the funders had no role in the study design; the collection, analysis, and interpretation of data; the writing of the report; or the decision to submit the article for publication. Survey interviewers visited eligible households and collected data on basic demographics. On a separate visit, nurses collected clinical information to calculate individual Framingham risk scores for first CVD events based on sex-specific multivariable risk functions including age, total and high-density lipoprotein cholesterol, systolic blood pressure, treatment for hypertension, smoking, and diabetes status. In addition, height and weight were measured for the calculation of body mass index and waist circumference for estimating central obesity (defined as ≥102 cm in men and ≥88 cm women).

M. G. Bissell, MD, PhD, MPH

National Academy of Clinical Biochemistry Laboratory Medicine Practice Guidelines for Use of Tumor Markers in Liver, Bladder, Cervical, and Gastric Cancers
Sturgeon CM, Duffy MJ, Hofmann BR, et al (Royal Infirmary of Edinburgh, UK; St Vincent's Univ Hosp, Dublin, Ireland; Univ of Toronto, Ontario, Canada; et al)
Clin Chem 56:e1-e48, 2010

Background.—Updated National Academy of Clinical Biochemistry Laboratory Medicine Practice Guidelines for the use of tumor markers in the clinic have been developed.

Methods.—Published reports relevant to use of tumor markers for 4 cancer sites—liver, bladder, cervical, and gastric—were critically reviewed.

Results.—α-Fetoprotein (AFP) may be used in conjunction with abdominal ultrasound for early detection of hepatocellular carcinoma (HCC) in patients with chronic hepatitis or cirrhosis associated with hepatitis B or C virus infection. AFP concentrations >200 μg/L in cirrhotic patients with typical hypervascular lesions >2 cm in size are consistent with HCC. After a diagnosis of HCC, posttreatment monitoring with AFP is recommended as an adjunct to imaging, especially in the absence of measurable disease.

Although several urine markers have been proposed for bladder cancer, none at present can replace routine cystoscopy and cytology in the management of patients with this malignancy. Some may, however, be used as complementary adjuncts to direct more effective use of clinical procedures.

Although carcinoembryonic antigen and CA 19-9 have been proposed for use gastric cancer and squamous cell carcinoma antigen for use in cervical cancer, none of these markers can currently be recommended for routine clinical use.

Conclusions.—Implementation of these recommendations should encourage optimal use of tumor markers for patients with liver, bladder, cervical, or gastric cancers.

▶ The authors present here to clinical chemists, clinicians, and other practitioners of laboratory and clinical medicine the latest update of the National Academy of Clinical Biochemistry (NACB) Laboratory Medicine Practice Guidelines for the use of tumor markers in liver, bladder, cervical, and gastric cancers. These guidelines are intended to encourage more appropriate use of tumor marker tests by primary care physicians, hospital physicians and surgeons, specialist oncologists, and other health professionals. Clinical practice guidelines are systematically developed statements intended to assist practitioners and patients in making decisions about appropriate health care for specific clinical circumstances. An explanation of the methods used when developing these guidelines has previously been published. As might be expected, many of the NACB recommendations are similar to those made by other groups, as is made clear from the tabular comparisons presented for each malignancy. The disciplines of all authors and statements of conflicts of interest, declared according to NACB requirements, are provided as required by *Clinical Chemistry*. All comments received about these guidelines, together with responses to these comments, are also recorded in the Comments Received Table in the Data Supplement that accompanies the online version of this report at http://www.clinchem.org/content/vol56/issue6. To prepare these guidelines, the literature relevant to the use of tumor markers was reviewed. Particular attention was given to reviews, including the few relevant systematic reviews, and to guidelines issued by expert panels. If possible, the consensus recommendations of the NACB panels reported here were based on available evidence, ie, were evidence based. NACB recommendations relating to general quality requirements for tumor marker measurements, including tabulation of important causes of false-positive tumor marker results that must also be taken into account (eg, heterophilic antibody interference, high-dose hooking) have previously been published. The conclusions are that alpha-fetoprotein (AFP) may be used in conjunction with abdominal ultrasound for early detection of hepatocellular carcinoma (HCC) in patients with chronic hepatitis or cirrhosis associated with hepatitis B or C virus infection. AFP concentrations > 200 µg/L in cirrhotic patients with typical hypervascular lesions > 2 cm in size are consistent with HCC. After a diagnosis of HCC, posttreatment monitoring with AFP is recommended as an adjunct to imaging, especially in the absence of measurable disease. Although several urine markers have been proposed for bladder cancer, none at present can replace routine cystoscopy and cytology in the management of patients with this malignancy. However, some may be used as complementary adjuncts to direct more effective use of clinical procedures. Although carcinoembryonic antigen and carbohydrate antigen 19-9 have been proposed for use in gastric cancer and squamous cell carcinoma antigen for use in cervical cancer, none of these markers can currently be recommended for routine clinical use.

M. G. Bissell, MD, PhD, MPH

Use of Cerebrospinal Fluid Biomarkers for Diagnosis of Incipient Alzheimer Disease in Patients with Mild Cognitive Impairment
Dean RA, Shaw LM (Eli Lilly and Company, Indianapolis, IN; Univ of Pennsylvania Med Ctr, Philadelphia)
Clin Chem 56:7-9, 2010

Background.—Alzheimer disease (AD) causes dementia in about 5.3 million people in the United States and about 35 million worldwide. Definitive diagnosis has only been possible postmortem, with antemortem diagnosis based on clinical symptoms, most of which are not specific to AD. Various clinical-, imaging-, and laboratory-based methods are being studied to determine which could not only distinguish AD from non-AD dementia but also permit the identification of asymptomatic persons and those whose mild cognitive impairment (MCI) is likely to develop into AD. Among these methods is the measurement of cerebrospinal fluid (CSF) concentrations of total tau (t-tau) and tau phosphorylated at threonine 181 (P-tau$_{181}$) to detect neuronal degeneration and the determination of CSF levels of a 42 amino acid isoform of amyloid (Aβ_{1-42}). Several studies show that combining these three assays can pinpoint persons who have clinically and pathologically diagnosed AD and identify persons with no symptoms or MCI that may progress to AD. A recent study confirmed the usefulness of these three CSF markers to detect incipient AD pathology and predict the risk for progression to dementia. It was limited by a lack of standardized clinical protocol for diagnosing MCI and for CSF collection, use of various immunoassay procedures with no external quality control or transformational procedures across laboratories, and a short 2-year follow-up period before classifying MCI persons as stable or progressing to AD.

Significance.—The study is significant because the results confirm that AD can be diagnosed biochemically long before clinical symptoms develop. In addition, using the three CSF biomarkers will improve the power of future prospective clinical trials by providing increased diagnostic certainty. Finally, detecting incipient AD early may improve the feasibility of secondary or primary prevention trials of various therapies for MCI patients or others with worrisome conditions.

Recommendations.—To achieve reliability of CSF measurements and biomarker assays, it was recommended that the lumbar puncture (LP) be done in the morning after an overnight fast to avoid diurnal variations and food intake effects. A small-gauge needle is recommended, and the technique should minimize the risk of meningeal tears, post-LP headache, and contamination of the CSF specimen. Polypropylene CSF collection and aliquot tubes will avoid surface interactions and variable loss of the biomarkers. Samples should be frozen at $-80\ °C$ quickly after collection. There should be well-characterized reference materials to standardize assays, optimize the analytical performance of commercially obtained immunoassay platforms and reagents, and minimize matrix interactions. Method-specific reference intervals or cutoffs are also suggested to account for variables such as age, gender, and education. To make tests more widely available, the access to LP must be increased, which will require changing the attitudes of physicians and the public toward the use of "spinal taps."

Conclusions.—The study recommends the standardization of CSF collection and handling procedures as well as analytic assays for the three CSF biomarkers. External proficiency programs are also recommended to ensure consistent performance across the various laboratories and time.

▶ Alzheimer disease (AD) is the most common cause of dementia. In the United States, AD is the sixth leading cause of death in Americans aged 65 years or older. In the United States, AD affects an estimated 5.3 million people and is expected to afflict approximately 35 million people worldwide by 2010. The global health economic impact of AD-related dementia is predicted to overwhelm social services in coming decades as a consequence of demographic aging. Definitive diagnosis of AD at postmortem examination of the brain reveals gross and microscopic evidence of neuronal atrophy and the presence of 2 histological hallmarks: amyloid β (Aβ)-containing plaques and neurofibrillary tangles. Antemortem diagnosis is based on the presence and progressive worsening of clinical symptoms. Clinical diagnosis is challenging because other causes of dementia are often difficult to differentiate from AD. Accordingly, researchers are actively evaluating a variety of clinical-, imaging-, and laboratory-based methods to distinguish AD and non-AD dementia through antemortem detection of AD pathology. These methods include MRI to quantify brain atrophy, fluorodeoxyglucose-positron emission tomography to characterize loss of metabolic function, positron emission tomography and single photon emission computed tomography to define amyloid plaque burden, measurement of cerebrospinal fluid (CSF) concentrations of total tau (t-tau) and tau phosphorylated at threonine181 (P-tau$_{181}$) to detect neuronal degeneration, and measurement of a 42-amino acid isoform of Aβ (Aβ$_{1-42}$) in CSF to detect abnormal trafficking of this peptide present in amyloid plaque. Several studies, including the Alzheimer's Disease Neuroimaging Initiative (ADNI), have provided compelling evidence that CSF t-tau, P-tau$_{181}$, and Aβ$_{1-42}$ measurements can identify individuals with clinically and pathologically diagnosed AD. Moreover, these studies suggest that these 3 CSF biomarkers can identify asymptomatic individuals and patients with mild cognitive impairment (MCI) likely to progress to AD. In a new study involving 750 patients with MCI, it has been demonstrated that biochemical evidence of incipient AD pathology based on measurements of CSF Aβ$_{1-42}$, t-tau, and P-tau$_{181}$ does indeed detect incipient AD pathology and predict the risk for progression to AD dementia.

M. G. Bissell, MD, PhD, MPH

Use of Saliva-Based Nano-Biochip Tests for Acute Myocardial Infarction at the Point of Care: A Feasibility Study

Floriano PN, Christodoulides N, Miller CS, et al (Univ of Texas at Austin; College of Dentistry Univ of Kentucky, Lexington; et al)
Clin Chem 55:1530-1538, 2009

Background.—For adults with chest pain, the electrocardiogram (ECG) and measures of serum biomarkers are used to screen and diagnose myocardial necrosis. These measurements require time that can delay therapy and affect prognosis. Our objective was to investigate the feasibility and utility of saliva as an alternative diagnostic fluid for identifying biomarkers of acute myocardial infarction (AMI).

Methods.—We used Luminex and lab-on-a-chip methods to assay 21 proteins in serum and unstimulated whole saliva procured from 41 AMI patients within 48 h of chest pain onset and from 43 apparently healthy controls. Data were analyzed by use of logistic regression and area under curve (AUC) for ROC analysis to evaluate the diagnostic utility of each biomarker, or combinations of biomarkers, in screening for AMI.

Results.—Both established and novel cardiac biomarkers demonstrated significant differences in concentrations between patients with AMI and controls without AMI. The saliva-based biomarker panel of C-reactive protein, myoglobin, and myeloperoxidase exhibited significant diagnostic capability (AUC = 0.85, $P < 0.0001$) and in conjunction with ECG yielded strong screening capacity for AMI (AUC = 0.96) comparable to that of the panel (brain natriuretic peptide, troponin-I, creatine kinase-MB, myoglobin; AUC = 0.98) and far exceeded the screening capacity of ECG alone (AUC approximately 0.6). En route to translating these findings to clinical practice, we adapted these unstimulated whole saliva tests to a novel lab-on-a-chip platform for proof-of-principle screens for AMI.

Conclusions.—Complementary to ECG, saliva-based tests within lab-on-a-chip systems may provide a convenient and rapid screening method for cardiac events in prehospital stages for AMI patients.

▶ Oral fluid assays have not yet been reported for the diagnosis of acute myocardial infarction (AMI). Furthermore, little is known about the salivary biomarker expression levels for the various cardiac indications. One challenge associated with oral fluids is that biomarker concentrations are often significantly lower than in serum counterparts, making measurement more challenging with traditional analytical approaches. Through the last decade, the authors' team has made sustained efforts to combine and adapt lab-on-a-chip (LaC), micro fluidic, microelectromechanical systems, and nano biochip tools for practical implementation of highly sensitive and accurate miniaturized sensors that are suitable for a variety of important applications, including multiplex analysis of minute amounts of bioanalytes in serum and saliva. These integrated test systems can complete all aspects of sample processing and separation and analyte detection, and are amenable to point-of-care (POC) applications. Chemically sensitized bead microreactors within the LaC system were recently applied for measurement of C-reactive protein (CRP) and other biomarkers of inflammation in saliva, demonstrating significantly lower detection level (by > 3 decade orders of magnitude) for CRP than high-sensitivity CRP ELISA methods, allowing for measurement of inflammatory biomarkers related to select disease states. The authors report here for the first time the measurement of salivary biomarkers associated with AMI and explore the possibility of using these new salivary biomarkers in novel nano biochip ensembles for screening chest pain patients for AMI. Their initial objective was to determine if serum biomarkers commonly associated with AMI diagnosis can be detected reliably using unstimulated whole saliva (UWS). Persons who did not have chest pain were recruited as controls for the first part of this study to demonstrate feasibility of measuring protein concentrations of both standard and novel biomarkers in saliva and serum. Choice of this control group was expected to amplify potential differences between salivary samples of AMI and non-AMI patients and thus allow for more efficient identification of potential biomarkers for use in subsequent larger studies.

M. G. Bissell, MD, PhD, MPH

Utility of Urine Myoglobin for the Prediction of Acute Renal Failure in Patients with Suspected Rhabdomyolysis: A Systematic Review

Rodríguez-Capote K, Balion CM, Hill SA, et al (McMaster Univ, Hamilton, Ontario, Canada)

Clin Chem 55.2190-2197, 2009

Background.—Urine myoglobin continues to be used as a marker of rhabdomyolysis, particularly to assess risk of developing acute renal failure and evaluate treatment success. We sought to determine the predictive validity of urine myoglobin (uMb) for acute renal failure (ARF) in patients with suspected rhabdomyolysis.

Methods.—We performed a broad systemic review of the literature from January 1980 to December 2006 using the search terms myoglobin$ AND (renal OR ARF OR kidney). Only primary studies published in English where uMb measurement was related to ARF were included.

Results.—Of 1602 studies screened, 52 met all selection criteria. The studies covered a wide spectrum of etiologies for rhabdomyolysis, dissimilar diagnostic criteria for ARF and rhabdomyolysis, and various methods of uMb measurement and were mostly case series (n = 32). There was poor reporting on the uMb method, and 17 studies failed to provide any information about the method. The reporting of clinical criteria for ARF with respect to timing, description, performance, and interpretation also lacked adequate detail for replication. Eight studies (total 295 patients) had data for 2-by-2 tables. Sensitivity of the uMb test was 100% in 5 of the 8 studies, specificity varied widely (15% to 88%), and CIs around these measures were high. Pooling of data was not possible because of study heterogeneity.

Conclusions.—There is inadequate evidence evaluating the use of uMb as a predictor of ARF in patients with suspected rhabdomyolysis.

▶ Rhabdomyolysis is a clinical and laboratory syndrome resulting from the breakdown of muscle fibers with release of muscle cell contents into plasma. Myoglobin (Mb), a 17-kDa single-chain oxygen-carrying hemoprotein, appears in the circulation within a few hours of skeletal or cardiac muscle damage and is rapidly filtered by the glomeruli and reabsorbed by the proximal tubules where it is catabolized. When the filtered load exceeds the reabsorptive capacity of the tubule, Mb spills over into the urine, coloring it red. Rhabdomyolysis can occur by direct muscle injury, ischemia, excessive muscular activity, drugs and toxins, infection, inflammatory myopathies, electrolyte and endocrine/ metabolic disorders, hereditary disorders, and temperature extremes. The complication of rhabdomyolysis is acute renal failure (ARF), and depending on the severity and duration of the renal dysfunction, it can lead to chronic renal failure, damage to the heart or nervous system, and death. The pathophysiology of Mb-induced ARF has not been fully elucidated, but 3 major mechanisms have been proposed, the combination of which contributes to the overall renal damage. One mechanism is physical obstruction of the renal tubule by Mb precipitation in association with Tamm-Horsfall protein under acidic conditions. Urate precipitation may also occur, which together leads to intraluminal casts, increased intratubular pressure, and subsequently decreased glomerular filtration rate. A second mechanism occurs via the heme group of Mb, which can enhance renal vasoconstriction and ischemia through activation of the cytokine cascade. The third proposed mechanism is oxidant injury through heme-induced reactive oxygen species, such as superoxide anion, hydrogen peroxide, or hydroxyl radicals, provoking direct oxidative damage to the renal tissue. To prevent the complication of ARF in cases of rhabdomyolysis, prophylactic treatment with mannitol, sodium bicarbonate, and fluids is given. The decision to treat is based on whether the patient is at risk of developing ARF; knowledge of the presence of urine Mb (uMb) may be helpful in making this decision. Several reviews and commentaries suggest that measurement of uMb is not helpful and should not be used owing to issues of Mb instability and poor test methodologies. Historically, the measurement of uMb was cumbersome and inaccurate. These early methods took advantage of the pseudo peroxidase activity of the heme moiety in Mb but required complete removal of hemoglobin in the urine, which was difficult to achieve. The development of immunometric assays for Mb allowed more specific measurement and the potential for better predictive ability, such as in establishing a cut point for development of ARF. Despite this method development, the older, less-specific methods continue to be used. To assess whether the measurement of uMb, by any method, aids the prediction of ARF in individuals suspected of having rhabdomyolysis, the authors conducted a systematic review of the literature.

M. G. Bissell, MD, PhD, MPH

17 Clinical Microbiology

A Mouse Model of Lethal Synergism Between Influenza Virus and Haemophilus influenzae

Lee LN, Dias P, Han D, et al (Torrey Pines Inst for Molecular Studies, San Diego, CA; et al)

Am J Pathol 176:800-811, 2010

Secondary bacterial infections that follow infection with influenza virus result in considerable morbidity and mortality in young children, the elderly, and immunocompromised individuals and may also significantly increase mortality in normal healthy adults during influenza pandemics. We herein describe a mouse model for investigating the interaction between influenza virus and the bacterium *Haemophilus influenzae*. Sequential infection with sublethal doses of influenza and *H. influenzae* resulted in synergy between the two pathogens and caused mortality in immunocompetent adult wild-type mice. Lethality was dependent on the interval between administration of the bacteria and virus, and bacterial growth was prolonged in the lungs of dual-infected mice, although influenza virus titers were unaffected. Dual infection induced severe damage to the airway epithelium and confluent pneumonia, similar to that observed in victims of the 1918 global influenza pandemic. Increased bronchial epithelial cell death was observed as early as 1 day after bacterial inoculation in the dual-infected mice. Studies using knockout mice indicated that lethality occurs via a mechanism that is not dependent on Fas, CCR2, CXCR3, interleukin-6, tumor necrosis factor, or Toll-like receptor-4 and does not require T or B cells. This model suggests that infection with virulent strains of influenza may predispose even immunocompetent individuals to severe illness on secondary infection with *H. influenzae* by a mechanism that involves innate immunity, but does not require tumor necrosis factor, interleukin-6, or signaling via Toll-like receptor-4.

▶ Infections with influenza virus cause mild to severe respiratory illness and may result in death in vulnerable human populations. On average, influenza causes 3 to 5 million cases of severe illness per year worldwide and over 200 000 hospitalizations and 36 000 deaths in the United States alone. Five percent to 20% of the US population is infected annually. While healthy adults typically experience only acute uncomplicated infection, influenza virus predisposes the lungs to bacterial coinfections, which cause significant additional morbidity, particularly in young children and elderly and immunocompromised individuals. Secondary bacterial infections may also significantly increase mortality in the population as a whole during influenza pandemics. For example, in the 1918 influenza pandemic, which killed approximately 50 million people worldwide, while infection with the virus alone could be lethal, most deaths appeared to result from secondary bacterial pneumonia. The most common bacterial agents mediating such secondary infections in the United States are *Streptococcus pneumoniae*, *Staphylococcus aureus*, and *Haemophilus influenzae*. *H influenzae* is a small Gram-negative coccobacillus that exists in capsulated or noncapsulated forms. *H influenzae* is a common cause of otitis media, acute sinusitis, bronchitis, pneumonia, and exacerbations of chronic obstructive pulmonary disease. A vaccine against *H influenzae* type b (Hib) has greatly reduced the incidence of invasive disease, such as meningitis, caused by this organism in children 5 years or younger. However, Hib invasive disease in children remains a problem in countries where the vaccine is not widely available. Furthermore, other encapsulated and nontypable *H influenzae* (NTHi) forms are increasing in frequency as causes of illness in young children. During the 1918 influenza pandemic, *H influenzae* was often isolated from the autopsied lungs of young adults, a subpopulation who do not usually die from influenza infection. Influenza also increases the susceptibility of newborn rats to *H influenzae*-induced meningitis and synergizes with the bacteria in the development of otitis media in the chinchilla. To investigate the pathobiological mechanisms further, the authors established a model of influenza and *H influenzae* coinfection in mice. Herein, they report that *H influenzae* synergizes with influenza virus to cause more severe disease in immunocompetent adult mice, leading to 100% lethality at doses that cause no mortality when the agents are given individually. The mechanism leading to disease exacerbation does not involve T- or B-cells and thus appears to be mediated by innate immunity. However, tumor necrosis factor, interleukin-6, and Toll-like receptor-4 are not essential for synergistic lethality in this model.

M. G. Bissell, MD, PhD, MPH

Abundance of Multiple High-Risk Human Papillomavirus (HPV) Infections Found in Cervical Cells Analyzed by Use of an Ultrasensitive HPV Genotyping Assay
Schmitt M, Dondog B, Waterboer T, et al (German Cancer Res Ctr (DKFZ), Heidelberg, Germany; et al)
J Clin Microbiol 48:143-149, 2010

PCR methods enable the detection of a large variety of human papillomavirus (HPV) genotypes that infect the anogenital tract. However, PCR with consensus primers, general primers, and, to a lesser extent, broad-spectrum primers may underrepresent the true prevalence of HPV, especially the true prevalence of multiple infections. We compared the rate of HPV positivity determined by a broad-spectrum PCR with primers BSGP5+ and BSGP6+ (BS-PCR) coupled to an established bead-based multiplex HPV genotyping (MPG) assay with the rate of HPV positivity determined by a multiplex PCR with type-specific primers (TS-PCR) coupled to a newly developed MPG assay for 735 selected cervical scraping samples. While the primers used for the BS-PCR are located within the L1 region of the HPV genome, the primers used for the TS-PCR target the E7 gene. The overall rates of positivity for the 19 HPV types included in both assays were 60.9% and 72.2% by the BS-PCR and the TS-PCR, respectively, and the two assays found multiple infections in 34.8% and 58.0% of the specimens, respectively. Both HPV detection assays allowed the semiquantitative detection of HPV types and identified the same dominant HPV type in 66.6% of the multiple infections. In conclusion, the TS-PCR-MPG assay significantly increased the rate of detection of HPV DNA and the number of infections with multiple HPV types detected and demonstrated that the prevalence of low-copy-number HPV infections in the anogenital tract may be strongly underestimated by conventional HPV amplification methods, especially in cases of multiple infections. As a consequence, PCR-TS-MPG appears to be highly suited for analysis of the significance of multiple infections in the development of cervical cancer and for the study the natural history and the latency of HPV.

▶ Human papillomaviruses (HPVs) are DNA viruses that infect cutaneous and mucosal epithelia. Until now, approximately 100 HPV genotypes have been fully characterized on the basis of the isolation of complete genomes, and there is evidence that a larger number exists. There are approximately 45 known mucosal HPV types, and these are further divided into 3 groups on the basis of their epidemiological association with cervical cancer: high-risk HPV (Hr-HPV) types (types 16, 18, 31, 33, 35, 39, 45, 51, 52, 56, 58, 59, 68, 73, and 82), putative high-risk HPV (pHr-HPV) types (types 26, 53, and 66), and low-risk HPV (Lr-HPV) types (types 6, 11, 40, 42, 43, 44, and 70). Hr-HPV types are causally associated with several malignant diseases, of which cervical cancer has particular significance, being the second most common cancer in women worldwide and is the main cancer of women in most developing countries. Hr-HPV type DNA has been detected in 99.7% of cervical cancer tissue specimens, and persistent infection with an oncogenic HPV type, particularly HPV type 16 (HPV-16) or HPV type 18 (HPV-18), is recognized as a necessary cause of cervical cancer. HPV genotyping is of importance for the study of the natural history of infections with one or several HPV types and the role of HPV persistence in the progression of cervical lesions and/or the monitoring of vaccine efficacy. Among HPV-positive women, 20% to 40% harbor in their cervices at least 2 types that were acquired simultaneously or successively. It remains controversial whether an infection with multiple types (referred here as a multiple infection) is a risk factor for the persistence of HPV and for cervical lesions. Moreover, it remains unknown whether women with quadruple infections, for example, are at higher risk than women with double infections. Interest in multiple HPV infections has recently increased as prophylactic vaccines against HPV types 6, 11, 16, and 18 are expected to also provide partial protection against related HPV types by cross-neutralizing antibodies. Therefore, it is important to accurately type all HPV infections present in 1 patient. It will also be of particular interest to study the long-term impact of vaccination on the established equilibrium in the distribution of HPV types within immunized populations. Therefore, the sensitive, reliable, and unbiased profiling of the individual HPV types in patients with multiple infections is important in order to learn more about the natural history of HPV and to evaluate the effect of HPV vaccination.

M. G. Bissell, MD, PhD, MPH

C. Diff Quik Chek Complete Enzyme Immunoassay Provides a Reliable First-Line Method for Detection of *Clostridium difficile* in Stool Specimens
Quinn CD, Sefers SE, Babiker W, et al (Vanderbilt Univ School of Medicine, Nashville, TN; Johns Hopkins Univ School of Medicine, Baltimore, MD)
J Clin Microbiol 48:603-605, 2010

We evaluated a single membrane device assay for simultaneously detecting both *Clostridium difficile* glutamate dehydrogenase (GDH) and toxin A/B antigens against a standard that combines two PCR assays and cytotoxigenic culture. Results showing dual GDH and toxin A/B antigen positives and negatives can be reported immediately as true positives and negatives, respectively. Specimens with discrepant results for GDH and toxins A/B, which comprised 13.2% of the specimens, need to be retested.

▶ Rapid and accurate diagnosis of *Clostridium difficile* infection (CDI) is crucial for patient care, infection control, and efficient surveillance. The well-accepted standard is cytotoxigenic culture, which is done by culturing *C difficile* from the stool and then performing a cytotoxin assay on the isolate. The cytotoxigenic culture is labor-intensive, subjective, and time-consuming, which has limited its wide use in the clinical setting. Enzyme immunoassays (EIAs) are the most common diagnostic laboratory methods used for rapid detection of *C difficile*-specific glutamate dehydrogenase (GDH) and/or toxin NB antigens in stool specimens. However, traditional EIAs lack sensitivity and specificity. Recently, a C. Diff Quik Chek Complete dual-antigen EIA (D-EIA; TechLab, Blacksburg, VA) became commercially available; this assay comprises rapid detection of both GDH antigen and toxin NB with one easy-to-use cartridge (Fig 1 in the original article). Previous studies based on 2 membrane-bound EIAs for GDH and toxins NB indicated that the single GDH testing was more sensitive than that for detection of *C difficile* toxins NB; however, false-positive results were recognized upon comparison with results for culture. It has been recommended that GDH be used as the first-line screening test, followed by cell culture for toxin testing. More than 700 000 patient visits occur each year, with approximately 35 000 patients being admitted at the Vanderbilt University Medical Center (VUMC). Approximately 9000 stool specimens were submitted for *C difficile* testing for the year 2008. Currently, the Premier toxin A and B EIA (NB EIA; Meridian Bioscience, Inc., Cincinnati, OH) is used in the clinical microbiology laboratory for detection of *C difficile* toxin in stool samples; this test uses a 96-well microtiter format to detect both toxins A and B. In this study, the authors validated the D-EIA in comparison to a standard that combines 2 polymerase chain reaction (PCR) assays and a cytotoxigenic culture. They did find that, while dual positive or negative results could be reported immediately, some 13% of the results were discrepant between GDH and toxin A/B antigen and needed to be repeated.

M. G. Bissell, MD, PhD, MPH

Comparison of PCR and Culture for Screening of Vancomycin-Resistant Enterococci: Highly Disparate Results for *vanA* and *vanB*

Mak A, Miller MA, Chong G, et al (McGill Univ Health Centre, Montreal, Quebec, Canada; Jewish General Hosp, Montreal, Quebec, Canada)
J Clin Microbiol 47:4136-4137, 2009

We compared PCR to conventional culture for the detection of vancomycin-resistant enterococci (VRE) in 30,835 rectal samples over a 3-year period. The positive and negative predictive values of *vanB* PCR were 1.42% and 99.9%, respectively. A positive *vanB* result by PCR is poorly predictive and necessitates culture for differentiation of VRE-positive and -negative individuals.

▶ Vancomycin-resistant enterococci (VRE) are multidrug-resistant colonizers of the gastrointestinal tract and have emerged as an important cause of nosocomial infections. Glycopeptide resistance is mediated by 6 different vancomycin resistance (Van) gene operons. *vanA* and *vanB* remain the most clinically relevant of the Van genes, as they are associated with transposons and may theoretically mediate horizontal transfer of vancomycin resistance to other organisms. Phenotypically, the *vanA* gene mediates high-level resistance to vancomycin and teicoplanin, while the *vanB* gene confers low to moderate-level resistance to vancomycin only. There are 3 subtypes of *vanB*: *vanB1*, *vanB2*, and *vanB3*. In addition to enterococci, the *vanB* genes have been described in a *Streptococcus mitis* strain isolated from blood and a *Streptococcus bovis* isolate as well as *Eggerthella lenta*, a Ruminococcus lactaris-like organism, and several *Clostridium* species isolated from human feces. The presence of *vanB*-containing organisms other than VRE in stool would decrease the specificity of VRE polymerase chain reaction (PCR) testing. In this study, the authors compared PCR with simultaneous selective culture for screening rectal swabs for VRE. They compared PCR with conventional culture for the detection of VRE in 30 835 rectal samples over a 3-year period. The positive and negative predictive values of *vanB* PCR were 1.42% and 99.9%, respectively. A positive *vanB* result by PCR is poorly predictive and necessitates culture for differentiation of VRE-positive and VRE-negative individuals.

M. G. Bissell, MD, PhD, MPH

Genomewide Association Study of Leprosy

Zhang F-R, Huang W, Chen S-M, et al (Shandong Provincial Inst of Dermatology and Venereology, Jinan, China)

N Engl J Med 361:2609-2618, 2009

Background.—The narrow host range of *Mycobacterium leprae* and the fact that it is refractory to growth in culture has limited research on and the biologic understanding of leprosy. Host genetic factors are thought to influence susceptibility to infection as well as disease progression.

Methods.—We performed a two-stage genomewide association study by genotyping 706 patients and 1225 controls using the Human610-Quad BeadChip (Illumina). We then tested three independent replication sets for an association between the presence of leprosy and 93 single-nucleotide polymorphisms (SNPs) that were most strongly associated with the disease in the genomewide association study. Together, these replication sets comprised 3254 patients and 5955 controls. We also carried out tests of heterogeneity of the associations (or lack thereof) between these 93 SNPs and disease, stratified according to clinical subtype (multibacillary vs. paucibacillary).

Results.—We observed a significant association $(P < 1.00 \times 10^{-10})$ between SNPs in the genes *CCDC122, C13orf31, NOD2, TNFSF15, HLA-DR,* and *RIPK2* and a trend toward an association $(P = 5.10 \times 10^{-5})$ with a SNP in *LRRK2*. The associations between the SNPs in *C13orf31, LRRK2, NOD2,* and *RIPK2* and multibacillary leprosy were stronger than the associations between these SNPs and paucibacillary leprosy.

Conclusions.—Variants of genes in the NOD2-mediated signaling pathway (which regulates the innate immune response) are associated with susceptibility to infection with *M. leprae* (Fig 2).

▶ Leprosy is a chronic infectious disease caused by *Mycobacterium leprae*. It affects the skin and peripheral nerves and can cause irreversible impairment of nerve function and consequent chronic disabilities. Despite a dramatic decrease in its prevalence over the past 2 decades (largely because of the worldwide introduction of multidrug therapy in 1982), leprosy remains a major public health problem and one of the most important preventable disabilities in many developing countries. It is therefore particularly unfortunate that research into the mechanisms underlying infection and clinical sequelae has been limited by the fact that *M leprae* infects only humans and cannot be cultured in vitro. The clinical disease of leprosy develops in a minority of infected persons, and it manifests as a spectrum of disease symptoms that result from interactions between the host's immune response and the bacterium. Tuberculoid and lepromatous leprosy are at opposite ends of the spectrum, each being associated with a relatively stable immune status of the host. Borderline categories of the disease, characterized by a variety of clinical manifestations, are associated with an unstable immune response to the bacilli. The

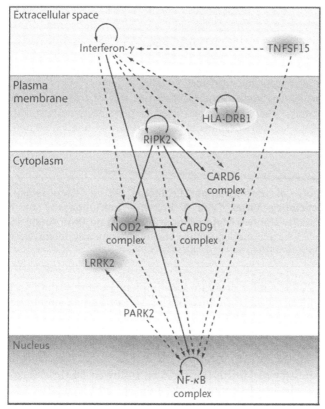

FIGURE 2.—A gene-interaction network of five genes conferring susceptibility to leprosy and five other genes. An Ingenuity Pathways Analysis of the seven susceptibility genes identified a single, closely connected network of interacting genes, including 5 of the 7 genes implicated in the development of leprosy in the genomewide association study (highlighted in red) and 30 additional genes. The network was unlikely to have been identified by chance (one-sided $P = 1.00 \times 10^{-15}$ by Fisher's exact test). Solid lines between genes represent known direct molecular interactions, and dashed lines, known indirect molecular interactions. CARD6 denotes caspase recruitment domain family member 6, CARD9 caspase recruitment domain family member 9, HLA-DRB1 major histocompatibility complex class II DR beta 1, LRRK2 leucine-rich repeat kinase 2, NF-κB nuclear factor κB, NOD2 nucleotide-binding oligomerization domain containing 2, RIPK2 receptor-interacting serine–threonine kinase 2, and TNFSF15 tumor necrosis factor (ligand) superfamily member 15. (Reprinted from Zhang F-R, Huang W, Chen S-M, et al. Genomewide association study of leprosy. *N Engl J Med.* 2009;361:2609-2618, with permission from Massachusetts Medical Society. All rights reserved.)

unusually low diversity of genomic sequences among *M leprae* strains makes it unlikely that differences in susceptibility or clinical manifestation are governed by the strain of *M leprae* or variation within each strain. Therefore, the immunologic response of the host is thought to play a critical role (Fig 2); multibacillary infection is associated with a type 2 helper T (Th2) cell response, whereas paucibacillary infection is associated with an immune response mediated by type 1 helper T (Th1) cells. Host genetic factors have been implicated in susceptibility to leprosy in studies of familial clustering, studies of twins, complex segregation analyses, and tests of association with the human leukocyte antigen (HLA) genes. Markers in several genes and genomic regions (eg, HLA-DR [the gene encoding major histocompatibility complex class II DR], PARK2-PACRG [genes encoding proteins related to Parkinson disease], LTA [the gene encoding lymphotoxin alpha], and chromosome 10p13) have been reported to be associated with susceptibility to leprosy or the development of a particular clinical form of the disease, but few of these associations have been replicated. The authors performed a genome-wide association study involving large numbers of patients with leprosy and unaffected persons.

M. G. Bissell, MD, PhD, MPH

Identification of Performance Problems in a Commercial Human Immunodeficiency Virus Type 1 Enzyme Immunoassay by Multiuser External Quality Control Monitoring and Real-Time Data Analysis
Kim J, CAHCLS Laboratories (Public Health Agency of Canada, Ottawa; et al)
J Clin Microbiol 47:3114-3120, 2009

In June 2005, a pilot program was implemented in Canadian laboratories to monitor the performance of the Abbott human immunodeficiency virus types 1 and 2 (HIV-1/2) gO enzyme immunoassay (EIA). Two different external quality control (QC) reagents and a "real-time" software analysis program were evaluated. In November 2005, higher-than-expected calibrator rate values in these kits were first reported at the Ontario Ministry of Health (Etobicoke), followed by the Alberta Provincial Public Health Laboratory (Edmonton and Calgary) and others. These aberrations were easily and readily tracked in "real time" using the external QC reagents and the software program. These high calibrator values were confirmed in Delkenheim, Germany, by Abbott, and a manufacturing change was initiated beginning with lot 38299LU00, which was distributed to laboratories in Canada in April 2006. However, widespread reports of calibrator failure by laboratories outside Canada were made in March 2006. In April 2006, Abbott Diagnostics initiated a level III investigation to identify the root cause, which was prolonged storage, under uncontrolled storage conditions, of the raw material used in the manufacture of the matrix cells. To the best of our knowledge, this is the first example of a program in Canada for serological testing that combines a common external QC reagent and a "real-time" software program to allow laboratories to monitor kit performance. In this case, external QC monitoring helped identify and confirm performance problems in the Abbott HIV-1/2 gO EIA kit, further highlighting the benefit of implementing such a program in a national or multilaboratory setting for laboratories performing diagnostic and clinical monitoring testing.

▶ Serological testing for human immunodeficiency virus (HIV)-specific antibodies by an enzyme immunoassay (EIA) remains the most practical method of screening for infection with HIV type 1 (HIV-I) and HIV-2. As an initial screening test, the HIV EIA remains an economical and convenient way of testing numerous samples at once. Significant improvements have been made in the HIV EIA so that the window period of the latest third-generation versions is quite sensitive (19 days [95% confidence interval, 15-23 days]). While the window period for HIV can be shortened several days by newer fourth-generation antibody-antigen assays and even further by nucleic acid testing, these technologies may not be practical or possible in resource-limited settings. Improvements to the HIV EIA have been the result of challenges. One of the best methods that an individual laboratory can use to ensure high quality in HIV testing is to enroll in external quality assessment schemes (EQAS), which provide a measure of proficiency testing (PT) on well-characterized panels composed of several challenging samples. These panels are typically sent out several times a year by PT providers. EQAS challenge the whole facility in addition to the specific laboratory. In addition to providing a measure of competency, EQA programs are required for medical laboratories seeking and maintaining accreditation. As an example, International Standards Organization (ISO) 15189 for medical laboratories now has specific requirements for pre-examination and postexamination procedures in addition to the examination phase itself. EQA programs are designed to help address all these areas. Furthermore, many standard-setting organizations, such as the ISO, require participation in third-party EQAS where possible. Problems identified by EQAS can then be addressed by process review, education, and/or other remedial actions. One weakness of EQAS, however, is their inability to identify problems that may have already happened or are about to happen. Even though test performance is one of the components measured during a given EQAS-PT round, a problem may never be identified or may be identified too late because of the usual lapse between PT panel shipments and the receipt of the final report. A method that complements PT by EQAS and addresses these weaknesses is quality control (QC) monitoring, in which an external reagent is tested at the same time that routine testing is performed, and the results can be followed over time to monitor kit performance. QC monitoring thus can measure precision or how well the assay reproduces the same test result under different operating conditions. Here the authors report findings from a program implemented since March 2005 in Canada in which (1) 2 different but common external QC reagents and (2) a real-time data analysis program were provided to Canadian laboratories performing HIV testing using the Abbott AxSYM HIV-1/2 gO EIA (Chicago, IL). Within 6 months of implementation, the program clearly identified performance problems with this assay that led to unacceptably high calibrator values, and Abbott Diagnostics conducted a high-level investigation resulting in the implementation of QC procedures in its manufacturing processes. One consequence of higher-than-normal signal-to-cutoff ratios is increased and unnecessary confirmatory testing of samples falsely reactive by HIV antibody testing.

M. G. Bissell, MD, PhD, MPH

Polymerase chain reaction screening for methicillin-resistant *Staphylococcus aureus* and contact isolation

Spence MR, Courser S, Dammel T (Kalispell Regional Med Ctr, MT)
Am J Infect Control 37:601-602, 2009

Background.—Methicillin-resistant *Staphylococcus aureus* (MRSA) infections are thought to now be endemic in some populations. The early identification of individuals admitted to the hospital who are harboring this organism is important for the timely implementation of appropriate control strategies. Our objective was to measure the prevalence of MRSA carriage in high-risk patients entering our hospital and to determine which of these patients screened for MRSA should be placed in contact precautions on admission.

Methods.—Between January 1, 2007, and December 31, 2007, we used polymerase chain reaction analysis, with a turnaround time of 4 hours or less, to screen for MRSA in a select group of patients entering our hospital.

Results.—We screened 1,568 patients and found 144 (9.2%) positive. Of the 1,568 patients, 170 (10.8%) were known to previously have been MRSA positive. Of these, 90 (52.9%) had negative screens.

Conclusion.—We used a rapid screening test to identify patients harboring MRSA. Our findings support that MRSA is harbored sporadically and patients do not have to be placed in contact isolation based on a history of previously being MRSA positive.

▶ Most individuals harboring methicillin-resistant *Staphylococcus aureus* (MRSA) are asymptomatically colonized with the organism. The colonization rates with MRSA vary depending on the demographics of the population and their risk factors, such as comorbidities and encounters with the health care system. In the absence of knowing which patients are harboring MRSA, colonized individuals can enter acute care facilities unrecognized and present a potential hazard for themselves and/or other patients. In view of this, some health care facilities have established MRSA screening programs for at-risk patients. Additionally, there is currently a recommendation that all individuals with a history of MRSA infection or carriage be placed in contact precautions upon readmission. Placing a patient with a history of MRSA infection or colonization in contact precautions upon readmission is a reasonable approach when one is using standard microbiologic culture techniques that require a minimum of 24 hours before the colonization status of the patient is known. However, with a rapid diagnostic technique to detect MRSA and a short turnaround time until the MRSA status is known, this may not be necessary. The authors' objectives for this investigation were to measure the prevalence of MRSA carriage in a group of high-risk individuals entering their facility and determine which ones needed to be placed in contact precautions based on the findings. They screened 1568 patients during calendar year 2007 with 144 being positive for MRSA. Patients were not rescreened during their admission or after discharge; therefore, it is not known whether the therapies they received during their stay resulted in their being recolonized. Nonetheless, they do know that none of the previously MRSA-colonized patients developed MRSA infections or were linked to a nosocomial MRSA infection during their stay. The authors conclude that with the use of polymerase chain reaction (PCR) screening for MRSA, patients with a history of MRSA infection need not be admitted under contact precautions.

M. G. Bissell, MD, PhD, MPH

Potential clinical utility of polymerase chain reaction in microbiological testing for sepsis

Lehmann LE, Alvarez J, Hunfeld K-P, et al (Univ Hosp Bonn, Germany; Univ Hosp Santiago de Compostela, Spain; Univ Hosp Frankfurt, Germany; et al)
Crit Care Med 37:3085-3090, 2009

Objectives.—To evaluate the potential improvement of antimicrobial treatment by utilizing a new multiplex polymerase chain reaction (PCR) assay that identifies sepsis-relevant microorganisms in blood.

Design.—Prospective, observational international multicentered trial.

Setting.—University hospitals in Germany (n = 2), Spain (n = 1), and the United States (n = 1), and one Italian tertiary general hospital.

Patients.—436 sepsis patients with 467 episodes of antimicrobial treatment.

Methods.—Whole blood for PCR and blood culture (BC) analysis was sampled independently for each episode. The potential impact of reporting microorganisms by PCR on adequacy and timeliness of antimicrobial therapy was analyzed. The number of gainable days on early adequate antimicrobial treatment attributable to PCR findings was assessed.

Measurements and Main Results.—Sepsis criteria, days on antimicrobial therapy, antimicrobial substances administered, and microorganisms identified by PCR and BC susceptibility tests.

Results.—BC diagnosed 117 clinically relevant microorganisms; PCR identified 154. Ninety-nine episodes were BC positive (BC+); 131 episodes were PCR positive (PCR+). Overall, 127.8 days of clinically inadequate empirical antibiotic treatment in the 99 BC+ episodes were observed. Utilization of PCR-aided diagnostics calculates to a potential reduction of 106.5 clinically inadequate treatment days. The ratio of gainable early adequate treatment days to number of PCR tests done is 22.8 days/100 tests overall (confidence interval 15–31) and 36.4 days/100 tests in the intensive care and surgical ward populations (confidence interval 22–51).

Conclusions. Rapid PCR identification of microorganisms may contribute to a reduction of early inadequate antibiotic treatment in sepsis (Fig 2).

▶ Sepsis is the second leading cause of death in the noncoronary intensive care unit. Early diagnosis, followed by prompt implementation of an appropriate treatment, improves the prognosis of septic patients. After early initiation of

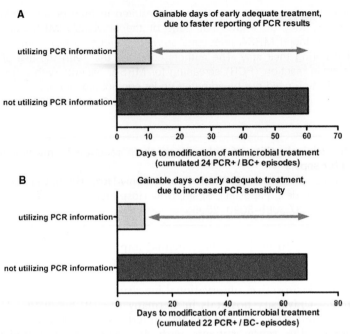

A

Gainable days of early adequate treatment,
due to faster reporting of PCR results

utilizing PCR information

not utilizing PCR information

0   10   20   30   40   50   60   70

Days to modification of antimicrobial treatment
(cumulated 24 PCR+ / BC+ episodes)

B

Gainable days of early adequate treatment,
due to increased PCR sensitivity

utilizing PCR information

not utilizing PCR information

0   20   40   60   80

Days to modification of antimicrobial treatment
(cumulated 22 PCR+ / BC- episodes)

FIGURE 2.—Potential impact of polymerase chain reaction (*PCR*) utilization on days of inadequate antimicrobial treatment. *A*, Episodes in which concurrently drawn PCR and blood culture (*BC*) pointed to an inadequately covered microorganism. *B*, Episodes in which PCR pointed to an inadequately covered microorganism, and another culture result and/or actual clinical course supported the potential clinical significance of the PCR result. (Reprinted from Lehmann LE, Alvarez J, Hunfeld K-P, et al. Potential clinical utility of polymerase chain reaction in microbiological testing for sepsis. *Crit Care Med.* 2009;37:3085-3090, with permission from the Society of Critical Care Medicine and Lippincott Williams & Wilkins.)

antimicrobial therapy, timely reassessment is important because inappropriate antibiotic therapy negatively influences, while adequate antibiotic therapy positively influences the outcome of patients with bacterial bloodstream infections (BSIs) and sepsis. Supplementing blood cultures for BSI testing by additional polymerase chain reaction (PCR)-based testing has been proposed. However, data for the clinical utility of PCR in microbiological testing for sepsis are still lacking. Here, in a model analysis, the authors retrospectively evaluate the potential clinical utility of supplemental PCR testing of patients with sepsis to determine the impact in terms of gainable days on early adequate antimicrobial treatment (Fig 2). They used covariate analysis to identify independent factors. The PCR method used was the Roche LightCycler SeptiFast PCR on ethylene-diamine tetraacetic acid whole blood.

M. G. Bissell, MD, PhD, MPH

Prospective Study of Vaginal Bacteria Flora and Other Risk Factors for Vulvovaginal Candidiasis

McClelland RS, Richardson BA, Hassan WM, et al (Global Health Univ of Washington, Seattle; et al)
J Infect Dis 199:1883-1890, 2009

Background.—It has been suggested that vaginal colonization with lactobacilli may reduce the risk of vulvovaginal candidiasis (WC), but supporting data are limited. Our objective was to determine the relationship between vaginal bacterial flora and VVC.

Methods.—We conducted a. prospective cohort analysis that involved 151 Kenyan sex workers. At monthly follow-up visits, VVC was defined as the presence of yeast buds, pseudohyphae, or both on a. wet preparation (including potassium hydroxide preparation) of vaginal secretions. Generalized, estimating equations were used to identify correlates of VVC.

Results.—Participants returned, for a median of 12 visits (interquartile range, 11–12 visits). VVC was identified at 162 visits, including 26 involving symptomatic VVC. Bacterial vaginosis was associated with fewer episodes of VVC (adjusted odds ratio [aOR], 0.29 [95% confidence interval {CI}, 0.16–0.50]). After excluding women with concurrent bacterial vaginosis, another possible cause of vaginal symptoms, the likelihood, of symptomatic VVC was higher among those who had had yeast identified on wet preparation of vaginal secretions during the past 60 days (aOR, 4.06 [95% CI, 1.12–14.74]) and those with concurrent vaginal *Lactobacillus* colonization (aOR, 3.75 [95% CI, 1.30–10.83]).

Conclusions.—Contrary to the commonly posited, hypothesis that vaginal *Lactobacillus* colonization has a protective effect, we found, that such colonization was associated with a nearly 4-fold increase in the likelihood of symptomatic VVC.

▶ Vulvovaginal candidiasis (VVC) affects up to 75% of reproductive-age women at least once. Nearly half will experience recurrences, and 5% to 8% have multiple episodes each year. In addition to discomfort and the costs associated with medication and health care visits, several prospective studies have suggested that VVC may increase a woman's risk of becoming infected with human immunodeficiency virus type 1 (HIV-I). Although not all studies have found this association, a meta-analysis published in 2001 also concluded that vaginal yeast infections are associated with a 2-fold increase in the risk of HIV-1 acquisition. Because of the high prevalence of this condition, VVC could contribute substantially to the population-level risk of HIV-1 infection. Numerous risk factors for VVC have been identified, but fundamental questions about the pathogenesis of this condition remain unanswered. It has been suggested that normal vaginal flora, consisting predominantly of *Lactobacillus* species, may protect against the development of VVC, but there are limited data to support this hypothesis. The objective of this prospective study, which was conducted in a population of Kenyan women at increased risk for HIV-1 infection, was to examine correlates of VVC and of the subset of cases of symptomatic VVC. The authors focused particular attention on the dynamic relationship between vaginal bacterial flora and vaginal yeast. Noting that both bacterial vaginitis and VVC have been associated with increased risk of HIV-1 infection in general, but vaginal colonization with hydrogen peroxide-producing *Lactobacillus* has been associated with a lower risk of acquiring HIV-1, they suggest that the optimal vaginal flora for minimizing this risk may include peroxide-producing *Lactobacillus* in the absence of VVC. Simply promoting *Lactobacillus* colonization may not reduce VVC. These conclusions are limited by the fact that they were unable to perform yeast culture, and relied on microscopy, which can give rise to false negatives and false positives.

M. G. Bissell, MD, PhD, MPH

Rapid Detection of Influenza A Pandemic (H1N1) 2009 Virus Neuraminidase Resistance Mutation H275Y by Real-Time Reverse Transcriptase PCR
Hindiyeh M, Ram D, Mandelboim M, et al (Chaim Sheba Med Ctr, Tel-Hashomer, Israel; et al)
J Clin Microbiol 48:1884-1887, 2010

The emergence of oseltamivir-resistant influenza A pandemic (H1N1) 2009 virus highlights the need for rapid oseltamivir resistance screening. We report the development and validation of high-throughput real-time reverse transcriptase PCR assays for the detection of the H275Y substitution in the neuraminidase 1 gene that can be accomplished in 3 to 4 h.

▶ The continuous spread of influenza A pandemic (H1N1) 2009 virus is compelling the use of the neuraminidase inhibitors (NAIs) oseltamivir (Tamiflu) and zanamivir (Relenza) to treat infected patients to minimize further spread of the virus. NAIs are the only available antivirals against this pandemic (H1N1) 2009 virus because adamantanes (amantadine and rimantadine) are completely ineffective. The extensive use of these NAIs, in particular oseltamivir, is creating an unprecedented selective pressure for the emergence and spread of drug-resistant viral strains. The World Health Organization (WHO) has recommended vigilant monitoring for oseltamivir-resistant viruses because the number of documented sporadic resistant cases is increasing, reaching nearly 100 cases worldwide by 15 December 2009. Recently, the US Centers for Disease Control and Prevention reported the first human-to-human transmission of oseltamivir-resistant pandemic (H1N1) 2009 virus in 2 summer campers receiving oseltamivir prophylaxis. In addition, the WHO has announced outbreaks of oseltamivir-resistant pandemic (H1N1) 2009 virus in 2 immunocompromised groups: one in North Carolina and the other in Wales, United Kingdom. In both outbreaks, human-to-human oseltamivir-resistant virus transmission was suspected. At least 2 mechanisms contribute to NA resistance in the seasonal influenza viruses H1N1 and H5NI (avian influenza). One mechanism involves reduction of the binding efficiency of virus hemagglutinin to its receptor. The other is associated with amino acid substitutions in and around the NA active site, of which the substitution at position 275 (histidine to tyrosine [H275Y]) is the most common. Sequence analysis of the hemagglutinin gene is not a reliable indicator of NA drug resistance phenotype, but H275Y substitution in the active site of the *NA-1* gene does indicate reduced binding affinity of the NAI oseltamivir. Recent reports characterizing the current oseltamivir-resistant pandemic (H1N1) 2009 virus confirmed the presence of the H275Y mutation. While phenotypic analysis of oseltamivir-resistant influenza A viruses is widely accepted as the gold standard methodology for detecting influenza virus drug resistance, genotypic analysis has been widely used to detect a point mutation (cytosine to thymine) at position 823 of the *NA-1* gene that results in a histidine-to-tyrosine substitution. The genotypic assays include sequencing part of the *NA* gene by using the Sanger dideoxy sequencing method or by pyrosequencing. These assays are labor-intensive, with a long turnaround time ranging from 24 to 72 h and require specialized equipment and human effort. Moreover, sequencing and pyrosequencing assays have reduced sensitivities for detecting low concentrations (<15%) of quasispecies present in a patient's sample. Therefore, high-throughput assays with short turnaround times are needed to expedite oseltamivir drug resistance detection. In this study, the authors validated 2 real-time reverse transcriptase polymerase chain reaction assays by utilizing TaqMan chemistry for the detection of the point mutation (cytosine to thymine) at position 823 of the *NA-1* gene of pandemic (H1N1) 2009 virus.

M. G. Bissell, MD, PhD, MPH

Two Distinct Clones of Methicillin-Resistant *Staphylococcus aureus* (MRSA) with the Same USA300 Pulsed-Field Gel Electrophoresis Profile: a Potential Pitfall for Identification of USA300 Community-Associated MRSA

Larsen AR, Goering R, Stegger M, et al (Statens Serum Institut, Copenhagen, Denmark; Creighton Univ Med Centre, Omaha, NE; et al)
J Clin Microbiol 47:3765-3768, 2009

Analysis of methicillin-resistant *Staphylococcus aureus* (MRSA) characterized as USA300 by pulsed-field gel electrophoresis identified two distinct clones. One was similar to community-associated USA300 MRSA (ST8-IVa, t008, and Panton-Valentine leukocidin positive). The second (ST8-IVa, t024, and PVL negative) had different molecular characteristics and epidemiology, suggesting independent evolution. We recommend *spa* typing and/or PCR to discriminate between the two clones.

▶ The methicillin-resistant *Staphylococcus aureus* (MRSA) clone USA300, having multilocus sequence type (MLST) ST8 and staphylococcal protein A (spa) type 008 and carrying staphylococcal cassette chromosome (SCC*mec*) IVa has disseminated in the United States as well as to other parts of the world. USA300 carries the *luk-PV* genes encoding Panton-Valentine leukocidin (PVL) has been identified in a variety of community populations and has been associated with skin and soft tissue infections (SSTI), as well as more severe infections, such as sepsis, pneumonia, and necrotizing fasciitis.

The identification of USA300 isolates is primarily based on pulsed-field gel electrophoresis (PFGE). Other genetic markers have also been suggested for identification of USA300 isolates, including (1) the *arcA* gene of the arginine catabolic mobile element (ACME), (2) sequencing of the direct repeat unit (*dru*) region, and (3) different USA300 specific multiplex polymerase chain reactions (PCRs) targeting *luk-PV* and a "signature" 6-AT-repeat sequence within the conserved hypothetical gene SACOL0058.

In Denmark, MRSA isolates have been consecutively typed by PFGE since 1999 with the addition of sequence-based methods, such as MLST and spa typing, on selected isolates since 2001. This process identified some of the first USA300 isolates in Europe but, surprisingly, also identified isolates with USA300 PFGE banding patterns but a different spa type. In this study, the authors investigated the epidemiology and genetic diversity of these isolates and USA300 and USA500 reference strains using PFGE, spa typing, MLST, SCC*mec* typing, *dru* typing, ACME, the 6-AT signature sequence, detection of *luk-PV*, and antimicrobial susceptibility testing (Neo-Sensitabs), as well as microarray analysis.

They suggest that reports of USA300 could include isolates with important genetic variations if PGFE, MLST, or SCC*mec* typing is the method used, as supported by findings of ACME- and PVL-negative USA300 isolates. USA300 MRSA identified solely by PGFE should be confirmed by at least 1 PCR analysis, which could be for *luk-PV* or a sequence based typing method, such as spa typing.

M. G. Bissell, MD, PhD, MPH

18 Hematology and Immunology

A Genomic Approach to Improve Prognosis and Predict Therapeutic Response in Chronic Lymphocytic Leukemia
Friedman DR, Weinberg JB, Barry WT, et al (Duke Univ Med Ctr, Durham, NC; et al)
Clin Cancer Res 15:6947-6955, 2009

Purpose.—Chronic lymphocytic leukemia (CLL) is a B-cell malignancy characterized by a variable clinical course. Several parameters have prognostic capabilities but are associated with altered response to therapy in only a small subset of patients.

Experimental Design.—We used gene expression profiling methods to generate predictors of therapy response and prognosis. Genomic signatures that reflect progressive disease and responses to chemotherapy or chemoimmunotherapy were created using cancer cell lines and patient leukemia cell samples. We validated and applied these three signatures to independent clinical data from four cohorts, representing a total of 301 CLL patients.

Results.—A genomic signature of prognosis created from patient leukemic cell gene expression data coupled with clinical parameters significantly differentiated patients with stable disease from those with progressive disease in the training data set. The progression signature was validated in two independent data sets, showing a capacity to accurately identify patients at risk for progressive disease. In addition, genomic signatures that predict response to chlorambucil or pentostatin, cyclophosphamide, and rituximab were generated and could accurately distinguish responding and nonresponding CLL patients.

Conclusions.—Thus, microarray analysis of CLL lymphocytes can be used to refine prognosis and predict response to different therapies. These results have implications for standard and investigational therapeutics in CLL patients.

▶ The practice of oncology continually faces 2 major challenges: determining which patients are at risk for progression or recurrence of disease and identifying the most effective therapeutic regimen for the individual patient. Obstacles to address these challenges include the complexity of the disease processes, individual differences and comorbidities, and the paucity of markers to guide the use of available treatments. However, examples such as the use of trastuzumab to treat human epithelial growth factor receptor (HER)2-positive breast cancer show that selecting therapies for patients based on tumor markers can improve overall response rates. Similarly, identifying predictors of sensitivity to cytotoxic agents that are able to select patients who will respond to these chemotherapeutic agents would directly affect current medical practice, wherein patients are often treated with one of several therapeutic regimens that, on a population basis, have equal efficacy. Chronic lymphocytic leukemia (CLL) displays a wide spectrum of aggressiveness. Even among those patients with low- or intermediate-risk disease at diagnosis, accurate determination of which patients will progress and require therapy is inexact. For those patients requiring therapy, there are a variety of treatment options varying in long-term efficacy and toxicity. Multiple factors, such as cytogenetic aberrations, immunoglobulin variable region heavy chain (IgV$_H$) mutational status, and CD38 and ZAP-70 expression, are increasingly used to help refine prognosis and guide patient care in the previously untreated CLL patient. However, at this time, only the interphase cytogenetic abnormality of 17p13 deletion has been consistently associated with poor response to purine analog-based therapy. Recent advances using genomic technology, particularly the use of gene expression profiling, has provided an opportunity to further address these issues. Previous studies have described the development of gene expression-based profiles that correlate with clinical outcomes or surrogates of outcome. These studies on gene expression differences include investigations of CLL and normal B cells, CLL with specific cytogenetic anomalies, and mutated versus unmutated IgV$_H$ status. Here, the authors describe the generation of gene expression signatures with improved capacity to predict which low- or intermediate-risk patients are most likely to progress with CLL and, at the same time, can predict response to a variety of treatment approaches.

M. G. Bissell, MD, PhD, MPH

A Single Tube, Four-Color Flow Cytometry Assay for Evaluation of ZAP-70 and CD38 Expression in Chronic Lymphocytic Leukemia
Hassanein NM, Perkinson KR, Alcancia F, et al (Duke Univ Med Ctr, Durham, NC)
Am J Clin Pathol 133:708-717, 2010

We describe a simple and robust flow cytometry assay for ZAP-70 and CD38 expression. The steps required to validate this assay in a clinical flow cytometry laboratory are described. Two criteria were used to characterize ZAP-70 expression into positive, negative, and indeterminate categories and applied to 111 cases of chronic lymphocytic leukemia (CLL) resulting in 29.7% positive, 56.8% negative, and 13.5% indeterminate cases. A sensitivity- specificity crossover plot between ZAP-70 and CD38 suggested a cutoff of 12.5% for defining CD38 positivity. ZAP-70+ cases were significantly more likely to be at a higher clinical stage and, together with CD38+ cases, were more likely to have unmutated

IgV$_H$. However, for individual patients, the concordance between these markers was not perfect. It may be necessary to evaluate several prognostic markers simultaneously in CLL, and availability of convenient assays for ZAP-70 and CD38 is desirable for optimal clinical decision making.

▶ Chronic lymphocytic leukemia (CLL) is characterized by the clonal expansion of mature-appearing lymphocytes that typically express CD19, CD5, and CD23. It is the most common leukemia in the United States and Europe. CLL is a heterogeneous disease with a median survival ranging from 2 to 20 years. Based on the anticipated and observed aggressiveness of CLL in a particular patient, the treatment may vary from observation alone to multiagent chemotherapy or allogeneic bone marrow or stem cell transplantation. Until about a decade ago, the clinical stage at diagnosis was the chief prognostic factor available for patients with CLL, but the correlation between clinical stage and aggressiveness of the disease was not ideal. Immunoglobulin heavy chain variable region (*IgV$_H$*) mutation status was first described as an independent prognostic marker in CLL in 1998 and 1999, and it is now well established that the lack of an *IgV$_H$* mutation in CLL correlates with a worse prognosis. Analysis of *IgV$_H$* mutation status is a relatively expensive and time-consuming test with restricted availability. Gene expression analysis of CLL cells revealed that messenger RNA (mRNA) for zeta-associated protein-70 (ZAP-70) is overexpressed in CLL compared with normal B cells. Further work showed that expression of ZAP-70 mRNA or protein may serve as a surrogate for *IgV$_H$* mutation status. By using flow cytometry, it was confirmed that leukemic cells without the *IgV$_H$* mutation express detectable intracellular ZAP-70 protein, whereas those with the *IgV$_H$* mutation do not. Several studies have identified CD38 expression by CLL cells as another marker of CLL prognosis. A simple, reliable, and convenient flow cytometric assay for ZAP-70 and CD38 is highly desirable. The authors present information regarding a single-tube assay using 4-color flow cytometry that can simultaneously examine the expression of CD38 and ZAP-70 in CLL cells. The results from 3 patients with CLL for these prognostic parameters were compared with the results of *IgV$_H$* mutation status, clinical stage at diagnosis, and cytogenetic abnormalities in a subset of the patients.

M. G. Bissell, MD, PhD, MPH

Cellular Plasticity of Inflammatory Myeloid Cells in the Peritoneal Foreign Body Response
Mooney JE, Rolfe BE, Osborne GW, et al (Univ of Queensland, St Lucia, Australia; et al)
Am J Pathol 176:369-380, 2010

Implantation of sterile foreign objects in the peritoneal cavity of an animal initiates an inflammatory response and results in encapsulation of the objects by bone marrow-derived cells. Over time, a multilayered tissue capsule develops with abundant myofibroblasts embedded in extra-cellular matrix. The present study used the transgenic MacGreen mouse to characterize the time-dependent accumulation of monocyte subsets and neutrophilic granulocytes in the inflammatory infiltrate and within the tissue capsule by their differential expression of the *csf1r*-EGFP transgene, F4/80, and Ly6C. As the tissue capsule developed, enhanced green fluores-cent protein-positive cells changed from rounded to spindle-shaped morphology and began to co-express the myofibroblast marker α-smooth muscle actin. Expression increased with time: at day 14, 11.13 ± 0.67% of tissue capsule cells co-expressed these markers, compared with 50.77 ± 12.85% of cells at day 28. The importance of monocyte/macro-phages in tissue capsule development was confirmed by clodronate-encapsulated liposome removal, which resulted in almost complete abrogation of capsule development. These results confirm the importance of monocyte/macrophages in the tissue response to sterile foreign objects implanted in the peritoneal cavity. In addition, the *in vivo* plasticity of peritoneal macrophages and their ability to transdifferentiate from a myeloid to mesenchymal phenotype is demonstrated.

▶ The tissue response to foreign materials, including biomaterials and medical devices, is known as the foreign body response and is universally characterized by inflammatory cell recruitment and subsequent encapsulation of the foreign material by fibrotic tissue. At the site of implantation, an array of inflammatory mediators (and signaling molecules), including cytokines, growth factors, extracellular matrix proteins, and matrix-degrading enzymes, create a dynamic microenvironment that mediates a defined sequence of events. In the initial acute inflammatory phase, neutrophils are recruited to the surface of the implanted materials, followed by lymphocyte and mononuclear cell involvement and foreign body giant cell formation (chronic inflammation). If the foreign material cannot be removed, resolution of these inflammatory responses occurs when a fibrous capsule has formed around it. Although the purpose of fibrous encapsulation is to isolate foreign material from the surrounding tissue, this fibrotic tissue, along with foreign body giant cells at the tissue/material inter-face, can significantly compromise the efficiency of medical devices or pros-theses and frequently leads to device failure. The authors' laboratory has observed a similar response to foreign material implanted in the peritoneal cavity. Within the first 3 to 5 days after implantation, the object is covered by rounded cells, many of which have a macrophage-like morphology and express the common leukocyte antigen Ly-5 (CD45). After 2 to 3 weeks, a tissue capsule comprising multiple layers of myofibroblasts and extracellular matrix and covered by a continuous layer of mesothelial cells surrounds the object. In contrast with the tissue surrounding foreign material at other anatomical sites, the tissue encapsulating free-floating foreign objects in the peritoneal cavity is avascular. On harvest, the tissue has been used as an autologous graft for replacement/repair of hollow smooth muscle organs, including blood vessels, bladder, vas deferens, and uterus. Over the ensuing 2 to 3 months, the grafted tissue undergoes further cell differentiation and tissue remodeling to assume the morphology and function of the host organ. In addition to providing a sterile location to develop myofibroblast-rich tissue for engineering purposes, the peritoneal cavity is a convenient site to investigate the involvement of myeloid cells in the inflammatory response. The mononuclear phagocyte system encompasses bone marrow precursors, peripheral blood monocytes, tissue macrophages, and dendritic cells, all of which express the macrophage colony-stimulating factor receptor (csf1r). Macrophage also express F4/80 and exhibit phenotypic and functional heterogeneity. Recently, blood monocytes have also been shown to exhibit heterogeneity in terms of expression of surface molecules such as Gr1 (Ly6C), chemokine receptors (CX3CR1), and migratory predisposition. Understanding the cellular processes involved in the foreign body response is central to the development of tissue engineering strategies using the resultant myofibroblast-rich tissue. It is also the key to maintaining the integrity and function of biomedical implants such as orthopedic implants, dental or breast implants, artificial organs, vascular grafts, heart valves, renal dialyzers, and controlled drug delivery systems. Thus, the aims of this study were to characterize the cells involved in the inflammatory response to foreign objects implanted in the peritoneal cavity and to determine whether monocyte/macrophages are the source of peritoneum-derived tissue capsule myofibroblasts.

M. G. Bissell, MD, PhD, MPH

Cutaneous type adult T-cell leukemia/lymphoma is a characteristic subtype and includes erythema/papule and nodule/tumor subgroups
Miyata T, Yonekura K, Utsunomiya A, et al (Aichi Cancer Ctr Res Inst, Nagoya, Japan; Kagoshima Univ Graduate School of Med and Dental Sciences, Japan; Imamura Bun-in Hosp, Kagoshima, Japan)
Int J Cancer 126:1521-1528, 2010

We first analyzed the genomic profile of cutaneous type adult T-cell leukemia/lymphoma (ATLL) in an attempt to clarify its clinical and biological characteristics. Genomic gains of 1p, 7q and 18q and loss of 13q were frequently detected. Gain of 1p36.33-32 or loss of 13q33.1-3 indicated poor prognosis. Among cases with generalized lesions, erythema/papule or nodule/tumor cases showed a distinct genomic profile, indicating that these 2 groups were biologically different and developed via different genetic pathways. Furthermore, cases with generalized nodule/tumor lesions tended to progress to aggressive ATLL (Fig 2).

▶ Adult T-cell leukemia/lymphoma (ATLL) is one of the most aggressive T-cell malignancies caused by human T-cell leukemia virus type 1 (HTLV-I). After several decades of latency, about 2.5% of carriers develop ATLL. ATLL has been clinically classified into 4 subtypes, 2 of which are aggressive ATLL (acute and lymphoma types) and 2 are indolent ATLL (chronic and smoldering types). Recently, it has been noticed that some indolent ATLL patients with cutaneous manifestation show a unique clinical course featuring lesions of

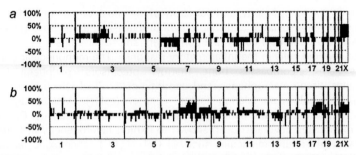

FIGURE 2.—Genome-wide frequencies of aberrations in the 2 groups of generalized type in cutaneous type ATLL patients. Horizontal axis shows 2193 BAC/PAC clones from chromosome 1 to 22 and X in order of p to q. Vertical axis shows frequency of aberration. Positive or negative direction indicates genomic gain or loss. (a) Erythema/papule group (cases with aberrations, $n = 6$) (b) Nodule/tumor group (cases with aberrations, $n = 8$). (Reprinted from Miyata T, Yonekura K, Utsunomiya A, et al. Cutaneous type adult T-cell leukemia/lymphoma is a characteristic subtype and includes erythema/papule and nodule/tumor subgroups. *Int J Cancer*. 2010;126:1521-1528.)

the skin only until the advanced stage. In this article, the authors use the name cutaneous type for these cases. Recently, new proposed diagnostic criteria for cutaneous type classify it as a new disease entity with low viral load in peripheral blood. However, the term cutaneous type has not been accepted in the clinical setting because half of all ATLL cases show cutaneous involvement. Following the current classification criteria, cutaneous type ATLL cases have to be classified into chronic or smoldering type. The authors previously reported that array comparative genomic hybridization (array CGH) of acute and lymphoma type ATLLs showed different genomic profiles and that each subtype has specific recurrent genomic aberrations. So far, however, no study has been conducted on the genomic profiles of cutaneous type ATLL. In the study, the authors analyzed these genomic profiles by means of array CGH and related their findings to the clinical features (Fig 2). Furthermore, they divided cutaneous type ATLL cases into localized and generalized types and tried to determine their characteristic genomic aberrations and clinical factors. They conducted this study with the following 3 aims: (1) to clarify the clinical picture of cutaneous type ATLL; (2) to identify a characteristic genomic profile; and (3) to determine the relationship between genomic aberrations and clinical features.

M. G. Bissell, MD, PhD, MPH

Diagnosis of Myelodysplastic Syndrome Among a Cohort of 119 Patients With Fanconi Anemia: Morphologic and Cytogenetic Characteristics

Cioc AM, Wagner JE, MacMillan ML, et al (Univ of Minnesota Masonic Cancer Ctr, Minneapolis)
Am J Clin Pathol 133:92-100, 2010

Predisposition to myelodysplastic syndrome (MDS) and acute leukemia is a hallmark of Fanconi anemia (FA). Morphologic criteria for MDS in FA are not well established, nor is the significance of clonal chromosomal abnormalities. We reviewed bone marrow samples of 119 FA patients: 23 had MDS, with the most common subtype refractory cytopenia with multilineage dysplasia. The presence of MDS was highly correlated with the presence of clonal abnormalities. Neutrophil dysplasia and increased blasts were always associated with the presence of a clone, in contrast with dyserythropoiesis. The most frequent clones had gains of 1q and 3q and/or loss of 7. Karyotype complexity also correlated with MDS. One third of patients with 3q as a sole abnormality had no MDS; patients with 3q and an additional abnormality all had MDS. The data provide a rationale for integrating cytogenetic findings with independently evaluated morphologic findings for monitoring bone marrow status in FA.

▶ Fanconi anemia (FA) is an inherited disorder associated with genomic instability, bone marrow failure (BMF), and predisposition to hematologic malignancies and/or solid tumors. Thirteen complementation groups have been identified, with 12 of the putative genes mapped to autosomal loci and the remaining gene to the X chromosome. The early life-threatening feature of FA is BMF, thought to result from excess apoptosis in stem and progenitor cells. The genetic instability and proapoptotic tendency then provide a selective force for the evolution of adapted hematopoietic stem cell clones that lead to acute myeloid leukemia (AML) and myelodysplastic syndrome (MDS). In published literature reviews and studies of patients enrolled in the International Fanconi Anemia Registry, leukemia was reported in 8% to 9% and MDS in 7% of patients. Analysis of the data for 754 patients from International Fanconi Anemia Registry demonstrated a cumulative incidence of 90% for BMF, 33% for hematologic malignancy (AML or MDS), and 35% for solid tumors by age 50. The diagnosis of a malignancy preceded the diagnosis of FA in more than one-third of the cases with cancer reported in the literature. MDS and AML are major predictors of clinical outcome in patients with FA. MDS is a particularly challenging diagnosis in FA owing to the frequent presence of dysplastic features, especially dyserythropoiesis, the complicating factor of hypocellularity, and the frequent administration of granulocyte colony-stimulating factor (G-CSF) resulting in hyposegmented neutrophils and circulating blasts. In addition, even among expert pathologists, it is difficult to reach a consensus on certain morphologic features such as megaloblastosis in erythroid precursors or hypogranularity in neutrophils. Neither the current World Health Organization nor the suggested pediatric classifications establish quantitative or qualitative criteria for MDS associated with constitutional/inherited abnormalities. Relevant to the development of MDS in FA is the emergence of abnormal cytogenetic clones in the bone marrow of patients. Previous studies have documented acquired clonal abnormalities in FA. However, incomplete characterization of the aberrations owing to limitations in available techniques, the absence of the more common recurring abnormalities in AML, the presence of background chromosomal instability generating nonclonal abnormalities, and the occasional report of transient clones have raised the issue of the clinical significance of these clonal abnormalities. More recently, it has been shown that a clone resulting in an extra copy of the distal long arm of chromosome 3 in FA is associated with a poor prognosis. Yet questions remain regarding the spectrum and clinical significance of clonal cytogenetic abnormalities. This study was undertaken to characterize the morphologic findings of MDS in FA and their relationship to cytogenetic findings. These results have led to the generation of an integrated approach to the diagnosis of MDS in FA.

M. G. Bissell, MD, PhD, MPH

Epstein-Barr virus–positive diffuse large B-cell lymphoma in elderly patients is rare in Western populations

Hoeller S, Tzankov A, Pileri SA, et al (Univ of Basel, Switzerland; Bologna Univ School of Medicine, Italy; et al)
Hum Pathol 41:352-357, 2010

In the currently published World Health Organization-Classification, the new entity of Epstein-Barr virus–positive diffuse large B-cell lymphoma of the elderly was introduced largely based on findings from East-Asian populations. Little is known about its frequency or characteristics in the West, especially in European populations. Using a tissue microarray approach, we identified 8 out of 258 diffuse large B-cell lymphoma cases fulfilling the World Health Organization criteria of an Epstein-Barr virus–positive diffuse large B-cell lymphoma of the elderly, suggesting an incidence of 3.1% in a European population. The median patient age was 65 years. The highest diagnostic sensitivity was only achieved by EBER in situ hybridization. No correlation between Epstein-Barr virus status and outcome was noted except in latency type 3 lymphomas, which had a very poor survival. Sixty-seven percent of Epstein-Barr virus–positive cases showed the presence of necrosis and 50% expressed the activation marker CD30. However, no morphological or immunohistochemical features reliably distinguished all Epstein-Barr virus–positive diffuse large B-cell lymphoma cases. Thus, to identify these Epstein-Barr virus–positive diffuse large B-cell lymphoma in the elderly, EBER in situ hybridization of all de novo diffuse large B-cell lymphoma cases of patients older than 50 years should be considered. In summary, Epstein-Barr virus–positive diffuse large B-cell lymphoma of the elderly is rare in Europeans older than 50 years. It can only be diagnosed by EBER-ISH, and its precise prognostic role is unclear. Whether routine testing of all diffuse large B-cell lymphoma patients older than 50 years can be recommended depends essentially on its clinical relevance. Future studies are needed to address this question.

▶ Epstein-Barr virus (EBV) is associated with a broad spectrum of lymphoproliferative diseases such as classical Hodgkin lymphoma, lymphomatoid granulomatosis, primary effusion lymphoma, plasmablastic lymphoma, Burkitt lymphoma, T-cell and natural killer cell lymphomas, and posttransplant lymphoproliferative disorders (PTLD). The recently published 4th edition of the World Health Organization (WHO) Classification of tumors of hematopoietic and lymphoid tissues included a new provisional entity, the EBV-positive diffuse large B-cell lymphoma (DLBCL) of the elderly. It is defined as an EBV-positive DLBCL of patients older than 50 years, without any known underlying immunosuppression or prior lymphoma. It is believed to be related to the senescence of the immune system. Such lymphomas are supposed to show an EBV latency type 2/3 pattern and are associated with a poorer prognosis compared with age-matched DLBCL without EBV infection, independent of the International Prognostic Index. However, most of the data that led to the introduction of this entity were derived from Asian patient populations and little is known about the situation in Western countries. The aims of this study were to (1) determine the frequency of EBV-positive DLBCL of the elderly in a representative large European population; (2) identify the optimal diagnostic approaches to determine EBV lymphoma association; (3) identify possible morphologic correlations to this diagnosis; and (4) assess the prognostic importance of this entity.

M. G. Bissell, MD, PhD, MPH

Expression of JL1 Is an Effective Adjunctive Marker of Leukemia Cutis

Park YS, Park SH, Park S-J, et al (Univ of Ulsan College of Medicine, Seoul, Korea; et al)
Arch Pathol Lab Med 134:95-102, 2010

Context.—Specific differentiation of leukemia cutis (LC) from nonleukemic dermatoses is crucial to ensure proper treatment for the disease. Because of the exceptionally variable histologic features of LC and the frequent nonleukemic dermatoses in leukemia patients, identification of leukemic cells that infiltrate skin lesions is important. Here, we introduce JL1, a novel leukemia-associated surface antigen, which is not expressed in mature human tissue but in cortical thymocytes and small subpopulations of bone marrow hematopoietic precursors.

Objectives.—To assess the expression pattern of JL1 in LC and compare it with other commonly used markers. Also, to evaluate the expression of JL1 in other cutaneous lesions that need differential diagnoses.

Design.—Immunohistochemical staining with anti-JL1 and other commonly used markers for LC was performed on paraffin-embedded skin biopsies from 32 cases of LC with acute lymphoblastic leukemia/lymphoma and acute myelogenous leukemia. Immunohistochemical staining score was evaluated in each case according to the proportion of positive tumor cells found. JL1 staining was also done on 96 reactive or neoplastic cutaneous lesions.

Results.—JL1 was detected in 7 of 11 acute lymphoblastic leukemia/lymphoma LC (63.6%) and 7 of 21 acute myelogenous leukemia LC (33.3%), with invariably high-staining scores. None of the other cutaneous lesions or normal tissues expressed JL1. The expression pattern of JL1 was not altered in 2 patients with follow-up biopsies.

Conclusions.—Our finding that JL1 is expressed exclusively and stably by leukemic cells suggests that it can be used as a useful adjunctive marker for initial diagnosis and follow-up biopsy of LC, particularly in cases of scarce infiltrates.

▶ Accurate and specific diagnosis of leukemia cutis (LC) is crucial because such patients experience more aggressive disease progression and require immediate local and systemic treatment. LC is strongly associated with extra-medullary leukemia and relapse in the bone marrow. Treatment of LC typically involves combination therapy comprising local treatments (eg, radiation therapy or electron beam radiation) and systemic chemotherapy. Histologic diagnosis of LC is fairly straightforward in cases of diffuse tumor cell infiltration, despite variable clinical and histopathologic features. However, because the incidence of nonleukemic dermatoses in leukemia patients is significantly higher than that of LC, it is difficult to make a specific diagnosis of LC when only a few leukemic infiltrates are present or leukemic cells display little atypism. Immunohisto-chemical markers are helpful in distinguishing leukemia cells from benign inflammatory cells of nonleukemic dermatosis in these situations. Therefore, immunohistochemical markers that are easy to interpret and that can effectively discriminate leukemic cells in routine paraffin-embedded formalin-fixed tissue should significantly aid in the diagnosis of LC with scant infiltrates. JL1 is a novel leukemia-associated surface glycoprotein that was initially described in immature double-positive (ie, CD4$^+$ CD8$^+$) T cells in the human thymic cortex. JL1 has been subsequently detected in a few subpopulations of bone marrow hematopoietic precursor cells but not in any other healthy human tissue. JL1 is also expressed in acute T-cell lymphoblastic leukemia cells, which are malignant counterparts of immature thymocytes. Interestingly, JL1 has been detected in other acute lymphoid and myeloid leukemias, regardless of their lineages. In view of its specific expression in leukemic cells, JL1 can potentially serve as an effective marker of leukemia with promising therapeutic potential. Although limited information is available on the biological functions of JL1, previous studies demonstrate that anti-JL1 antibodies induce homo-typic aggregation of thymocytes and play an important role in the positive selection of thymocytes. If JL1 were expressed exclusively on leukemic cells of LC, but not on any other skin lesions, it would be a good adjunctive diag-nostic marker for LC with scant infiltrates. The authors assessed JL1 expression patterns via immunohistochemical staining on formalin fixed paraffin-embedded human skin biopsy specimens from 32 patients diagnosed with LC. To establish whether JL1 expression is specific for leukemic cells, they assessed immunoreactivity in other skin lesions, including those obtained from patients with Sweet syndrome, graft-versus-host disease, cutaneous neoplasms, and other inflammatory conditions.

M. G. Bissell, MD, PhD, MPH

Immunophenotypic Variations in Mantle Cell Lymphoma

Gao J, Peterson L, Nelson B, et al (Northwestern Univ Feinberg School of Medicine, Chicago, IL)
Am J Clin Pathol 132:699-706, 2009

Mantle cell lymphoma (MCL) expresses pan-B-cell antigens and is usually CD5+/CD10–/CD23–/FMC7+. In this study, we evaluated 52 patients with confirmed diagnoses of MCL and identified variant immuno-phenotypes in 21 patients (19/48 classical and 2/4 variant MCLs), including CD5– in 6 (12%) of 52, CD10+ in 4 (8%) of 50, CD23+ in 10 (21%) of 48, and FMC7- in 4 (11%) of 37 cases. Three cases showed variations in 2 antigens, including CD5–/CD23+, CD10+/FMC7–, and CD23+/FMC7–; they were all classical MCLs. One blastoid variant MCL was CD23+, and one was FMC7–. Evaluation for proliferation index by immunohistochemical analysis for Ki-67 demonstrated no significant difference between MCLs with variant immunophenotypes and MCLs with typical immunophenotypes. The high proliferation index (>60%) was exclusively seen in the blastoid and pleomorphic variants. Our results indicate that immunophenotypic variations are common in MCL, and recognizing the variability is important for accurate subclassification of B-cell lymphoma.

▶ Mantle cell lymphoma (MCL) accounts for approximately 3% to 10% of non-Hodgkin lymphomas and predominantly occurs in men of advanced age. Morphologically, classical MCL is characterized by a monomorphic proliferation of small- to medium-sized lymphocytes with irregular nuclei and inconspicuous nucleoli. Several morphologic variants have been recognized, such as blastoid and pleomorphic variants, which are associated with more aggressive clinical behavior. Virtually all MCLs harbor t(11;14)(q13;q32) translocation, which juxtaposes the *CCND1* gene encoding cyclin D1 to an enhancer of the immuno-globulin heavy chain (IgH) gene, leading to an overexpression of cyclin D 1. Therefore, cyclin D 1 has been widely used as an immunohistochemical marker for MCL. Flow cytometric immunophenotyping also serves an important role in the diagnosis of MCL. Typically, MCLs are positive for pan-B-cell antigens (CDI9, CD20, and CD22) and usually are CD5+, CD 10–, CD23–, and FMC7 +. However, variations from the typical immunophenotype have been observed, some of which could be misleading and cause diagnostic difficulties, particularly when the morphologic features are not classical or the biopsy specimen is small. These cases could be misdiagnosed as other types of B-cell lymphomas, such as follicular lymphoma or chronic lymphocytic leukemia/small lymphocytic lymphoma (CLL and SLL). Therefore, recognizing the variability of immunophenotype in MCL is important for diagnostic workup of patients with lymphoma. Clinically, MCL is considered an aggressive neoplasm with a median survival of 3 to 4 years. However, in a subset of patients, the disease may follow an indolent course, and patients may survive more than 10 years. It has been recognized in earlier studies that proliferation of the tumor, as evaluated by the mitotic index or the proliferation-associated antigen Ki-67, was the best predictor of survival in patients with MCL. Recent studies have demonstrated that it remains an important prognostic marker in the era of anti-CD20 therapy and is independent of other clinical factors. Previous reports on unusual immunophenotypes in MCL are about patients with single antigen variation, and the data on correlation of variant immunophenotypes with morphologic features, proliferation of the tumor, or clinical outcome are rare. In this study, flow cytometric analysis was performed to investigate the types and frequencies of the variant immunophenotypes in a cohort of 52 patients with confirmed diagnoses of MCLs. The findings were correlated with morphologic features, immunohistochemical results, and proliferation index of the tumor to investigate whether MCLs with variant immunophenotypes differ in morphologic features or biologic behavior from MCLs with typical immunophenotypes.

M. G. Bissell, MD, PhD, MPH

Multi-Step Aberrant CpG Island Hyper-Methylation Is Associated with the Progression of Adult T-Cell Leukemia/Lymphoma
Sato H, Oka T, Shinnou Y, et al (Okayama Univ, Japan; et al)
Am J Pathol 176:402-415, 2010

Aberrant CpG island methylation contributes to the pathogenesis of various malignancies. However, little is known about the association of epigenetic abnormalities with multistep tumorigenic events in adult T cell leukemia/lymphoma (ATLL). To determine whether epigenetic abnormalities induce the progression of ATLL, we analyzed the methylation profiles of the *SHP1, p15, p16, p73, HCAD, DAPK, hMLH-1,* and *MGMT* genes by methylation specific PCR assay in 65 cases with ATLL patients. The number of CpG island methylated genes increased with disease progression and aberrant hypermethylation in specific genes was detected even in HTLV-1 carriers and correlated with progression to ATLL. The CpG island methylator phenotype (CIMP) was observed most frequently in lymphoma type ATLL and was also closely associated with the progression and crisis of ATLL. The high number of methylated genes and increase of CIMP incidence were shown to be unfavorable prognostic factors and correlated with a shorter overall survival by Kaplan-Meyer analysis. The present findings strongly suggest that the multistep accumulation of aberrant CpG methylation in specific target genes and the presence of CIMP are deeply involved in the crisis, progression, and prognosis of ATLL, as well as indicate the value of CpG methylation and CIMP for new diagnostic and prognostic biomarkers.

▶ Adult T-cell leukemia/lymphoma (ATLL) is an aggressive malignant disease of CD4-positive T lymphocytes caused by infection with human T-lymphotropic virus type I (HTLV1). HTLV-1 causes ATLL in 3% to 5% of infected individuals after a long latent period of 40 to 60 years. Advanced acute ATLL has a poor prognosis. ATLL is divided into 4 stages: smoldering, chronic, lymphoma, and acute types. The smoldering and chronic types are indolent, but the acute and lymphoma types are aggressive ATLL characterized by resistance to chemotherapy and a poor prognosis. Such a long latent period suggests that a multistep leukemogenic/lymphomagenic mechanism is involved in the development of ATLL, although the critical events in the progression have not been characterized. The pathogenesis of HTLV-1 has been investigated intensively in terms of the viral regulatory protein HTLV-1 Tax or Rex, which is supposed to play key roles in the HTLV-1 leukemogenesis/lymphomagenesis and the recently discovered HTLV-1 basic leucine zipper factor. The authors and others have reported the progression mechanism of ATLL from various genetic aspects, including specific chromosome abnormalities, changes of characteristic HTLV-1 Tax and Rex protein expression pattern, and aberrant expression of the *SHP1, p53, MEL1S, DRS,* and ASY/Nogo genes, although the detailed mechanism triggering the onset and progression of ATLL is yet elucidated. On the other hand, epigenetic aberration processes have been recognized as playing another important role in carcinogenesis. The aberrant hypermethylation of CpG islands within the promoter and 5′-regions of genes is the most widely studied epigenetic abnormality in cancer and is associated with loss of gene function. Target genes of aberrant hypermethylation of CpG islands seem to be tumor type-specific, and current efforts are concentrated on finding ways to exploit the diagnostic and therapeutic implications of these abnormalities. A comprehensive knowledge of the methylation profile of a given tumor may provide important information for risk assessment, diagnosis, monitoring, and treatments.

M. G. Bissell, MD, PhD, MPH

Phenotyping Studies of Clonotypic B Lymphocytes From Patients With Multiple Myeloma by Flow Cytometry

Conway EJ, Wen J, Feng Y, et al (The Methodist Hosp and The Methodist Hosp Res Inst, Houston, TX; Huazhong Univ of Science and Technology, Wuhan, China; et al)
Arch Pathol Lab Med 133:1594-1599, 2009

Context.—Clonotypic B lymphocytes, monoclonal B lymphocytes sharing identical, rearranged IGH-CDR3 sequences with the patient's myeloma cells, have been detected in the peripheral blood of patients with multiple myeloma. These cells have been postulated to act as a therapy-resistant tumor reservoir that drives recurrence.

Objective.—To characterize clonotypic B lymphocytes for future investigation of their role in myeloma pathogenesis.

Design.—Harvests of cryopreserved peripheral blood stem-cells from 20 myeloma patients were enriched for clonotypic B lymphocytes. Cytoplasmic immunoglobulin light chain and surface immunophenotype were analyzed by flow cytometry. *IGH-CDR3* gene-rearrangement pattern was performed to determine clonality. Posttransplant remission rate was compared with the percentage of clonotypic B lymphocytes.

Results.—Clonotypic B lymphocytes expressing $CD34^{\pm}$, $CD38^{+}$, $CD184^{+}$, $CD31^{\pm}$, $CD50^{\pm}$, $CD138^{-}$, $CD19^{-}$, $CD20^{-}$, and the same immunoglobulin light chain as the patients' known myeloma cells were identified in 12 of 20 patients (60%). Progenitor B lymphocytes expressing similar surface immunophenotype but opposite light chains were identified in the same patients. Polymerase chain reaction for IGH rearrangement showed clonal rearrangement pattern in clonotypic lymphocytes but not in B lymphocytes expressing light chains opposite to myeloma cells. There was no statistically significant correlation between the percentage of clonotypic B lymphocytes and response to autologous transplant.

Conclusions.—Clonotypic B lymphocytes expressing CD34, but not CD19, were identified in stem cell harvests from patients with myeloma and could represent progenitor cells of neoplastic plasma cells. However, the same or similar immunophenotyping can be detected in both clonotypic B lymphocytes and benign progenitor B cells, suggesting clonality analysis might be needed to determine clonotypic B lymphocytes in patients with myeloma. Further studies are warranted to study the role of clonotypic B lymphocytes in the pathogenesis of myeloma.

▶ Multiple myeloma (MM) is the second most common hematologic cancer in the United States, representing 10% of all hematopoietic malignancies, and the most common hematopoietic malignancy in African Americans; 19 900 new cases of MM are diagnosed yearly, with nearly 11 000 deaths. Although a number of novel agents have been introduced in the treatment of MM, it remains an incurable disease even with myeloablative chemotherapy and autologous peripheral blood stem cell (PBSC) transplantation. The concept of clonotypic B lymphocytes (CBLs), also known as precursors of neoplastic plasma cells, in MM is widely accepted. CBLs have been identified in patients with MM and are monoclonal and share identical rearranged CDR3 sequences with the patient's myeloma cells. CBLs show somatic mutations of *IgH* gene in a nonrandom fashion, without intraclonal variation, suggesting a postgerminal center B-cell origin. Evidence, including oncogene expression, DNA aneuploidy, stem cell-like characteristics, and the clonal homogeneity, suggests that most of these B cells are malignant or premalignant and may represent precursors of neoplastic plasma cells. It is proposed that these B cells originate outside the marrow (lymph nodes and other lymphoid organs) and give rise to plasma cells only after migration to the bone marrow, which provides a microenvironment suitable for terminal plasma-cell differentiation. CBLs similar to those in MM are also detected in monoclonal gammopathy of undetermined significance, although at a lower frequency. Although the concept of CBL is widely accepted, their number and phenotypic characteristics remain an issue of controversy. CBL has been described as $CD19^{+}$, $CD38^{+}$, $CD10^{+}$, $CD11b^{+}$, $CD34^{+}$ (HPCA-1), variable $CD20^{+}$, $PCA-I^{+}$, $CD45RO^{+}$, variable $CD45^{+}$, and $CD56^{+}$. Cells expressing these markers have been shown to be present in significant amounts at 0.15×10^{9}/L (SD, 0.02; range, 9%-95% of peripheral blood B cells). The authors' preliminary studies, and studies of others, have detected far fewer CBLs in patients with MM. Furthermore, different phenotypic expression patterns, particularly regarding the expression of CD19 and CD34, have been reported in CBLs. It has been suggested that the CBLs, which are not eradicated by chemotherapy, are responsible for incurability in MM. Bone marrow neoplastic plasma cells in MM are usually depleted by chemotherapy, but recent studies have shown that the CBLs survive despite intensive chemotherapy and remain at high levels even during transient remissions. Higher numbers of CBL have been observed in peripheral blood from patients with progressive disease or early relapse after high-dose chemotherapy and PBSC transplant. In vitro, these cells have been shown to express the multidrug-resistance protein (P-glycoprotein) encoded by *MDR1* gene and exhibit a very efficient drug export capacity leading to resistance to multiple chemotherapeutic agents. The main goal of this study was to characterize the CBLs in patients with MM using a comprehensive panel of surface markers.

M. G. Bissell, MD, PhD, MPH

White Blood Cell Count Predicts All-Cause Mortality in Patients with Suspected Peripheral Arterial Disease
Arain FA, Khaleghi M, Bailey KR, et al (Mayo Clinic, Rochester, MN)
Am J Med 122:874.e1-874.e7, 2009

Objective.— We investigated whether markers of inflammation—white blood cell (WBC) count, C-reactive protein (CRP), and lipoprotein-associated phospholipase A2—are associated with mortality in patients referred for noninvasive lower-extremity arterial evaluation.

Methods.—Participants (n = 242, mean age 68 years, 54% men) were followed for a median of 71 months. Ankle-brachial index (ABI), WBC count, plasma CRP, and lipoprotein-associated phospholipase A2 were measured at the start of the study. Factors associated with all-cause mortality were identified using Cox proportional hazards.

Results.—During the follow-up period, 56 patients (25%) died. Factors associated with higher mortality were greater age, history of coronary artery disease/cerebrovascular disease, lower ABI, higher serum creatinine, and higher WBC count/plasma CRP. In stepwise multivariable regression analysis, ABI, serum creatinine, WBC count, and CRP were associated significantly with mortality. Patients in the top tertile of WBC count and CRP level had a relative risk of mortality of 3.37 (confidence interval [CI], 1.56-7.27) and 2.12 (CI, 0.97-4.62), respectively. However, only the WBC count contributed incrementally to prediction of mortality. Inferences were similar when analyses were limited to patients with peripheral arterial disease (ABI < 0.9, n = 114).

Conclusion.—WBC count, but not plasma CRP level, provides incremental information about the risk of death in patients referred for lower-extremity arterial evaluation and in the subset of these patients with peripheral arterial disease.

▶ Peripheral arterial disease affects approximately 8 million people in the United States and is associated with a 3-fold higher risk of all-cause mortality and a 6-fold higher risk of cardiovascular-related mortality independent of conventional risk factors. Peripheral arterial disease is a surrogate of systemic atherosclerosis and is considered a coronary artery disease risk equivalent. Inflammation is suspected of playing a central role in the development and progression of systemic atherosclerosis. Markers of inflammation, including white blood cell (WBC) count, C-reactive protein (CRP), and lipoprotein associated phospholipase A2, are associated with increased risk of myocardial infarction, peripheral arterial disease, and stroke. There is also evidence that inflammatory markers are associated with higher mortality and adverse cardiovascular outcomes in patients with known atherosclerotic vascular disease. The authors hypothesized that in patients with suspected peripheral arterial disease who are referred for noninvasive lower-extremity arterial evaluation, the WBC count and plasma levels of CRP and lipoprotein-associated phospholipase A2 would be associated with mortality in the intermediate term. They investigated whether markers of inflammation—WBC count, CRP, and lipoprotein-associated phospholipase A2—are associated with mortality in patients referred for noninvasive, lower extremity arterial evaluation. Participants (n = 242, mean age 68 years, 54% men) were followed for a median of 71 months. Ankle-brachial index (ABI), WBC count, plasma CRP, and lipoprotein-associated phospholipase A2 were measured at the start of the study. Factors associated with all-cause mortality were identified using Cox proportional hazards. During the follow-up period, 56 patients (25%) died. Factors associated with higher mortality were greater age, history of coronary artery disease/cerebrovascular disease, lower ABI, higher serum creatinine, and higher WBC count/plasma CRP. In stepwise multivariable regression analysis, ABI, serum creatinine, WBC count, and CRP were associated significantly with mortality. Patients in the top tertile of WBC count and CRP level had a relative risk of mortality of 3.37 (confidence interval (CI), 1.56-7.27) and 2.12 (CI, 0.97-4.62), respectively. However, only the WBC count contributed incrementally to the prediction of mortality. Inferences were similar when analyses were limited to patients with peripheral arterial disease (ABI < 0.9, n = 114). WBC count, but not plasma CRP level, provides incremental information about the risk of death in patients referred for lower extremity arterial evaluation and in the subset of these patients with peripheral arterial disease.

M. G. Bissell, MD, PhD, MPH

19 Transfusion Medicine and Coagulation

Analysis of sample-to-cutoff ratios on chemiluminescent immunoassays used for blood donor screening highlights the need for serologic confirmatory testing
Kiely P, Walker K, Parker S, et al (Infectious Disease Screening Laboratory, Melbourne, Brisbane, Australia)
Transfusion 50:1344-1351, 2010

Background.—High sample-to-cutoff (s/co) ratios on hepatitis C virus antibody (anti-HCV) screening immunoassays (IAs) are indicative of confirmed-positive results and, according to some reports, can be used to determine anti-HCV status without the need for confirmatory testing. The purpose of this study was to determine whether s/co ratios on hepatitis B surface antigen (HBsAg), antibody to human immunodeficiency virus Types 1 and 2 (anti-HIV-1/2), anti-HCV, and antibody to human T-lymphotropic virus Types I and II (anti-HTLV-I/II) chemiluminescent immunoassays (ChLIAs) can be used to discriminate between biologic false-reactive (BFR) and confirmed-positive results.

Study Design and Methods.—In a blood donor population the s/co ratio distributions for BFR and confirmed-positive results were compared for the Abbott PRISM HBsAg, HIV O Plus, HCV, and HTLV-I/II ChLIAs to determine the extent of overlap between the two distributions for each assay.

Results.—The s/co ratio distributions for BFR and confirmed results overlapped in the range of 10.00 to 60.00, 1.00 to 6.00, 3.00 to 15.00, and 1.00 to 100.00 for the PRISM HIV O Plus, HCV, HTLV-I/II, and HBsAg assays, respectively.

Conclusion.—Although high s/co ratios were predictive of confirmed-positive results in all four assays, a number of confirmed-positive samples gave low values while some biologic false-positive samples showed high values. As the s/co ratio distributions for BFR and confirmed-positive results overlapped for all four PRISM assays, this study highlights the importance of serologic confirmatory testing and the need for caution when using screening IA results to assign a final donor status.

▶ A number of reports have shown that relatively high sample-to-cutoff (s/co) ratios on screening immunoassays (IAs) for antibodies to hepatitis C virus (anti-HCV) are predictive of confirmed-positive results in both blood donors and nondonor populations. As well, it has been suggested that an anti-HCV status can be assigned solely on the basis of screening IA s/co ratios. The purpose of this study was to compare the s/co ratio distributions of biologic false-reactive (BFR) results with confirmed-positive results for 4 chemiluminescent IAs (ChLIAs) in a blood donor population. For each assay, the extent of s/co ratio overlap between BFR and confirmed-positive results was analyzed to determine whether ChLIA s/co ratios were reliably predictive of the final donor status. Although high s/co ratios were predictive of confirmed-positive results in all 4 assays, a number of confirmed-positive samples gave low values, while some biologic false-positive samples showed high values. As the s/co ratio distributions for BFR and confirmed-positive results overlapped for all 4 PRISM assays, this study highlights the importance of serologic confirmatory testing and the need for caution when using screening IA results to assign a final donor status.

M. G. Bissell, MD, PhD, MPH

Automated Assay for Fondaparinux (Arixtra) on the Dade Behring BCS XP
Sanfelippo MJ, Tillema VB (Marshfield Clinic, WI)
Am J Clin Pathol 132:608-612, 2009

An assay for fondaparinux (Arixtra) is described based on a modified commercial assay for heparin. The assay is automated on a Dade Behring BCS XP (Siemens Healthcare Diagnostics, Deerfield, IL) and uses the inhibition of activated factor X to quantitate the drug. The assay was unaffected by platelet contamination or the presence of warfarin. The assay was affected by the antithrombin level, and the value obtained in the assay decreased significantly when the antithrombin level was less than 60%. The assay is, however, not specific for fondaparinux. Specimens containing unfractionated or low-molecular-weight heparin will yield results by this assay that will not be an accurate estimation of concentration.

▶ Fondaparinux (Arixtra) is a pentasaccharide with anticoagulant activity by reason of its ability to accelerate the inactivation of activated factor X (Xa) by antithrombin. Fondaparinux has a long half-life and rarely requires monitoring because of its very predictable anticoagulant activity. The only patients for whom monitoring is required are elderly patients and patients with compromised renal function. When monitoring is required, common laboratory tests, such as the prothrombin time and the activated partial thromboplastin time are of no use because fondaparinux has a minimal effect on both test systems. Fondaparinux can be monitored by measuring its anti-Xa activity in a test system similar to the one used for monitoring unfractionated and low-molecular-weight heparins in which factor Xa is present in excess to which plasma specimen containing fondaparinux is added. The formation of the inactive antithrombin-fondaparinux complex is allowed to proceed to endpoint and the remaining factor Xa is determined by reaction with a chromogenic substrate that liberates paranitroaniline when hydrolyzed. The change in absorbance at 405 nm relates directly to the concentration of Xa and inversely to that of fondaparinux. Because fondaparinux inactivates Xa at a different rate than either unfractionated heparin or low-molecular-weight heparin, the assay must be calibrated using fondaparinux. As the use of this drug becomes broader, requests for monitoring will increase. Although there are reference laboratories that are assaying fondaparinux, a simple automated assay will allow hospital laboratories to provide an in-house assay with a reasonably short turnaround time. This article describes an assay that is automated on a common laboratory instrument. In addition, the authors evaluated the requirement for antithrombin in the test plasma to obtain an accurate level of fondaparinux in the assay, finding that it is affected by reduced levels, although it is not affected by the presence of warfarin or platelets in the specimen. They also evaluated commercial calibration plasma and control material.

M. G. Bissell, MD, PhD, MPH

Demographic variations in blood donor deferrals in a major metropolitan area

Shaz BH, James AB, Hillyer KL, et al (Emory Univ, Atlanta, GA; American Red Cross Blood Services Southeast Division, Douglasville, GA; Westat, Rockville, MD; et al)

Transfusion 50:881-887, 2010

Background.—Presenting blood donors are screened to ensure both their safety and that of the recipients of blood products. Donors with identified risks are deferred from donating blood either temporarily or permanently. Minorities are underrepresented as donors in the United States and this may in part be a result of increased donor deferral rates in minorities compared to white individuals.

Study Design and Methods.—Data consisted of deferred and successful blood donor presentations to the American Red Cross Southern Region in the metropolitan Atlanta area in 2004 to 2008. Bivariate and multivariate analyses were conducted by race/ethnicity, age group, and sex.

Results.—A total of 586,159 voluntary donor presentations occurred in 2004 to 2008, of which 79,214 (15.6%) resulted in deferral. In the age 16 to 69 years subset (98.3% of the presentations), deferred presentations were mostly women (78.2%). The most common reason for donor deferral was low hemoglobin (62.6%). The donor deferral rate varied by race/ethnicity, age, and sex: whites (11.1%), Hispanics (14.1%), and African Americans (17.9%); 16- to 19-year-olds (17.0%) and 50- to 59-year-olds (11.7%); and females (20.0%) and males (6.2%). Compared to whites and Hispanics, African American females had the highest deferral rate in each age group.

Conclusions.—Minorities are disproportionately impacted by blood donor deferrals. Methods to decrease blood donor deferral rates among African Americans are needed.

▶ In the United States, blood donation rates, expressed as the number of donated products per population, of African Americans are approximately 30% of that of whites. The reason for this difference is not known; one hypothesis is that the prevalence of medical comorbidities may reduce the number of African Americans that are eligible to donate. If the donation rate could be determined based on individuals who are eligible to give blood the rates for African Americans may not be dissimilar to other groups. Donor eligibility criteria are designed to protect both the donor and the recipient. The Food and Drug Administration's Code of Federal Regulations and the MBE Standards for Blood Banks and Transfusion Services define these criteria. Conventional methods for calculating blood donor eligibility have used only age adjustment; therefore, it was calculated that 60% of the total United States population was eligible to donate. Recently, Riley and coworkers published estimates of the donor pool based on an exclusion adjusted method and estimated that only 38% of the population is likely to be eligible. Their model did not capture demographic factors such as sex, race/ethnicity, and seasonality, which may further limit the number of eligible donors within each of these groups. The proportion of a population that is eligible to donate may differ for various racial and ethnic populations based on additional assumptions not included by Riley and coworkers including race-based medical comorbidities. Indeed, in African Americans, there is a higher incidence of sickle-cell disease, cancer, hypertension, diabetes, renal disease, human immunodeficiency virus/acquired immunodeficiency syndrome, and anemia. Furthermore, the mean hemoglobin value of African Americans is between 0.5 and 0.7 g/dL lower than that of whites, even when controlled for selected variables, including iron deficiency, age, sex, hemoglobinopathies, and socioeconomic factors. In addition, iron-deficiency anemia is more prevalent among minorities, especially women. Therefore, African Americans may have higher deferral rates than whites, which may in turn result in lower blood donation rates. Another important factor in lower blood donation rates secondary to deferral is that individuals who present to donate and are temporarily deferred return less frequently for subsequent donation than those who were successfully able to donate; this is especially true for those presenting for the first time. The purpose of this study was to evaluate donor deferral rates and the reasons for deferrals by race/ethnicity, sex, and age in a metropolitan area. An understanding of these rates is necessary to better understand the discrepancy in donation rates among African Americans, Hispanics, and whites.

M. G. Bissell, MD, PhD, MPH

Development and validation of a SYBR Green I–based real-time polymerase chain reaction method for detection of haptoglobin gene deletion in clinical materials

Soejima M, Tsuchiya Y, Egashira K, et al (Kurume Univ Hosp, Japan)
Transfusion 50:1322-1327, 2010

Background.—Anhaptoglobinemic patients run the risk of severe anaphylactic transfusion reaction because they produce serum hapto-globin (Hp) antibodies. Being homozygous for the Hp gene deletion (HP^{del}) is the only known cause of congenital anhaptoglobinemia, and clinical diagnosis of HP^{del} before transfusion is important to prevent anaphylactic shock. We recently developed a 5′-nuclease (TaqMan) real-time polymerase chain reaction (PCR) method.

Study Design and Methods.—A SYBR Green I–based duplex real-time PCR assay using two forward primers and a common reverse primer followed by melting curve analysis was developed to determine HP^{del} zygosity in a single tube. In addition, to obviate initial DNA extraction, we examined serially diluted blood samples as PCR templates.

Results.—Allelic discrimination of HP^{del} yielded optimal results at blood sample dilutions of 1:64 to 1:1024. The results from 2231 blood samples were fully concordant with those obtained by the TaqMan-based real-time PCR method.

Conclusion.—The detection rate of the HP^{del} allele by the SYBR Green I–based method is comparable with that using the TaqMan-based method. This method is readily applicable due to its low initial cost and analyzability using economical real-time PCR machines and is suitable for high-throughput analysis as an alternative method for allelic discrimination of HP^{del} (Fig 1).

▶ Anaphylaxis is a severe nonhemolytic transfusion reaction, and determination of its causes is urgently needed. The absence of a serum protein such as immunoglobulin A or haptoglobin (Hp) is one factor that can lead to anaphylactic transfusion reactions due to production of serum antibodies against it. At

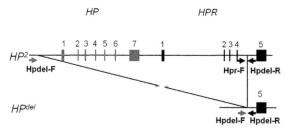

FIGURE 1.—Structures of the HP^2, and HP^{del} alleles and relative positions of the Hpdel-F, Hpr-F, and Hpdel-R primers. (Reprinted from Soejima M, Tsuchiya Y, Egashira K, et al. Development and validation of a SYBR Green I–based real-time polymerase chain reaction method for detection of haptoglobin gene deletion in clinical materials. *Transfusion.* 2010;50:1322-1327.)

present, a homozygous deletion of the Hp gene (Hp^{del}, Fig 1) is the only known cause of anhaptoglobinemia. Hp binds hemoglobin to prevent both iron loss and kidney damage during hemolysis. Humans have a genetic polymorphism of the protein because of 2 codominant alleles, Hpl and Hp2, that give rise to the 3 major phenotypes, Hpl, Hp2-l, and Hp2. Because of its polymorphic nature, Hp has been used as a genetic marker for identification of individuals and determination of parentage. Anomalous inheritance of the Hp phenotypes was encountered during determinations of parentage, and Hp^{del} was identified by genetic analyses of 1 such family in Japan. The Hp^{del} allele lacks an approximately 28-kb segment of Chromosome 16 extending from the promoter region of the Hp gene to Intron 4 of the Hp-related gene. Two different methods have been demonstrated to be useful for the detection of anhaptoglobinemia. One is detection of Hp^{del} allele by polymerase chain reaction (PCR) or Southern blotting and the other is quantification of Hp protein by enzyme-linked immunosorbent assay (ELISA). The ELISA method is sensitive and able to discriminate efficiently between anhaptoglobinemia and hypohaptoglobinemia. However, this method requires confirmation of the presence of Hp^{del} by a PCR-based method. A duplex PCR method allows determination of the zygosity of Hp^{del}. Using this method, frequencies of the Hp^{del} allele were examined in several human populations. This allele has been found only in East and Southeast Asian populations (Chinese, Korean, Japanese, Mongols, Thais, and Indonesians) but not in African, West and South Asian, and European populations so far. Detection of homozygotes for Hp^{del} before blood transfusion or blood component infusion is important to prevent severe side effects of transfusion because washed red blood cells and platelet concentrate are effective in preventing the transfusion-related anaphylactic reactions. Although isolation of genomic DNA, conventional PCR, and gel electrophoresis are routine methods in research and molecular biology laboratories, they are not suitable for large-scale analysis or diagnosis before transfusion in the clinical laboratory because they require laborious post-PCR processing steps. Real-time PCR is a high-throughput, rapid, and sensitive method that has become common. It also eliminates post-PCR processing of PCR products, which reduces the chance of carryover contamination. Recently, the authors established a diagnostic method for detection of Hp^{del} by a 5'-nuclease assay using dual-labeled (TaqMan) probes. This method is highly specific because of the sequence-specific hybridization of the probe and is cost effective when many samples are treated simultaneously, such as screening for anhaptoglobinemic patients in a blood donor pool or for large-scale screening in various populations. However, if only a few samples are examined in the clinical laboratory, the initial cost is high because 2 dual-labeled probes are necessary for determination of zygosity. In addition, multichannel real-time PCR machines, which are expensive compared with single-channel real-time PCR machines, are required to perform this system. To resolve this problem, they developed a SYBR Green I-based real-time PCR method for detection of Hp^{del}. SYBR Green I, an intercalating dye that binds to double-stranded DNA, is used to detect the accumulated PCR product. Because an increase in the fluorescent signal is detected not only by specific amplification of the product but also by the primer dimer or nonspecific amplified product, dissociation curve analysis is required to confirm the specificity of the PCR product. In addition, to reduce the time and cost of genomic DNA isolation, they examined serially diluted blood samples as PCR templates instead of genomic DNA.

M. G. Bissell, MD, PhD, MPH

First transmission of human immunodeficiency virus Type 1 by a cellular blood product after mandatory nucleic acid screening in Germany
Schmidt M, Korn K, Nübling CM, et al (Johann Wolfgang Goethe Univ, Frankfurt, Germany; Univ Hosp Erlangen, Germany; the Paul-Ehrlich-Institut, Langen, Germany; et al)
Transfusion 49:1836-1844, 2009

Background.—In February 2007, a 63-year-old man underwent surgery. Retrospective testing with nucleic acid testing (NAT) showed that the patient was human immunodeficiency virus Type 1 (HIV-1) positive 10 days after transfusion. The transfusion-transmitted infection had been identified by a donor-related lookback started in April 2007 after anti-HIV seroconversion.

Methods.—Sequence analysis was performed in the gag-pol region as well as in the V3 loop env region. Archived plasma from the transmitting donation was investigated for the individual-donation NAT with the Roche COBAS AmpliPrep/COBAS TaqMan HIV-1 test (Roche CAP/CTM HIV-1 test) and for HIV antigen/antibody combination testing (Abbott Architect). Additional testing was done on the donor's follow-up sample and on the recipient's sample.

Results.—The Roche CAP/CTM HIV-1 test failed to detect viral RNA by minipool NAT in the index donation (April 2007) as well as in the donation that caused the infection (January 2007). Phylogenetic analysis showed a very high genetic similarity among viral sequences from both donor and recipient, proving the HIV-1 transmission by sequence data.

Conclusion.—This case represents the first documented HIV-1 transmission by transfusion of red blood cells after mandatory introduction of HIV-1 NAT for blood screening in Germany. Low viral load and mismatches in the primer/probe region might explain the detection failure of the NAT screening assay. A certain risk remains that new virus variants contain mutations at positions critical for amplification or detection of viral genomes. An option to reduce the risk of a detection failure by NAT is the simultaneous use of several conserved regions as amplification targets.

► In the 1980s and early 1990s, approximately 50% of all German hemophilia patients were infected with human immunodeficiency virus type I (HIV-I) by contaminated plasma derivatives. To improve blood safety, the German Red Cross (GRC) blood donor services developed in-house minipool nucleic acid testing (MP-NAT; pools of 96) systems for blood donor screening. The MP-NAT systems were introduced in 1997 on a voluntary basis for HIV-I, hepatitis

C virus (HCV), and hepatitis B virus (HBV) and in 2000 for hepatitis A virus and parvovirus BI9. Blood donor screening by NAT was mandated in Germany for HCV in 1999 and for HIV-I in 2004 with an analytical sensitivity of at least 5000 IU/mL and 10 000 IU/mL for HCV and HIV-I, respectively. The efficiency of MP-NAT after screening more than 31 million blood donations by GRC from 1997 to 2005 was reported on. Seven HIV-I NAT-only-positive window phase donations were detected by MP-NAT. Based on a mathematical model developed by Glynn and colleagues, the residual risk of acquiring a transfusion-associated HIV-I infection was calculated at 1 in 4.3 million. At the inception of MP-NAT screening, 1 HIV-I breakthrough infection by RNA-screened blood occurred in 1998. The design of the GRC early in-house NAT system used was primarily optimized for the detection of HIV-I M subtype B, which is the most common HIV-I subtype in Germany. Subtype A, present in this breakthrough transmission, was detected with lower efficiency due to mismatches in the primer-binding region. Therefore, the design of the HIV-I polymerase chain reaction (PCR) assay at the affected test site was changed to detect all currently known HIV-I M subtypes. From this time on, no transfusion-associated HIV-I infection was reported by GRC blood service until the occurrence of this case in 2007. This article reports the first HIV-I breakthrough infection in Germany after MP-NAT was mandated by the German authorities in 2004. Time period linkage and sequence analysis in 2 HIV genome regions, in the conserved gag and pol regions and in the hypervariable env region, confirmed the transfusion-related transmission. Additional experimental data demonstrate new opportunities for simultaneous amplification and detection in 2 conserved genome regions.

M. G. Bissell, MD, PhD, MPH

Implementation of a Rapid Whole Blood D-Dimer Test in the Emergency Department of an Urban Academic Medical Center: Impact on ED Length of Stay and Ancillary Test Utilization
Lee-Lewandrowski E, Nichols J, Van Cott E, et al (Massachusetts General Hosp and Harvard Med School, Boston)
Am J Clin Pathol 132:326-331, 2009

Overcrowding and prolonged patient length-of-stay (LOS) in emergency departments (EDs) are growing problems. We evaluated the impact of implementing a rapid whole blood quantitative D-dimer test (Biosite Triage, Biosite Diagnostics, San Diego, CA) in our ED satellite laboratory on 252 patients before vs 211 patients after implementation. All patients also underwent testing with the existing central laboratory method (VIDAS D-dimer, bioMérieux, Durham, NC). D-dimer turnaround time (from blood draw to result) decreased approximately 79% (~2 hours vs 25 minutes). The mean ED LOS declined from 8.46 to 7.14 hours ($P = .016$). Hospital admissions decreased 13.8%, ED discharges increased 7.3%, and the number of patients admitted for observation increased 6.4% ($P = .005$). No difference in the utilization of radiologic studies was observed

($P =.86$). At 3 months' follow-up, none of the after-implementation patients with negative D-dimer results were admitted for subsequent venous thromboembolic disease. The rapid D-dimer test was associated with a shorter ED LOS and fewer hospital admissions.

▶ Emergency department (ED) overcrowding and prolonged patient length of stay (LOS) are increasing problems in most American hospitals. One factor influencing ED efficiency is the availability of ancillary services, including the turnaround time for laboratory tests required to triage, diagnose, and make decisions concerning patient disposition. However, there are relatively few data concerning the impact of rapid point-of-care testing (POCT) on ED operations, including patient LOS. Testing for D-dimer is commonly used in the ED for the exclusion of venous thromboembolic (VTE) disease in low-risk patients. Traditionally, testing has been performed in the central laboratory, preferably using a quantitative enzyme-linked immunosorbent assay (ELISA). Current evidence indicates that for excluding VTE disease in low-risk patients, including deep venous thrombosis (DVT) and pulmonary embolism (PE), a negative D-dimer ELISA test effectively excludes VTE disease in a manner comparable with a lung scan or duplex ultrasonography. One of the more commonly used D-dimer ELISA assays is the bioM6rieux (Durham, NC) VIDAS D-dimer test. This assay was the first D-dimer ELISA to be accepted by the US Food and Drug Administration for the exclusion of VTE disease in low-risk patients One problem with this assay is that the test turnaround time is relatively slow (approximately 40 minutes, including sample processing); in addition, the instrument is poorly suited for POCT applications. Furthermore, the preanalytic time required to get a sample from an ED to the laboratory can be quite long, even when a pneumatic tube is available, averaging 42% of the total turnaround time in 1 study. In a crowded ED experiencing pressure to minimize patient LOS, the relatively long turnaround time of central laboratory testing may be a significant problem. In this study, the authors evaluated the impact of implementing a rapid whole blood quantitative D-dimer test in their ED satellite laboratory at the Massachusetts General Hospital, Boston. They hypothesized that the availability of a rapid whole blood D-dimer test would decrease the time needed to evaluate patients suspected of having VTE disease and thus permit more rapid decisions concerning appropriate disposition. Furthermore, they wanted to evaluate whether the availability of the rapid test would impact use of follow-up radiologic studies or the rate of admission to our observation unit or general medical beds.

M. G. Bissell, MD, PhD, MPH

Paired crossover study of two plateletpheresis systems concerning platelet product quality and donor comfort
Flesch BK, Adamzik I, Steppat D, et al (Univ Hosp Schleswig-Holstein, Kiel, Germany; Fenwal Inc, Lake Zurich, IL)
Transfusion 50:894-901, 2010

Background.—Two plateletpheresis cell separator systems were compared in a paired crossover study with respect to the product quality, the number of platelet (PLT) units per donation, and the donor comfort.

Study Design and Methods.—Forty-four female and 47 male donors were distributed to three body weight groups. Double PLT units with 6×10^{11} PLTs were collected from three Fenwal Amicus Crescendo (AC) and three CaridianBCT Trima Accel (TA) machines. Each donor made one donation on each randomly assigned system and answered a questionnaire on the subjective donor comfort. The answers were scored from 5 (best) to 1 (worst).

Results.—Based on 182 donations, with 91 donations on AC and TA separators each, 179 runs resulted in double PLT units and three ($2 \times AC$, $1 \times TA$) in single units. The white blood cell counts were below 1×10^6 in all but eight therapeutic units ($8 \times TA$; mean, 1.98×10^6). The mean PLT yield (AC 6.00×10^{11}, TA 5.98×10^{11}), the collection rate, and the PLT extraction coefficient did not significantly differ between the two devices. Differences of the donor comfort over all groups were only observed for the loudness of the instrument (4.63 AC vs. 4.24 TA, $p < 0.001$) and the subjective impression of the run time (4.24 AC vs. 4.48 TA, $p < 0.05$). Male donors greater than 88 kg preferred the TA instruments concerning the impact of the needle, run time, overall experience ($p < 0.01$ each), and willingness to donate on the same instrument again ($p < 0.05$).

Conclusions.—Only minor differences were observed despite the fact that the AC separators are run with two needles and the TA with one needle.

▶ Single-donor plateletpheresis products are preferred, especially for patients at high risk (eg, hematology or oncology patients awaiting hematopoietic progenitor cell transplantation) or for immunized patients. Apheresis systems based on different technical concepts and enabling single- or double-needle donations were developed by different manufacturers. For blood donation services, the product quality and the donor comfort are the most important aspects. Recent apheresis systems enable the simultaneous donation of platelet (PLT) and plasma products and the production of double or even triple therapeutic PLT units from 1 donation. The total PLT count, the residual white blood cell (WBC) count, and the absence of PLT aggregates are the variables contributing to the product quality, while the entire procedure handling time, the loudness, and the impact of the needle are concerning the user friendliness and donor comfort. Because blood donation centers are dependent on the willingness of their donors to give blood voluntarily and repeatedly, donor comfort is an essential criterion. The aim of this randomized crossover study was to compare the apheresis instruments of 2 manufacturers concerning donor preferences and quality criteria as well.

M. G. Bissell, MD, PhD, MPH

Rapid screening of granulocyte antibodies with a novel assay: flow cytometric granulocyte immunofluorescence test

Nguyen XD, Flesch B, Sachs UJ, et al (Heidelberg Univ, Mannheim, Germany; Univ Hosp Schleswig-Holstein, Kiel, Germany; Justus-Liebig-Univ Giessen, Germany; et al)

Transfusion 49:2700-2708, 2009

Background.—White blood cell (WBC)-associated antibodies can lead to severe pulmonary transfusion reactions (transfusion-related acute lung injury [TRALI]). Investigation of a large number of blood donor samples using the standard granulocyte immunofluorescence test (GIFT) and granulocyte agglutination test (GAT) proved to be difficult to perform due to the time-consuming process and the large quantity of test cells required. This study describes the novel flow cytometric GIFT (Flow-GIFT) method for a rapid detection of granulocyte antibodies by flow cytometric analysis.

Study Design and Methods.—A total of 141 sera were analyzed for the presence of granulocyte antibodies that were previously associated with suspected TRALI. As test cells whole blood samples from human neutrophil antigen (HNA)-typed donors were isolated using cell sedimentation in a ficoll density gradient. WBCs were incubated with the respective serum and binding of antibodies to the test cells was detected using fluorescein isothiocyanate–conjugated anti-human antibody. Standard GIFT and GAT were performed as reference methods.

Results.—Seven sera containing anti-HNA-3a, CD16, and HLA Class I were negative in the standard GIFT and eight sera containing anti-HNA-2a, anti-CD16, and anti-HLA Class I were not detected in the GAT. The novel Flow-GIFT was able to detect all granulocyte antibodies, which were only detectable in a combination of standard GIFT and GAT. In serial dilution tests, the Flow-GIFT detected the antibodies at higher dilutions than the reference methods GIFT and GAT.

Conclusion.—The Flow-GIFT method permits rapid detection of granulocyte antibodies requiring fewer donor test cells. This method is ideal for automation and will potentially open the way for screening of granulocyte antibodies in a large donor population.

▶ Granulocyte alloantibodies can lead to febrile transfusion reactions or severe pulmonary transfusion reactions (transfusion-related acute lung injury [TRALI]). Occasionally, these antibodies cause serious symptoms that may be fatal to recipients, especially when granulocyte antibodies specific for the human neutrophil antigen 3a (HNA-3a) are involved. The pathogenesis of

TRALI includes the infusion of specific antibodies from the donor directed against antigens (HLA Class II or HNA) present on the recipient's white blood cells (WBCs) resulting in granulocyte activation, complement activation, neutrophil sequestration, and activation in the lung, culminating in endothelial damage, capillary leak, and acute lung injury. The granulocyte immunofluorescence test (GIFT) and the granulocyte agglutination test (GAT) have been introduced as the reference methods for the detection of granulocyte antibodies in the past. Recently, flow cytometry has also been established as a sensitive method for the detection of granulocyte-bound immunoglobulins. However, these methods require the isolation of granulocytes frequently coming along with a high cell loss due to the cell isolation using ficoll density centrifugation. Thus, the investigation of a large number of blood donor samples using the standard GIFT and GAT proved to be difficult to perform because of the time-consuming process and the large number of test cells required. The combination of both methods is at present necessary to detect all relevant antibodies to HNA, particularly HNA-3a antibodies that can be reliably detected only by GAT. Luminex-based multiplex fluorescent bead platform has also been developed to test for HLA antibodies. This system has been further developed to also detect neutrophil antibodies. However, anti-HNA-3a cannot be detected by this system because this antigen is intended for coating, which is not available on the beads. In this study, the authors developed a new flow cytometric GIFT (Flow-GIFT) method for the rapid detection of granulocyte antibodies without the necessity for an additional GAT. For the isolation process they used a ficoll density gradient without a centrifugation step to avoid a high cell loss.

M. G. Bissell, MD, PhD, MPH

Screening of single-donor apheresis platelets for bacterial contamination: the PASSPORT study results

Dumont LJ, Kleinman S, Murphy JR, et al (Dartmouth Med School, Lebanon, NH; Univ of British Columbia, Vancouver, Canada; Natl Jewish Health, Denver, CO; et al)

Transfusion 50:589-599, 2010

Background.—The PASSPORT study was an FDA-mandated surveillance of outdated 7-day apheresis platelets (APs) to assess the bacterial culture release test (RT) performance and the chance of transfusing APs containing viable bacteria compared to untested 5-day APs.

Study Design and Methods.—Aerobic and anaerobic culture bottles were inoculated with 4 to 5 mL from APs 24 to 36 hours postcollection. APs were released after 24 hours if no growth was observed. Released APs were recalled for RT positives, and clinical services were notified. Day 8 APs were recultured (surveillance test [ST]). Initially positive RTs and STs were confirmed by AP reculture.

Results.—A total of 388,903 RTs were accrued September 2005 through January 2008 from 52 regional blood centers: RT-positive APs interdicted before transfusion, 76 true positive (TP; 195/million; 95%

AP Storage Days

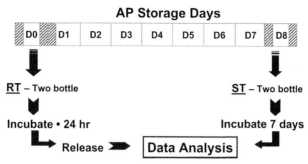

FIGURE 1.—PASSPORT flow: APs were collected on Day 0, sampled for two-bottle RTs 24 to 36 hours after collection, and released to inventory as 7-day PLTs if BTA negative after 24 hours on test (one center labeled only for 5-day shelf life, see text). All centers participated in the RT phase. APs not transfused at the end of Day 7 were resampled for surveillance cultures. Cultures were held up to 7 days. See text for details. (Reprinted from Dumont LJ, Kleinman S, Murphy JR, et al. Screening of single-donor apheresis platelets for bacterial contamination: the PASSPORT study results. *Transfusion*. 2010;50:589-599.)

confidence interval [CI], 154-244/million) and 57 indeterminate (IN); and RT-positive APs transfused, 14 TP and 242 IN. There were 14 reported septic transfusion reactions (STRs) from 13 AP collections (23 units) transfused on Days 3 through 7; three STRs were from Day 6 or 7 APs. There were two false-negative RTs causing STRs in three patients. No deaths were reported. STs had four TPs of 6039 tested (662/million; 95% CI, 180-1695/million).

Conclusions.—RT culturing prevents issuance of some bacterially contaminated APs. ST culture data and clinical reports suggest that this screening fails to detect all contaminated units. No fatalities were reported related to AP transfusion. Additional actions or testing may be required to further reduce the residual STR risk of RT APs, even with a 5-day storage limitation (Fig 1).

▶ Before routine bacterial culture testing of platelets (PLTs), transmission of bacteria in blood components was the highest risk transfusion-transmitted infectious disease. The incidence of contamination has been reported between 0.3 and 1 per 1000 units (300-1000/million), while the risk of a clinical septic transfusion reaction was between 75 and 402 per million for single-donor PLTs and PLTs from whole blood, respectively. Bacterial contamination of PLTs for transfusion has historically been one of the leading causes of morbidity and mortality associated with transfusion. This risk has been one of the important determinants of the maximum storage time permitted for room temperature-stored PLTs. Because of concerns over bacterial proliferation in room temperature-stored PLTs, the US Food and Drug Administration (FDA) reduced the permissible storage time of PLTs from 7 to 5 days in the mid-1980s. In 2005, the FDA cleared leukoreduced PLTs collected by apheresis (AP) from 3 companies for storage through 7 days at room temperature based on acceptable PLT performance. To implement storage of AP for up to 7 days, the FDA required a postmarketing surveillance study to assess the field performance of the bacterial screening method used as a release test (RT) for APs. CaridianBCT, Inc (formerly Gambro BCT, Inc), initiated the study and was later joined by Fenwal, Inc (formerly Baxter, Inc). This report will present the outcomes of the Post Approval Surveillance Study of Platelet Outcomes, Release Tested (Fig 1). In 2003, the American Association of Blood Banks issued Standard 5.1.5.1 requiring 100% testing of all PLT products for bacteria by March 2004. In response, many blood collection organizations implemented 100% bacterial screening of AP as a quality control (QC) test using the bioMerieuxBacT/ ALERT Microbial Detection System (BTA; bioMerieux, Durham, NC), a widely used system in North America and Europe both for diagnostic clinical microbiology and for the testing of PLT products. This system had been cleared by FDA for the QC testing of leukoreduced PLTs. The authors surveyed the first 20 months of experience from several US blood suppliers that tested 4-mL APs in the aerobic bottle. Their primary objective in this postmarketing surveillance study was to demonstrate that 7-day APs when tested using the BTA would not present a greater risk of a detectable bacterially contaminated PLT unit than 5-day APs untested for bacterial contamination. They also estimated the sensitivity of the 2-bottle RT, estimated the prevalence of bacterial contamination for untested and for 2-bottle BTA-tested APs, determined the performance contribution of the anaerobic bottle to the BTA, and assessed the need for anaerobic culturing in this application.

M. G. Bissell, MD, PhD, MPH

Urinary di-(2-ethylhexyl)phthalate metabolites in athletes as screening measure for illicit blood doping: a comparison study with patients receiving blood transfusion
Monfort N, Ventura R, Latorre A, et al (IMIM-Hosp del Mar, Barcelona, Spain; Universitat Pompeu Fabra, Barcelona, Spain; Hosp del Mar, Barcelona, Spain)
Transfusion 50:145-149, 2010

Background.—Subjects submitted to intravenous (IV) blood transfusions for medical reasons or blood doping to increase athletic performance are potentially exposed to the plasticizer di-(2-ethylhexyl) phthalate (DEHP) found in IV bags. Exposure to DEHP has been evaluated by measuring DEHP metabolites in selected groups of subjects.

Study Design and Methods.—Urinary DEHP metabolites, mono-(2-ethylhexyl)phthalate, mono-(2-ethyl-5-hydroxyhexyl)phthalate (MEHHP), and mono-(2-ethyl-5-oxohexyl)phthalate (MEOHP) were measured in a control group with no explicit known exposure to DEHP (n = 30), hospitalized patients receiving blood transfusions (n = 25), nontransfused hospitalized patients receiving other medical care involving plastic materials (n = 39), and athletes (n = 127). Patients were tested in the periods 0 to 24 and 24 to 48 hours after exposition.

Results.—Urinary concentrations of all three DEHP metabolites were significantly higher in patients receiving blood transfusion than in nontransfused patients and the control group, except for MEHHP and

MEOHP in the period 24 to 48 hours. Samples from four athletes showed increased concentrations of DEHP metabolites comparable to urinary concentrations of patients receiving blood transfusion.

Conclusion.—Elevated concentrations of urinary DEHP metabolites represent increased exposure to DEHP. High concentrations of DEHP metabolites present in urine collected from athletes may suggest illegal blood transfusion and can be used as a qualitative screening measure for blood doping.

▶ Bags storing blood or blood concentrates for transfusion contain plasticizers to assure appropriate container properties of polyvinyl chloride (PVC). In many blood bag materials, and in some countries only exclusively, the plasticizer is di-(2-ethylhexyl)phthalate (DEHP). It is known that DEHP leaks into the bag's contents and therefore subjects submitted to transfusions are exposed to DEHP. This fact is highly relevant, given the hypothesized toxic effects of exposure to plasticizers in general, and to DEHP in particular, including endocrine disruption and potential carcinogenicity. DEHP is also released from a variety of PVC products, and the general population has residual levels of DEHP and its metabolites. Concentrations of DEHP metabolites in urine have been used to evaluate exposure to DEHP for epidemiologic purposes. Metabolism of DEHP involves hydrolysis to mono-(2-ethylhexyl)phthalate and subsequent oxidation to mono-(2-ethyl-5-hydroxyhexyl)phthalate and mono-(2-ethyl 5-oxohexyl)phthalate. Those metabolites are excreted in urine mainly as conjugates with glucuronic acid. The urinary presence of DEHP metabolites could be also useful to detect blood transfusion use in sports. The detection of blood transfusions in antidoping control is limited so far by the fact that usually urine is the only biologic fluid available for testing, while the existing blood doping detection methods are based on blood analysis. Even in heavy testing programs, such as the Olympic Games, only a small number of samples correspond to blood, implying some subjective decisions on which sports are to be tested or not for blood transfusion. In addition, the existing blood methods mainly discriminate toward allogeneic (homologous) blood transfusion practices. Accordingly, a method able to suspect on the possibility of either allogeneic or autologous blood doping addressed to all urine controls would be an enormous deterrent step forward. Subsequently, suspicious subjects after urine analysis could be targeted for more definitive forensic or clinical evidences of blood transfusion. In this article, the authors compare the urinary concentrations of DEHP metabolites in the general population, in patients subjected to clinical care or to blood transfusions, and in the athlete population. It is shown that DEHP metabolites, in addition to its most common use to evaluate environmental exposure, could be used in sports drug testing as alert markers of the potential misuse of blood transfusion.

M. G. Bissell, MD, PhD, MPH

Validation of a hospital-laboratory workstation for immunohematologic methods

Schoenfeld H, Pretzel KJ, von Heymann C, et al (Charité–Universitätsmedizin Berlin, Germany; Univ Muenster, Germany)
Transfusion 50:26-31, 2010

Background.—The FREELYS Nano system (Diagast) is a manual workstation for ABO/D grouping, Rh phenotyping, K typing, and antibody screening (ABS) for immunoglobulin G (IgG) antibodies only and works with the erythrocyte-magnetized technology (EMT). The principle of EMT is based on magnetization of red blood cells and avoids centrifugation and washing steps.

Study Design and Methods.—A total of 304 samples were tested with our routine blood bank methods, 100 samples for ABO/D grouping, 196 samples (100 at first evaluation, 96 at second evaluation) for Rh phenotyping and K typing (PK7200, Olympus), and 108 samples for ABS (DiaMed). All samples were tested in parallel with the FREELYS Nano.

Results.—We found a 100% concordance between the observed (FREELYS Nano) and the expected (Olympus PK7200) results for ABO/D grouping in all 100 samples. For Rh phenotyping and K tests, in 24 of 100 samples false-positive reactions were observed in the first evaluation by the FREELYS Nano. After changing the test kit batch for Rh phenotyping by the manufacturer, a complete concordance in Rh phenotyping and K tests was observed in a second evaluation. For ABS, the FREELYS Nano showed in 4 of 108 samples (3.7%) false-negative reactions for IgG antibodies (two anti-K, one anti-E, one anti-C^w), and one (0.9%) false-positive reaction.

Conclusions.—The FREELYS Nano is reliably suited to ABO/D grouping, Rh phenotyping, and K testing. The rate of false-negative reactions for IgG antibodies should be reduced.

▶ The authors recently reported about the evaluation of a fully automated application (QWALYS 2, Diagast, Loos, France) for immunohematologic routine methods using the new erythrocyte-magnetized technology (EMT) for ABO/D blood grouping, Rh phenotyping, K typing, and antibody screening (ABS) for unexpected immunoglobulin G (IgG) antibodies. The principle of EMT is based on magnetization of red blood cells and avoids centrifugation and washing steps. This new method was recently described in detail. This article describes the validation of a new manual workstation, the FREELYS Nano system (Diagast), which uses EMT as well. The FREELYS Nano system is a manual workstation for ABO/D blood grouping, Rh phenotyping, K typing, and ABS for IgG antibodies only and works with the EMT. A total of 304 samples were tested with the authors' routine blood bank methods, 100 samples for ABO/D grouping, 196 samples (100 at first evaluation and 96 at second evaluation) for Rh phenotyping and K typing (PK7200, Olympus), and 108 samples for ABS (DiaMed). All samples were tested in parallel with the FREELYS Nano. They found a 100% concordance between the observed

(FREELYS Nano) and the expected (Olympus PK7200) results for ABO/D grouping in all 100 samples. For Rh phenotyping and K tests, in 24 of 100 samples false-positive reactions were observed in the first evaluation by the FREELYS Nano. After changing the test kit batch for Rh phenotyping by the manufacturer, a complete concordance in Rh phenotyping and K tests was observed in a second evaluation. For ABS, the FREELYS Nano showed in 4 of 108 samples (3.7%) false-negative reactions for IgG antibodies (2 anti-K, 1 anti-E, and 1 anti-C^W) and 1 (0.9%) false-positive reaction. The FREELYS Nano is reliably suited to ABO/D grouping, Rh phenotyping, and K testing. The rate of false-negative reactions for IgG antibodies should be reduced.

M. G. Bissell, MD, PhD, MPH

20 Cytogenetics and Molecular Pathology

A Commercial Real-Time PCR Kit Provides Greater Sensitivity than Direct Sequencing to Detect *KRAS* Mutations: A Morphology-Based Approach in Colorectal Carcinoma
Angulo B, García-García E, Martínez R, et al (Universidad San Pablo-CEU, Madrid, Spain)
J Mol Diagn 12:292-299, 2010

KRAS mutation testing has become a standard procedure in the management of patients with carcinomas. The most frequently used method for *KRAS* testing is direct sequencing of PCR products. The development of commercial real-time quantitative PCR kits offers a useful alternative since they are in theory much more sensitive than direct sequencing and they avoid post-PCR handling. We present our experience as a reference center for the study of *KRAS* mutations, comparing direct sequencing and the use of a commercial real-time quantitative PCR kit, as well as determining the sensitivity of both procedures in clinical practice. The TheraScreen K-RAS Mutation Kit identified mutations in 75 (44%) of the 170 tumors. Three cases were tested positive using TheraScreen K-RAS Mutation Kit and negative by direct sequencing. We then compared the sensitivity of the kit and that of direct sequencing using 74 mutant tumors. The kit was able to detect the presence of a mutation in a 1% dilution of the total DNA in 13.5% of the tumors and, in 84%, *KRAS* mutation was identified at a dilution of 5%. Sequencing was able to detect *KRAS* mutations when the mutant DNA represented 10% of the total DNA in 20/74 (27%) of the tumors. When the mutant DNA represented 30% of the total DNA, sequencing could detect mutations in 56/74 (76%).

▶ *KRAS* mutation testing has become a standard procedure in the management of patients with carcinomas. Patients with colorectal carcinoma (CRC) who carry mutations in *KRAS* gene do not benefit from the administration of antiepidermal growth factor receptor (anti-EGFR) monoclonal antibodies, as a primary, secondary, or tertiary-line treatment. Therefore, testing *KRAS* gene mutations should be taken into account before therapy selection for all patients with CRC in the near future. Likewise, there is also an increasing need to study the mutations in the *KRAS* gene in patients with pulmonary adenocarcinomas, as this is a primary marker of resistance to tyrosine kinase inhibitors of EGFR. This necessity is creating some important logistical problems worldwide because there is currently no standardized test approved by the US Food and Drug Administration. In accordance with a recent review, 2 CE-marked *KRAS* mutation test kits currently exist in Europe for diagnostic use: TheraScreen (DxS Ltd.) and KRAS LightMix (by TIB Mol Biol). At present, the most frequently used method to test KRAS mutation is the direct sequencing of polymerase chain reaction (PCR) products. This method has 2 key disadvantages: its low sensitivity (20%-50%) and the important risk of contamination when handling the products of the PCR reaction. The development of commercial real-time quantitative PCR kits may offer a useful alternative because they are, in theory, much more sensitive than direct sequencing and they avoid the post-PCR handling. Interestingly, one of these assays was used in one of the metastatic CRC phase 3 trial, which led to the approval of panitumumab in patients with wild-type *KRAS* tumors by the European Medicines Agency. Indeed, using this kit in the context of a clinical trial was so successful that it has received public recognition in a high-impact journal. The development of biomarker-assessing kits opens a new era not only in CRC but also in future approval of other drugs and/or indications. However, despite this approval of a drug associated to a biomarker that was studied by a specific method, it is noteworthy that the same approach has not been universally accepted in clinical practice. In this article, the authors present their experience as a reference center for the study of *KRAS* mutations, comparing direct sequencing and the use of a commercial real-time PCR kit as well as determining the true sensitivity of both procedures by serial dilution.

M. G. Bissell, MD, PhD, MPH

A New Chromosome X Exon-Specific Microarray Platform for Screening of Patients with X-Linked Disorders

Bashiardes S, Kousoulidou L, van Bokhoven H, et al (the Cyprus Inst of Neurology and Genetics, Nicosia; Radboud Univ Nijmegen Med Centre, The Netherlands; et al)
J Mol Diagn 11:562-568, 2009

Recent studies and advances in high-density oligonucleotide arrays have shown that microdeletions and microduplications occur at a high frequency in the human genome, causing various genetic conditions including mental retardation. Thus far little is known about the pathways leading to this disease, and implementation of microarrays is hampered by their increasing cost and complexity, underlining the need for new diagnostic tools. The aim of this study was to introduce a new targeted platform called "chromosome X exon-specific array" and to apply this new platform to screening of 20 families (including one blind positive control) with suspected X-linked mental retardation, to identify new causative X-linked mental retardation genes. The new microarray contains of 21,939 oligonucleotides covering 92.9% of all exons of all genes on chromosome X. Patient screening resulted in successful identification of the blind positive control included in the sample of 20 families, and one of the remaining 19 families was found to carry a 1.78-kilobase deletion involving all exons of pseudogene *BRAF2*. The *BRAF2* deletion segregated in the family and was not found in 200 normal male samples, and no copy number variations are reported in this region. Further studies and focused investigation of X-linked disorders have the potential to reveal the molecular basis of human genetic pathological conditions that are caused by copy-number changes in chromosome X genes.

▶ Mental retardation (MR) is a devastating clinical disorder that affects 2% to 3% of the human population, causing serious handicap in children and young adults. It is characterized by cognitive impairment (intelligence quotient [IQ] lower than 70) and by functional deficits in adaptive behavior, such as daily living skills, social skills, and communication. Recent studies have shown that microdeletions and microduplications can be the cause of MR; however, so far, little is known about the exact interactions on the gene and protein level that lead to the occurrence of the disease. Approximately 15% of inherited MR cases are linked to chromosome X, with as many as 82 relevant X chromosomal genes cloned so far. New MR genes are usually identified through investigation of clinically affected individuals by using high-resolution screening techniques for detection of copy number alterations, followed by linkage studies and expression profiling. Candidate genes may carry a causative mutation segregating in the family or be disrupted in isolated patients. Current data show that approximately 40% of causative mutations on chromosome X identified so far are copy number alterations. According to latest estimations there are at least 50 MR-causative X-chromosomal genes that are as yet unidentified. Therefore, there is clearly an immediate need to further understand and characterize the genetic causes of X-linked MR (XLMR). In response to the increased interest in chromosome X aberrations, different chromosome X-specific DNA microarrays were developed and applied for screening of XLMR families in search for new causative mutations. As microarray-based copy number assessment techniques are gaining popularity among diagnostic laboratories and researchers, their implementation is hampered by the cost and by other limitations, such as the number of features (microarray elements), increasing the overall complexity of the array. Targeted platforms could be an alternative solution, which would provide the ability to overcome the above limitations. Array-based exon-specific analysis for 162 exons of 5 disease genes has been described and implemented in screening of patients with known mutations in the relevant disease loci, demonstrating the potential of a more focused strategy. Similarly to other exon arrays, the purpose of the chromosome X exon-specific array was to detect copy number changes within gene exons. The rationale behind the development of this new platform is the hypothesis that there is still a large number of genes on chromosome X that play a role in XLMR and are as yet unidentified. Recognizing that copy number variations in intergenic regions may often be pathogenic, altering the regulation of genes located in the region, the focus of this study was to search for new XLMR genes targeting gene exons and not intergenic regions. The introduction of a new array-based targeted screening system is currently motivated by the need for increased efficiency and specificity in chromosome X gene copy number assessment, reduced complexity, cost-effectiveness of the analysis, and easier translation of a copy number alteration to a functional abnormality.

M. G. Bissell, MD, PhD, MPH

A Quantitative ELISA Assay for the Fragile X Mental Retardation 1 Protein
Iwahashi C, Tassone F, Hagerman RJ, et al (Univ of California Davis; Univ of California Davis Health System, Sacramento; et al)
J Mol Diagn 11:281-289, 2009

Non-coding (CGG-repeat) expansions in the fragile X mental retardation 1 (*FMR1*) gene result in a spectrum of disorders involving altered neurodevelopment (fragile X syndrome), neurodegeneration (late-onset fragile X-associated tremor/ataxia syndrome), or primary ovarian insufficiency. While reliable and quantitative assays for the number of CGG repeats and *FMR1* mRNA levels are now available, there has been no scalable, quantitative assay for the *FMR1* protein (FMRP) in non-transformed cells. Using a combination of avian and murine antibodies to FMRP, we developed a sensitive and highly specific sandwich enzyme-linked immunosorbent assay (ELISA) for FMRP in peripheral blood lymphocytes. This ELISA method is capable of quantifying FMRP levels throughout the biologically relevant range of protein concentrations and is specific for the intact FMRP protein. Moreover, the ELISA is well-suited for replicate protein determinations across serial dilutions in non-transformed cells and is readily scalable for large sample numbers. The FMRP ELISA is potentially a powerful tool in expanding our understanding of the relationship between FMRP levels and the various *FMR1*-associated clinical phenotypes.

▶ Fragile X syndrome (OMIM #300624), the most common heritable form of intellectual impairment and the leading known single-gene form of autism, is nearly always caused by lowered (or absence of) expression of the fragile X mental retardation 1 (FMR1) protein (FMRP) in individuals who harbor *FMR1* alleles in the full mutation range (>200 CGG repeats) or high premutation range (premutation, 55-200 CGG repeats). Most individuals with a premutation allele have intelligence quotients (IQs) that fall within the normal range, although some children experience attention deficit hyperactivity disorder and autism spectrum disorders. Moreover, in adults, there is an increased risk of primary ovarian insufficiency, emotional problems including depression and anxiety, and the late-onset neurodegenerative disorder fragile X-associated tremor/ataxia syndrome. Although reduction or loss of FMRP is generally believed to be the basis for fragile X syndrome and many of the neurodevelopmental problems in the upper premutation range, quantitative comparisons of molecular FMRP and clinical phenotypes are generally lacking because of the absence of a quantitative measure of the protein. Thus far, the main approaches for measuring protein levels have been indirect, involving immunohistochemical staining of peripheral blood lymphocytes or hair roots. Given the central importance of FMRP to the presence and severity of the clinical phenotype in fragile X syndrome, a method for accurately and rapidly quantifying FMRP levels is necessary. To this end, the authors have developed a sandwich enzyme-linked immunosorbent assay (ELISA) for FMRP that precisely determines levels of the protein in circulating lymphocytes in humans. The assay is sensitive to small changes in protein levels, targets intact FMRP specifically, and is a reliable method for the measurement of FMRP in blood. Of course, the caveat of measuring a peripheral protein level for a central nervous system disorder remains to be completely resolved. Not withstanding this concern, a truly quantitative measure of FMRP will allow a better assessment of its importance in various clinical settings.

M. G. Bissell, MD, PhD, MPH

Clinical Laboratory Analysis of Immunoglobulin Heavy Chain Variable Region Genes for Chronic Lymphocytic Leukemia Prognosis

Szankasi P, Bahler DW (Associated Regional and Univ Pathologists (ARUP), Salt Lake City, UT; Univ of Utah, Salt Lake City)
J Mol Diagn 12:244-249, 2010

Chronic lymphocytic leukemia (CLL) is the most common leukemia affecting adults in the western world. The clinical course of CLL is highly variable: cases that express mutated immunoglobulin heavy chain variable regions (IgV_H) typically have a more indolent clinical course compared with those with unmutated IgV_H. The use of the V_H3-21 variable region has also been found to confer a poor prognosis, independent of mutation status. Here we describe an assay for the identification of the expressed V_H segment and its mutation status in CLL. This test uses whole blood-derived RNA and PCR primers annealing to the leader regions and the joining region segments. This approach allows more accurate determination of the IgV_H mutation status relative to using framework region specific V_H primers. An additional primer specific for the leader region of the V_H3-21 segment is described and is shown to be necessary to identify this diagnostically important variable region. We successfully analyzed 99 of 103 samples, including five expressing the V_H3-21 variable region. Approximately 5% of cases had complement determining region 3 sequences similar to previously reported cases, and overrepresentation of the V_H1-69 segment was observed among unmutated cases. These results confirm the proper functioning and high success rate of this valuable prognostic for CLL designed for the use in a clinical laboratory setting.

▶ Chronic lymphocytic leukemia (CLL) is a neoplasm of small mature B-cells and the most common leukemia affecting adults in the United States and Europe. Almost all cases of CLL express CD5 along with pan-B-cell markers such as CD19 and show other characteristic immunophenotypic features that can be easily identified by flow cytometry analysis. Many patients are asymptomatic in early-stage disease at diagnosis and are now often identified through routine blood testing. However, the clinical course of CLL is highly variable with many cases behaving indolently with little effect on survival and others behaving aggressively with patients succumbing to their disease after only a few years. Because traditional staging methods cannot predict the clinical course of disease in patients with early stage CLL, the identification of biological prognostic markers to potentially help guide treatment decisions has assumed increased importance. One of the earlier biological markers reported to correlate with CLL clinical course was the somatic mutation status of the expressed immunoglobulin (Ig) heavy chain variable region gene segment (V_H). Cases that express mutated V_H gene segments (less than 98% homology to the germline counterparts) typically have a more favorable clinical course than those expressing unmutated V_H segments (98% or greater homology to the germline segment). Subsequent studies confirmed these findings and also that usage of the V_H3-21 gene segment confers a poor prognosis, regardless of the IgV_H mutation status. The basis for the prognostic significance of V_H mutational status and expression of V_H3-21 is still unclear but likely relates to signaling differences mediated by surface Ig, the CLL antigen receptor. The importance of direct antigen receptor stimulation in the development and growth of CLL is also supported by studies revealing preferential use of certain V_H gene segments and cases from different patients with nearly identical V_H and V_L genes, including the highly variable complement determining region 3 (CDR3). Expression of ZAP-70 and CD38 have been found to correlate with the Ig gene mutation status, and measurement of these markers by flow cytometry is used as a surrogate for IgV_H mutation status. Several recurrent cytogenetic abnormalities present in CLL typically identified by fluorescence in situ hybridization have also been shown to have prognostic significance such as presence of deletions in the long arms of chromosomes 13 (del[13q14.10]), 11 (del[11q]), and 6 (del[6q]) and deletions in the short arm of chromosome 17 (del[17 p]). However, recent studies have shown that V_H mutational status still has prognostic significance in CLL independent of cytogenetic findings. The authors describe a method for the accurate determination of the identity and mutation status of the IgV_H segment expressed in CLL. Their assay has high sensitivity and several features that help with implementation in a routine clinical laboratory.

M. G. Bissell, MD, PhD, MPH

Direct DNA Amplification from Crude Clinical Samples Using a PCR Enhancer Cocktail and Novel Mutants of Taq

Zhang Z, Kermekchiev MB, Barnes WM (DNA Polymerase Technology Inc, St Louis, MO)
J Mol Diagn 12:152-161, 2010

PCR-based clinical and forensic tests often have low sensitivity or even false-negative results caused by potent PCR inhibitors found in blood and soil. It is widely accepted that purification of target DNA before PCR is necessary for successful amplification. In an attempt to overcome PCR inhibition, enhance PCR amplification, and simplify the PCR protocol, we demonstrate improved PCR-enhancing cocktails containing nonionic detergent, L-carnitine, D-(+)-trehalose, and heparin. These cocktails, in combination with two inhibitor-resistant Taq mutants, OmniTaq and Omni Klentaq, enabled efficient amplification of exogenous, endogenous, and high-GC content DNA targets directly from crude samples containing human plasma, serum, and whole blood without DNA purification. In the presence of these enhancer cocktails, the mutant enzymes were able to tolerate at least 25% plasma, serum, or whole blood and as high as 80% GC content templates in PCR reactions. These enhancer cocktails also improved the performance of the novel Taq mutants in real-time PCR amplification using crude samples, both in SYBR Green fluorescence detection and TaqMan assays. The novel enhancer mixes also facilitated DNA amplification from crude samples with various commercial Taq DNA polymerases.

▶ A major problem with polymerase chain reaction (PCR)-based diagnostic tests of blood samples is the false-negative or low-sensitivity reactions caused by PCR inhibitors. Blood samples are extensively used for PCR-based diagnosis of microbial infection, genetic disease, forensic analysis, and blood banking. Prenatal genetic diagnosis using maternal plasma or serum has been developed recently. However, when these techniques are applied to blood samples, it must be considered that PCR inhibitors in the specimens may lead to possible false-negative or reduced sensitivity despite advanced DNA purification methods. For example, even after DNA purification steps are used before PCR, a 14% false-negative rate has been observed for hepatitis B virus detection, most probably due to incomplete removal of PCR inhibitors. PCR inhibition is a common concern in detection of various pathogens, such as herpes, varicella, Epstein-Barr, polyoma, and cytomegalovirus viruses, bacteria, and fungi. Inhibition of RT-PCR in plasma samples has been reported to occur at a frequency of 0.34% to 2.4% of the tests in patients infected with human immunodeficiency virus and hepatitis C virus, respectively. Among the most potent PCR inhibitors reported are hemoglobin/heme, leukocyte DNA, and an immunoglobulin G fraction, in addition to anticoagulants, such as ethylenediamine tetraacetic acid, sodium citrate, and heparin, which also inhibit PCR. Other known inhibitors are bilirubin, bile salts, and lactoferrin. Researchers have been trying to find additives to PCR that can relieve the inhibition and enhance amplification. The known PCR enhancers, however, usually cover only 1 aspect of the problem by working on GC-rich targets of purified DNA template or relieving the inhibition. As an alternative to the various time- and labor-consuming pre-PCR procedures needed with blood, the authors recently reported inhibition-resistant mutants of Taq DNA polymerase, OmniTaq (Taq-22) and Omni Klentaq (Klentaq-10), which can tolerate the major PCR inhibitors found in blood and soil. Here they report a novel PCR enhancer cocktail (PEC), which improves the performance of the Taq mutants, allowing direct amplification of targets from whole blood, serum, or plasma present in the final PCR volume at least at 25%, without DNA purification. This could especially benefit PCR applications in which the target concentration is low and a larger input amount of the crude sample is necessary for successful detection. With this enzyme enhancer combination they were also able to amplify endogenous and exogenous, non-GC-rich and GC-rich targets directly from crude samples without DNA extraction. PEC was also efficient with most commercial Taq enzymes, although it performed optimally with the OmniTaq and Omni Klentaq enzymes, especially with crude blood. Therefore, the novel PCR enhancer combined with these mutants or other commercial Taqs should simplify, speed up, and lower the cost of important clinical, forensic, and environmental PCR-based tests.

M. G. Bissell, MD, PhD, MPH

Evaluation of 13q14 Status in Multiple Myeloma by Digital Single Nucleotide Polymorphism Technology
Hanlon K, Harries LW, Ellard S, et al (Royal Devon and Exeter NHS Foundation Trust, Exeter, UK; Peninsula Med School, Exeter, UK)
J Mol Diagn 11:450-457, 2009

Chromosome 13q deletions are common in multiple myeloma and other cancers, demonstrating the importance of this region in tumorigenesis. We used a novel single nucleotide polymorphism (SNP)-based technique, digital SNP (dSNP), to identify loss of heterozygosity (LOH) at chromosome 13q in paraffin-embedded bone marrow biopsies from 22 patients with multiple myeloma. We analyzed heterozygous SNPs at 13q for the presence of allelic imbalances and examined the results by sequential probability ratio analysis. Where possible, dSNP results were confirmed by fluorescence *in situ* hybridization. Using dSNP, we identified 13q LOH in 16/18 (89%) (95% Confidence Interval; 65%, 99%) patients without the need for neoplastic cell enrichment. In 8/16 (50%) cases, either partial or interstitial patterns of LOH were observed. Both fluorescence *in situ* hybridization and dSNP data proved concordant in just 3/9 cases. Five of the six discrepancies showed LOH by dSNP occurring beyond the boundaries of the fluorescence *in situ* hybridization probes. Our findings show that dSNP represents a useful technique for the analysis of LOH in archival tissue with minimal infiltration of neoplastic cells. The high-resolution screening afforded by the dSNP technology allowed for the identification of complex chromosomal rearrangements, resulting in either partial or interstitial LOH. Digital SNP represents an attractive approach for the investigation of tumors not suitable for genomic-array analysis.

▶ Multiple myeloma (MM) is a postgerminal center B-cell malignancy characterized by the accumulation of plasma cells in the bone marrow, chromosomal instability, and chromosomal translocations involving the immunoglobulin heavy chain locus. This disorder is estimated to account for 10% of all hematological malignancies and has an extremely variable prognosis, with survival ranging from a few months to more than 10 years. Despite recent advances in gene expression profiling, the molecular mechanisms underlying the development of MM remain unclear. Cytogenetic instability is a key feature of MM, and chromosomal abnormalities are detectable in most cases. Several recurrent abnormalities have emerged that appear to influence disease development and progression. These include gains of chromosome regions 1q, 9q, and 11q, losses of chromosome regions 6q, Xp, and Xq, and translocations involving 14q32. Deletion of chromosome 13q is one of the most frequent cytogenetic abnormalities associated with MM, occurring in 40% to 50% of cases. Most deletions involve entire chromosomes or chromosome arms, although partial and interstitial deletions have also been described. Where interstitial deletions are present, they most commonly involve chromosome band 13q14 to 13q 21. The presence of chromosome 13q deletions has been suggested to be an adverse prognostic factor in MM. The authors report here the novel application of digital single nucleotide polymorphism (dSNP) analysis for the characterization of 13q loss of heterozygosity (LOH) status in a panel of 22 MM cases. They have previously shown that dSNP compares well with established molecular techniques, including fluorescence in situ hybridization (FISH) and multiplex ligation-dependent probe amplification, for the detection of the chromosome aberrations resulting in LOH. dSNP allows detection of LOH through the direct counting of alleles. The technique relies on the identification of heterozygous SNPs in patient samples and the subsequent separation of the heterozygous alleles through the serial dilution of patient DNA. Polymerase chain reaction (PCR) amplification of the heterozygous alleles is performed and the allelic frequencies counted. Deviation from the expected 50:50 ratio for heterozygous alleles represents LOH at that specific locus and is highly suggestive of a deletion. Sequential probability ratio testing confirms the significance of such deviations. dSNP technology is applicable to both fresh and archival material and can be used on samples regardless of proliferative state. The aim of this study was to use a panel of SNP probes to characterize 13q14 LOH status in archival tissue from a cohort of 22 patients with MM.

M. G. Bissell, MD, PhD, MPH

FISH Diagnosis of Acute Graft-Versus-Host Disease Following Living-Related Liver Transplant

Kanehira K, Riegert-Johnson DL, Chen D, et al (Mayo Clinic, Rochester, MN)
J Mol Diagn 11:355-358, 2009

Acute graft-versus-host disease (GVHD) is an uncommon but often fatal complication following liver transplant. We describe a GVHD case in which a female patient with primary biliary cirrhosis underwent a living-related liver transplant from her son. The human leukocyte antigen typing of the donor was homozygous at all loci. The recipient's human leukocyte antigen type was haplo-identical to that of the donor. A bone marrow aspirate performed for pancytopenia revealed a severely hypoplastic marrow. Fluorescent *in situ* hybridization (FISH) using X- and Y-chromosome probes demonstrated that 80% of marrow cells were of donor origin. Comparison of Giemsa-stained cell morphology and FISH showed that the erythroid precursor cells were predominantly of male pattern (XY). This report is one of only a few studies that prove the migration of a donor's hematopoietic stem cells to a recipient's bone marrow. We demonstrated that FISH analysis using sex chromosome probes is useful to confirm a diagnosis of GVHD following organ transplantation from a donor of the opposite sex. We also showed that donor hematopoietic stem cells in a liver graft can migrate to the recipient's bone marrow. We suggest that FISH is a rapid and reliable test for confirming the diagnosis of GVHD in a peripheral blood or skin biopsy sample.

▶ Acute graft-versus-host disease (GVHD) following liver transplantation is a rare complication with a high mortality rate. GVHD occurs when immuno-competent donor lymphocytes originating from the transplanted organ undergo activation and clonal expansion, reacting against the recipient antigens. The clinical course begins with fever or skin rash as an early sign, followed by pancytopenia, overwhelming sepsis, and death. The diagnosis of GVHD is a major challenge and thus the condition often goes unrecognized. Detection of donor lymphocytes in peripheral blood or bone marrow in high level (> 1%) is a key to early detection of GVHD. A 49-year-old white female with hilar cholangiocarcinoma associated with primary biliary cirrhosis received a living-related liver transplant from her son. She received 2 units of leuko-cyte-reduced packed red blood cells for operative blood loss. Post-transplant immunosuppression was with mycophenolate mofetil, tacrolimus, and predni-sone. Her post-transplant course was complicated by multiple embolic strokes 6 days after transplantation. Four weeks after transplantation, she developed pancytopenia with nadir blood counts of hemoglobin 8.0 g/dL, platelets 4×10^9/L, and leukocytes 0.2×10^9/L. Treatment with granulocyte colony-stimulating factor was begun but there was no improvement in blood counts. Six weeks after transplant, she developed diarrhea and an erythematous maculo-papular skin rash on her back. The rash was biopsied and pathological findings were consistent with GVHD. CT of the abdomen showed thickened loops of small intestine. The patient was diagnosed with GVHD and was treated with methylprednisolone. She developed acute respiratory failure, worsening gastro-intestinal symptoms, and died 46 days after transplantation. The authors demonstrated that FISH analysis using sex chromosome probes is useful to confirm a diagnosis of GVHD following organ transplantation from a donor of the opposite sex. They also showed that donor hematopoietic stem cells in a liver graft can migrate to the recipient's bone marrow. They suggest that FISH is a rapid and reliable test for confirming the diagnosis of GVHD in a peripheral blood or skin biopsy sample.

M. G. Bissell, MD, PhD, MPH

One Hundred Twenty-One Dystrophin Point Mutations Detected from Stored DNA Samples by Combinatorial Denaturing High-Performance Liquid Chromatography
Torella A, Trimarco A, Blanco FdelV, et al (Seconda Università degli Studi di Napoli, Italy; et al)
J Mol Diagn 12:65-73, 2010

Duchenne and Becker muscular dystrophies are caused by a large number of different mutations in the dystrophin gene. Outside of the deletion/duplication "hot spots," small mutations occur at unpredictable positions. These account for about 15 to 20% of cases, with the major group being premature stop codons. When the affected male is deceased, carrier testing for family members and prenatal diagnosis become difficult and expensive. We tailored a cost-effective and reliable strategy to discover point mutations from stored DNA samples in the absence of a muscle biopsy. Samples were amplified in combinatorial pools and tested by denaturing high-performance liquid chromatography analysis. An anomalous elution profile belonging to two different pools univocally addressed the allelic variation to an unambiguous sample. Mutations were then detected by sequencing. We identified 121 mutations of 99 different types. Fifty-six patients show stop codons that represent the 46.3% of all cases. Three non-obvious single amino acid mutations were considered as causative. Our data support combinatorial denaturing high-performance liquid chromatography analysis as a clear-cut strategy for time and cost-effective identification of small mutations when only DNA is available.

▶ Duchenne muscular dystrophy (DMD [MIM 310200]) and Becker muscular dystrophy (BMD [MIM 300376]) are allelic inherited disorders of muscle. They affect males in > 99% of cases, being transmitted as X-linked recessive traits. The DMD gene spans 2.2 million bp of genomic DNA on the X chromosome, and the 14-kb transcript encodes a full-length protein (dystrophin) of 427 kd (Dp427 m). Both DMD and BMD arise due to mutations at the dystrophin gene locus, which comprises 79 exons and 8 tissue-specific promoters. The most common mutations are large intragenic deletions or duplications, encompassing one or more exons, but point mutations are about 15% to 20% of cases, with the major group being premature stop codons. Patients and their families not only confer great value to mutation detection for genetic counseling but also to therapeutic options, since there are claims of novel mutation-targeted treatments. Unfortunately, very often muscle biopsies are not possible because the affected family member is deceased. The authors have tailored a cost-effective and reliable strategy to discover point mutations from DNA samples. Based on the sensitivity of denaturing high-performance liquid chromatography (DHPLC) to detect mutations, especially in A/T-rich sequences, such as the dystrophin gene, they developed a combinatorial DHPLC approach to screen pooled samples.

M. G. Bissell, MD, PhD, MPH

Rapid Genotyping of Single Nucleotide Polymorphisms Influencing Warfarin Drug Response by Surface-Enhanced Laser Desorption and Ionization Time-of-Flight (SELDI-TOF) Mass Spectrometry
Yang S, Xu L, Wu HM (Ohio State Univ, Columbus)
J Mol Diagn 12:162-168, 2010

Warfarin exhibits significant interindividual variability in dosing requirements. Different drug responses are partly attributed to the single nucleotide polymorphisms (SNPs) that influence either drug action or drug metabolism. Rapid genotyping of these SNPs helps clinicians to choose appropriate initial doses to quickly achieve anticoagulation effects and to prevent complications. We report a novel application of surface-enhanced laser desorption and ionization time-of-flight mass spectrometry (SELDI-TOF MS) in the rapid genotyping of SNPs that impact warfarin efficacy. The SNPs were first amplified by PCR and then underwent single base extension to generate the specific SNP product. Next, genetic variants displaying different masses were bound to Q10 anionic protein-Chips and then genotyped by using SELDI-TOF MS in a multiplex fashion. SELDI-TOF MS offered unique properties of on-chip sample enrichment and cleanups, which streamlined the testing procedures and eliminated many tedious experimental steps required by the conventional MS-based method. The turn-around time for genotyping three known warfarin-related SNPs, *CYP2C9*2*, *CYP2C9*3*, and *VKORC1 3673G>A* by SELDI-TOF MS was less than 5 hours. The analytical accuracy of this method was confirmed both by bidirectional DNA sequencing and by comparing the genotype results ($n = 189$) obtained by SELDI-TOF MS to reports from a clinical reference laboratory. This new multiplex genotyping method provides an excellent clinical laboratory platform to promote personalized medicine in warfarin therapy.

▶ A great deal of effort has been devoted to developing accurate, rapid, and cost-effective technologies for single-nucleotide polymorphism (SNP) analysis to advance clinical diagnosis and therapeutics. There are several technological platforms for the determination of SNPs. A typical genotyping approach is to first increase the number of SNPs that will be analyzed. In most instances, polymerase chain reaction amplification of a desired SNP-containing region is performed initially to introduce specificity and increase the number of allele-specific molecules. Afterward, amplified DNA fragments containing a specific SNP are measured by a device based on mass or another biochemical property. Mass spectrometry (MS) is a widely used method for the mass determination of various biomolecules such as peptides, proteins, oligosaccharides, and oligonucleotides. In this approach, the analyte is detected as a measurable peak with a specific mass/charge ratio. MS has been successfully used in SNP genotyping. For instance, matrix-assisted laser desorption/ionization time-of-flight MS, a commonly used platform of MS, has been reported for detection of hereditary thrombotic risk factors. The surface-enhanced laser desorption and ionization time-of-flight MS (SELDI-TOF MS) is a unique type of MS that involves matrix array technology. The most important feature comes from the different matrices or chips that are available to isolate or enrich a specific analyte before mass analysis. Several kinds of chips are available, each coated with a specific chemical matrix. Examples include immobilized metal affinity capture chips, cation or anion exchange chips, or chips with hydrophobic properties. Therefore, it is possible to preselect a chip (based on the properties of target analytes), enrich a target molecule, remove unwanted elements such as salt, and then detect it by using an MS. Conceivably, the unique features of SELDI-TOF MS make it the most plausible device for genotype testing because it can rapidly and efficiently isolate the targeted oligonucleotides (analytes) from other reaction reagents and therefore greatly improve the detection process. Warfarin (Coumadin) is an anticoagulant that disrupts the process of vitamin K recycling. Vitamin K is an essential cofactor for the posttranslational modification of several clotting factors, including factors II, VII, IX, and X, and the anticoagulant proteins C and S. In this study, we used SELDI-TOF MS and developed a novel approach for rapid genotyping of SNPs that are known to influence warfarin sensitivity or warfarin metabolism.

M. G. Bissell, MD, PhD, MPH

Serum DNA Motifs Predict Disease and Clinical Status in Multiple Sclerosis

Beck J, Urnovitz HB, Saresella M, et al (Chronix Biomed Goettingen, Germany; Laboratory of Molecular Medicine and Biotechnology, Milan, Italy; et al)
J Mol Diagn 12:312-319, 2010

Using recently available mass sequencing and assembly technologies, we have been able to identify and quantify unique cell-free DNA motifs in the blood of patients with multiple sclerosis (MS). The most common MS clinical syndrome, relapsing-remitting MS (RRMS), is accompanied by a unique fingerprint of both inter- and intragenic cell-free circulating nucleic acids as specific DNA sequences that provide significant clinical sensitivity and specificity. Coding genes that are differentially represented in MS serum encode cytoskeletal proteins, brain-expressed regulators of growth, and receptors involved in nervous system signal transduction. Although coding genes distinguish RRMS and its clinical activity, several repeat sequences, such as the L1M family of LINE elements, are consistently different in all MS patients and clinical status versus the normal database. These data demonstrate that DNA motifs observed in serum are characteristic of RRMS and disease activity and are promising as a clinical tool in monitoring patient responses to treatment modalities.

▶ Although multiple sclerosis (MS) remains a clinical diagnosis, the definitive standard for the confirmation of diagnosis and the clinical assessment of MS disease activity is T1-weighted gadolinium (Gd)-enhanced magnetic resonance imaging (MRI). Gd-MRI supplies information about current disease activity by highlighting areas of breakdown in the blood-brain barrier that indicate inflammation. Areas of inflammation appear as active lesions. T1-weighted images also show black holes, which are thought to indicate areas of permanent damage. T2-weighted MRI scans are used to provide information about disease burden or lesion load. The high costs of randomized clinical trials in MS are directly associated with the requirement of frequent Gd-MRI scans to assess clinical activity as a function of pharmaceutical intervention and optimal dose assessment. Gd carries significant risk for some patients. In 2007, the US Food and Drug Administration issued a black box warning for the use of Gd (http://www.fda.gov/Drugs/DrugSafety/PostmarketDrugSafetyInformationforPatientsandProviders/ucm142884.htm, last accessed October 13, 2009). This warning was based on research that linked the use of Gd as an image enhancement aid for MRI to the development of nephrogenic systemic fibrosis, a debilitating and potentially fatal disease. The development of new therapies for MS is hindered by the lack of a low-cost minimally invasive diagnostic assay to monitor disease activity. The high cost per patient of Gd-MRI prohibits the number of patients studied in randomized controlled clinical trials and the rate at which important questions can be tested. High per patient costs make it prohibitively expensive to study the comparative effectiveness of a treatment, prevention, or diagnostic regimen as it transitions from clinical trial to the larger venue of clinical practice. The cost for maximizing disease control in clinical practice has adverse economic consequences for the uninsured patient as well as societal effects on the health insurance industry and on local, state, and federal governments. The basic sequence data reported here from mass sequence and assembly technology provide significant promise that the differential frequencies of specific DNA motifs in patients with relapsing-remitting MS can be translated into a rapid serum-based diagnostic assay for MS and assessment of its clinical activity.

M. G. Bissell, MD, PhD, MPH

Trends in Down's syndrome live births and antenatal diagnoses in England and Wales from 1989 to 2008: analysis of data from the National Down Syndrome Cytogenetic Register
Morris JK, Alberman E (Queen Mary Univ of London, UK)
BMJ 339:b3794, 2009

Objectives.—To describe trends in the numbers of Down's syndrome live births and antenatal diagnoses in England and Wales from 1989 to 2008.

Design and Setting.—The National Down Syndrome Cytogenetic Register holds details of 26488 antenatal and postnatal diagnoses of Down's syndrome made by all cytogenetic laboratories in England and Wales since 1989.

Interventions.—Antenatal screening, diagnosis, and subsequent termination of Down's syndrome pregnancies.

Main Outcome Measures.—The number of live births with Down's syndrome.

Results.—Despite the number of births in 1989/90 being similar to that in 2007/8, antenatal and postnatal diagnoses of Down's syndrome increased by 71% (from 1075 in 1989/90 to 1843 in 2007/8). However, numbers of live births with Down's syndrome fell by 1% (752 to 743; 1.10 to 1.08 per 1000 births) because of antenatal screening and subsequent terminations. In the absence of such screening, numbers of live births with Down's syndrome would have increased by 48% (from 959 to 1422), since couples are starting families at an older age. Among mothers aged 37 years and older, a consistent 70% of affected pregnancies were diagnosed antenatally. In younger mothers, the proportions of pregnancies diagnosed antenatally increased from 3% to 43% owing to improvements in the availability and sensitivity of screening tests.

Conclusions.—Since 1989, expansion of and improvements in antenatal screening have offset an increase in Down's syndrome resulting from rising maternal age. The proportion of antenatal diagnoses has increased most strikingly in younger women, whereas that in older women has stayed relatively constant. This trend suggests that, even with future improvements in screening, a large number of births with Down's syndrome are still likely, and that monitoring of the numbers of babies born with Down's syndrome is essential to ensure adequate provision for their needs (Fig 3).

▶ Between 1989 and 2008 two changes occurred that influenced the number of diagnosed Down syndrome pregnancies, despite no change in the overall number of births in England and Wales. First was the considerable increase in maternal age, which is a major known risk factor for Down syndrome. Second was the increase in antenatal diagnoses of Down syndrome, which included nonviable fetuses who would not have survived to term and therefore remained undiagnosed. In the early years of the period from 1989-2008, the major indication for invasive antenatal diagnosis was a maternal age of 37 years or older. Since the mid-1990s, maternal serum testing and measurement of fetal nuchal

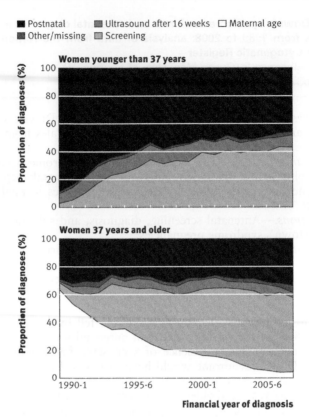

FIGURE 3.—Reasons for Down's syndrome diagnoses according to year of diagnosis for women younger than 37 years and women 37 years and older. (Reprinted from Morris JK, Alberman E. Trends in Down's syndrome live births and antenatal diagnoses in England and Wales from 1989 to 2008: analysis of data from the National Down Syndrome Cytogenetic Register. *BMJ.* 2009;339:b3794, reproduced with permission from the BMJ Publishing Group Ltd.)

translucency were successful screening tests, and antenatal screening has achieved higher rates of correct predictions and higher coverage year on year. In 2001, the UK National Screening Committee advised that all pregnant mothers should be offered one of the available screening tests for Down syndrome, and their recommendations for 2007-2010 are that these tests should have a positive rate of less than 3% and a detection rate of more than 75%. This report describes the effects of the changes in maternal age and advances in screening on the incidence of live births with Down syndrome and on the number of antenatal diagnoses between 1989 and 2008 in England and Wales (Fig 3).

M. G. Bissell, MD, PhD, MPH

Article Index

Chapter 1: Outcomes Analysis

Chapter 2: Breast

Chapter 3: Gastrointestinal System

Chapter 4: Hepatobiliary System and Pancreas

Chapter 5: Dermatopathology

Chapter 6: Lung and Mediastinum

Chapter 7: Cardiovascular

Chapter 8: Female Genital Tract

Chapter 9: Urinary Bladder and Male Genital Tract

Chapter 10: Kidney

Chapter 11: Head and Neck

Chapter 15: Laboratory Management and Outcomes

Chapter 16: Clinical Chemistry

Chapter 17: Clinical Microbiology

Chapter 18: Hematology and Immunology

Chapter 19: Transfusion Medicine and Coagulation

Chapter 20: Cytogenetics and Molecular Pathology

Author Index

A

Adams JM, 21
Adams P, 147
Adamzik I, 310
Adsay NV, 13
Aishima S, 47
Akerboom S, 22
Alberman E, 333
Alcancia F, 286
Alsharif M, 195
Altavilla G, 171
Alvarado-Cabrero I, 139, 141
Alvarez J, 279
Amer H, 149, 160
Amin MB, 139, 141
Ang DSC, 254
Angulo B, 319
Aponte SL, 129
Apple SK, 216
Arain FA, 299
Arber N, 43
Argenyi ZB, 61
Ariyan CE, 58
Auprich M, 124
Azuma K, 192

B

Babiker W, 272
Bahler DW, 323
Bailey KR, 299
Baker PM, 105
Balciza C, 240
Balion CM, 267
Banaei N, 218
Bangarulingam SY, 223
Bankowski MJ, 146
Barnes WM, 325
Barry WT, 285
Bashiardes S, 320
Batal I, 161
Beck AH, 39
Beck J, 331
Bekeris LG, 7
Beltraminelli H, 64
Bentz JS, 194, 219
Berden AE, 156
Bergeron C, 87
Bhanot U, 48
Bianchi DW, 115
Bishop JA, 199
Bjornsson E, 223
Blanca A, 132

Blanco FdelV, 329
Boer F, 22
Bowers JN, 80
Brait M, 167
Brill LB II, 53
Brimo F, 159
Brodsky V, 235
Busam KJ, 92
Busatto G, 171

C

Çağlı K, 76
Canoz O, 153
Cao J-z, 178
Cardona DM, 80
Carinelli SG, 101
Carlo-Demovich J, 195
Carmack SW, 42
Carpi A, 184
Carter G, 26
Catasus L, 99
Caudill JL, 16
Cerroni L, 64
Chang SS, 121
Chatterjee M, 129
Chen D, 328
Chen S-M, 274
Chen X, 213
Chen Y, 126
Chen Y-B, 130
Chen Z, 123
Cheok PY, 33
Chew I, 101
Chida Y, 260
Chong G, 273
Christodoulides N, 266
Chute DJ, 204
Cioc AM, 290
Clarke BA, 96
Clark PE, 121
Cohen Tervaert TW, 157
Compton SP, 165
Conway EJ, 297
Cornell LD, 149, 160
Courser S, 278
Crothers BA, 194

D

Dal Cin P, 228
Dammel T, 278
Dancer JY, 151
D'Angelo E, 99

Dargan P, 255
Dean RA, 264
de Boer IH, 252
de Bruijne M, 19
de la Garza GO, 181
Demetris AJ, 74
Deshpande C, 67
Deshpande V, 44
Dias P, 269
Di Bonito L, 196
Dicato M, 43
Dickerson JM, 21
Dissanayake D, 255
Diwan AH, 56
Dondog B, 270
Dowsett M, 25
Duffy MJ, 262
Dumont LJ, 312
Dunn EJ, 245
Dustin SM, 200

E

Egashira K, 305
Ellard S, 326
Enders F, 223
Epstein JI, 130
Erickson-Johnson M, 226

F

Falcón-Escobedo R, 30
Fallenberg E, 28
Fan Y-S, 56
Feng Y, 297
Ferrario F, 156
Filali-Mouhim A, 110
Flesch BK, 310, 311
Floriano PN, 266
Folkins AK, 97
France DJ, 9
French JD, 188
Fretwell DL, 188
Friedman DR, 285
Fukase M, 112
Fung ET, 257

G

Gao F, 26
Gao H, 135
Gao J, 295
García-García E, 319

Printed and bound by CPI Group (UK) Ltd, Croydon, CR0 4YY

08/05/2025

01864677-0011